Hippocrates,
*On the Art of Medicine*

# Studies in Ancient Medicine

*Edited by*

John Scarborough

Philip J. van der Eijk
Ann Ellis Hanson
Joseph Ziegler

VOLUME 39

*The titles published in this series are listed at brill.nl/sam*

# Hippocrates,
# *On the Art of Medicine*

*By*

Joel E. Mann

BRILL

LEIDEN · BOSTON
2012

*Cover illustration*: Hippocrates of Kos (ca. 460–370 BC) is considered the most famous physician of antiquity. Original woodcut published by Otto Spamer, Leipzig and Berlin, 1882.

Library of Congress Cataloging-in-Publication Data

Mann, Joel Eryn, 1975-
Hippocrates, On the art of medicine / by Joel E. Mann.
pages cm. – (Studies in ancient medicine, ISSN 0925-1421 ; volume 39)
Includes bibliographical references and index.
ISBN 978-90-04-22413-1 (hardback : alk. paper) 1. Hippocrates. Peri technes.
2. Medicine–Philosophy. I. Hippocrates. Peri technes. English & Greek. II. Title. III. Title: On the art of medicine.

R126.H7P5736 2012
610.1–dc23

2011048130

This publication has been typeset in the multilingual "Brill" typeface. With over 5,100 characters covering Latin, IPA, Greek, and Cyrillic, this typeface is especially suitable for use in the humanities. For more information, please see www.brill.nl/brill-typeface.

ISSN 0925-1421
ISBN 978 90 04 22413 1 (hardback)
ISBN 978 90 04 22429 2 (e-book)



This book is printed on acid-free paper.

For Josephine

CONTENTS

# PREFACE

Few have much experience with the so-called Hippocratic *Corpus*, that farrago of over seventy ancient Greek medical treatises that come down to us under the name of Hippocrates. Credit for my first exposure is due to a graduate seminar on medicine and rhetoric led by Lesley Dean-Jones. My interest at the time lay chiefly in sophistic rhetoric and Pre-Socratic philosophy, and I was surprised at how much of both were to be found in the *Corpus*, especially in the treatise known as περὶ τέχνης, *de Arte*, or, as I call it in the title to this book, *On the art of medicine*. I was further surprised at how little scholarly attention had been devoted to *de Arte*. The major studies (Gomperz 1910, Vegetti 1964, Jori 1996) were extremely valuable, but I had the feeling that much more was left to say. Missing was scholarship that preserved the insights of earlier studies while applying the methods of analytic philosophy that have proven so fruitful to the study of ancient thought in the past several decades.

Such is the aim of the present commentary. It does not aim to give the "last word" on *de Arte*. It does not aim to replace Gomperz' learned literary analysis or Vegetti's comprehensive comparison of *de Arte* to other Hippocratic works. Much less does it aim to invalidate the observations afforded by Jori's "Continental" treatment of the text. Instead, I operate under the conviction that *de Arte*, as a work of sophistic rhetoric and Pre-Socratic philosophy, is driven by argument, and the tools of Anglo-American analytic philosophy are particularly well suited to teasing out the tangles of the often very dense and technical arguments we encounter in *de Arte*.

And while I still consider this Hippocratic treatise a scintillating specimen of sophistic rhetoric and Pre-Socratic philosophy, I must confess, too, that I have come to better understand *de Arte* as a medical work. Some have thought that its contribution to ancient medical knowledge is unimpressive, and in a narrow sense that may be true. But a close reading of the whole treatise—and especially of its second half—reveals an author familiar with the peculiar challenges, both theoretical and practical, that doctors faced in the ancient world. The cogence of its basic argument, that medicine 'is' and is powerful, cannot be appreciated without taking seriously its medical content.

This commentary itself would not have 'been' without the help of a great many people, starting first with Lesley Dean-Jones and Jim Hankinson, who supervised my dissertation on *de Arte*, as well as the other members of the dissertation committee, Paul Woodruff, Alex Mourelatos, and Michael Gagarin. I owe much to the guidance and encouragement of the editors of Brill's *Studies in Ancient Medicine* series, especially Philip van der Eijk and John Scarborough, and Elizabeth Craik deserves thanks for patiently tolerating my inquiries. A spontaneous conversation with Monte Johnson about τὸ αὐτόματον saved me from some crucial omissions in the commentary. Special thanks goes to the Loeb Classical Library Foundation for awarding me a research fellowship for the 2008–2009 academic year, which allowed me to take a leave of absence from teaching. Thanks, too, to St. Norbert College and its faculty and students for allowing me to take that leave. Certain of my colleagues deserve special recognition for their willingness to review drafts of the commentary, notably Ravi Sharma, Betsy Baumann, Don Abel, and Diane Legomsky. My students Alex Hilke and, especially, Getty Lustila, helped me in preparing the final manuscript. Finally, I must thank my parents, James and Evelyn Mann, and my wife, Josephine Dobson, for their support at many crucial points along the way. I hope, when all is printed and done, that it was worth it.

Joel Mann
De Pere, Wisconsin
November 2010

# A NOTE ON THE TEXT AND CITATIONS

My translation of *de Arte* is based (with kind permission) on the text of Jacques Jouanna's Budé edition (1988), with minor changes as noted in the commentary. Occasionally, I draw on the texts in Jori 1996, Heiberg 1927, Reinhold 1865, Ermerins 1862, and Daremberg 1855, and I frequently discuss emendations suggested in Diels 1914. Comparison of the language of *de Arte* to that of other texts in the *Corpus* was made inestimably easier by Maloney and Frohn 1986.

References to *de Arte* contain the chapter and sentence number. Wherever possible I cite works from the Hippocratic *Corpus* by way of their Budé editions. Exceptions include *Vict.* and *Nat. Hom.*, which use editions from the *Corpus Medicorum Graecorum* ('CMG') series by Joly and Jouanna, respectively; and *Loc. Hom.* and *Gland.*, for which I use editions by Craik. Citations include the page and line numbers of the relevant text as well as the volume and page number of the Littré equivalent ('L.'). For all other Hippocratic works, I refer simply to the Littré edition of 1861 by volume, page, and line number. I cite Galen using volume, page, and line numbers of the Kühn edition as well as Deichgräber 1930. For all other ancient medical literature, I strive to use the standard editions.

References to fragments and testimonia from pre-Socratic philosophy are made according to the usual conventions for citing the chapter and fragment numbers from Diels-Kranz (e.g., DK 31 B21). However, for Empedocles I use Inwood 1992, and for Antiphon's fragments, I use Pendrick's meticulous 2002, with a few exceptions as noted. Extended quotes from Plato use the translations given in Cooper 1997; from Aristotle, Barnes 1984. Fragments from Hellenistic philosophers are identified using their assigned numbers in Long and Sedley 1987. Unless otherwise noted, abbreviations follow the conventions used in Liddell, Scott, and Jones, *A Greek-English Lexicon* ('LSJ') and the Thesaurus Linguae Graecae *Canon of Greek Authors and Works*.

# INTRODUCTION

## 1. Technē *and Medicine in Ancient Greece*

Any comprehensive study of the Hippocratic treatise περὶ τέχνης, or *de Arte* (often *On the art*, or, as I render it in the title, *On the art of medicine*), must begin from the Greek notion of *technē*. The long and disputed history of the concept prevents me from giving a full synopsis of its development, much of which would in any event prove superfluous for understanding the present text.[1] *De Arte* does not, for example, presuppose the theories of *technē* present in Plato or Aristotle; it is not clear that it presupposes any systematic theory at all. Rather, it is written as a response to an attack both on art generally and on medicine in particular. The question is whether art, and then medicine, exists. As we shall see, *de Arte* remains distinct from the Platonic debate insofar as it assumes at every step that medicine, if it exists, is a *technē*. This point is never at issue. (Our author perhaps gestures feebly at it in c. 5, where he asserts that a distinction between correctness and incorrectness are essential to any *technē*. But there is no evidence that he countenances the possibility that medicine could *be* and yet not *be an art*.) The Platonic question, on the other hand, is not whether *technē* or rhetoric exists, but whether rhetoric is a genuine *technē*. It is this question that more naturally leads to theoretical reflection on the nature of *technē* (see further my comments on c. 2).

However, *de Arte* is not therefore without value as a testament to early theoretical ideas about *technē*. The critics of medicine have for the art certain expectations that they claim it fails to fulfill. Inevitably, in tracing our author's response to such critics, we will hit upon some of these expectations and the reasons for them. And our author will of course question some of the expectations themselves. Thus, we will be able to gain some insight into early theoretical ideas related to *technē* and technical activity, though these shall by no means constitute a systematic theory.

[1] Concerning *technē* as treated in the Classical period, with ample references to the continued debate in the Hellenistic, Heinimann 1961, Hutchinson 1988, and Hankinson 1995a have proven invaluable to my research. Roochnik 1996 and Schiefsky 2005 make important contributions as well.

The guiding aims of *de Arte* are polemical, not theoretical, and we should adjust our own expectations accordingly.

We can, nonetheless, develop a general sense for Greek views on *technē* during the period when *de Arte* was written. The various accounts of human progress we find in fifth-century literature tend to credit the arts with enabling human beings to triumph over the adversity of their natural situation (see my notes on 1.2). Thus, in Aeschylus' *Prometheus Bound* (442–506), Prometheus describes with apparent pride how human beings use the arts he taught them, including medicine, to predict future events and devise precautions against impending catastrophe. This capacity for grasping and manipulating their environment sets humans apart from the other animals (cf. *Protagoras* 321cff.), and the arts become thereby emblematic of human intelligence and ingenuity, which uncover connection and correlation where *tuchē*, or chance, once reigned supreme. The opposition of *technē* to *tuchē* develops in the fifth century (e.g., Euripides, *IT* 89: λαβόντα δ' ἢ τέχναισιν ἢ τύχῃ τινί,) into a classic antithesis that resurfaces in Plato (*Gorgias* 448c) and Aristotle (*Metaph.* 981a1 ff.; *EN* 1105a21–26, 1140a1–23). What is accomplished through art cannot be a matter of chance or luck, though determining what exactly that entails becomes central to defending the integrity of *technē*, not least for the Hippocratic writers (see especially *VM* 118.10–119.1 = L. 1.570; *Morb.* I 6.140; *Loc. Hom.* 85.25–35 = L. 6.342), including the author of *de Arte* (cc. 4–6). For *tuchē* takes many forms. It may be fate, as in Gorgias' *Helen* (DK 82 B11 6), or, absent its supernatural aura, merely the outcome, whether harmful or beneficial, of one's course of action (*Loc. Hom.* 85.25–35 = L. 6.342). It may be the random coincidence of causal chains, as Democritus might have held (Aristotle, *Ph.* 196a24–27), or the incidental intersection of teleological causal processes, as Aristotle himself argued (*Ph.* 197a36–37). Alternatively, *tuchē* may be a real discontinuity in the causal nexus, a genuine indeterminacy, as it probably was for Epicurus (LS 18G 6), or sometimes simply a product of ignorance, namely, ignorance of the causes relevant to an agent's situation (*VM* 132.18–133.6).

Chance in this last sense will seem especially pertinent to the practitioner of a *technē* who purports to achieve his aims by knowing, understanding, and ultimately controlling the relevant causal processes. How much must one know, and how reliable or precise must one's knowledge be, in order to be considered expert? In short, how successful must an expert be? Surely, an expert can be depended on to achieve the aim of his *technē* with some regularity (Roochnik 20), but it is hardly surprising that the Greeks, with their keen sense for the tragic, were aware that not even the most expert could eliminate contingency and uncertainty from human affairs. Consider Solon's observation that

> another man, who has learned the works of Athena and Hephaestus, skilled in many *technai*, makes his living with his hands. Another who has been taught his gifts by the Olympian Muses knows a measure of longed-for wisdom.
>
> Another man lord Apollo, whose works are known far and wide, makes a seer. This man, with whom the gods keep company, recognizes the distant that approaches; no omen or sacrifice will hinder what is fated.
>
> Others are doctors and have the job of the healer, master of many remedies. To these there is no end. It is often that a minor pain turns into major suffering, and no doctor can relieve it by administering soothing remedies. But at other times he immediately makes well the one suffering from evil, unyielding diseases by touching him with his hands.
>
> Indeed, it is Fate who brings good and evil to mortals, and no one escapes the gifts of the immortal gods. And there is risk in everything that is done, and no one knows, when something is started, how it will turn out.
>
> (West 13.49–66)

Though Solon is pessimistic, he is not skeptical of the arts or their usefulness. Medicine may not offer perfect protection from disease or death, but surely it improves the patient's odds. Nevertheless, the limitations of medicine, including the acceptable levels and sources of failure, became a subject of some controversy for the Hippocratics and others (see Appendix § 3). This much, at least, was uncontroversial: the true craftsman should know, within reason, the outcomes of events that fall within the purview of his art. But what it means to 'know,' and what factors determine such knowledge, is not always clear.

Knowledge of the future, in particular, was important to the art of medicine, and the ability to prognosticate carries much weight in Hippocratic estimations of technical prowess (most famously, at *Prog.* 2.110; cf. *de Arte* 6.4, 12.2).[2] Moreover, a doctor will know also how to intervene in cases where he judges there is something that can be done to restore a patient to health. Thus, it is crucial for a *technē* to have not only a clear domain (e.g., health and sickness of the human body, including its anatomy and physiology and the various factors affecting it) but also a beneficial and well defined goal, or *telos*, within that domain (e.g. making particular sick bodies healthy). The Hippocratics describe the *telos* of medicine variously, and *de Arte* offers as its definition of medicine an account of the proper goals of the *technē*, to which I will return in detail (see notes on 3.2). For many Hippocratics,

---

[2] See further Nutton 2004, 88 ff., as well as Edelstein 1967, 65–85.

including our author, this 'knowing how' to achieve the appropriate goal is of a piece with knowledge of future outcomes; to know how to treat a febrile patient is to know what would be the outcome of subjecting his or her body to various possible treatments. So possessing a *technē* is not just a matter of knowing all there is to know about bodies, boats, or boots, but rather of organizing a relevant part of this knowledge around some positive aim. This provides for the craftsman a standard for his activity: he knows what measures will achieve his goal (these would be constitutive of τὸ ὀρθόν, or 'the correct') and which will not (τὸ μὴ ὀρθόν, 'the incorrect'; see also notes on 5.5–6).

While the capacity to discover what is correct in an art may be in some sense innate, the knowledge itself is not. It must be discovered and passed on through teaching. This is already evident in Aeschylus' *Prometheus Bound*, where Prometheus repeatedly praises himself for discovering the arts and explaining them clearly to human beings (487: ἐγνώρις' αὐτοῖς). Euripides, writing later in the same century, argues that manliness can be taught (ἡ δ' εὐανδρία διδακτός, *Supp.* 913–914) as a *technē*, or perhaps as a necessary part of the soldier's *technē*. Teaching requires that there be teachers, who are skilled in the art, and students, who have the status of laypersons before undergoing training. In fact, the Greek intuition seems to have demanded more. The arts were thought to be specialized to the extent that there would be for every art a distinct class of skilled practitioners, apart from mere laypersons.

For something to count as a *technē*, then, not everybody could be proficient at it. This is addressed by the author of *VM* (123.9–12 = L. 1.578) and by Protagoras in Plato's dialogue of that name (322c–e), both of whom argue that the restriction should be relaxed for basic dietetics and the political art respectively. In the mythic Protagorean account, we get little explanation of the restriction beyond the remark that having only a few medical experts around is sufficient to care for an entire community. The author of *VM*, on the other hand, concedes that it is reasonable to withhold technical status from dietetics because all are knowledgeable in it 'through the necessity of use' (διὰ τὴν χρῆσίν τε καὶ ἀνάγκην, a hendiadys), though it matches against this concession the assertion that dietetics nevertheless represents a great discovery indicative of much investigation and art. The thought may be that while dietetics fails the test of *technē* on the letter of the specialist-layperson criterion, it fulfills it in spirit by satisfying the implicit requirement that a *technē* be suitably complicated and non-obvious. This in turn suggests that technical knowledge and practice were regarded by the Greeks as complex, requiring a real commitment to training on the part of those desiring to learn.

These, then, are the predominant intuitions in play around the Greek notion of *technē* as it developed in the fifth century: 1) art involves control, by cognitive or intellectual means, over the whims of chance and demands of nature; 2) technical activity is goal-directed, and the goal of an art determines its domain; 3) expertise in an art is sufficiently difficult so as to require specialized training, resulting in, at least for most arts, a class of specialists in the field. All three intuitions are important to the arguments marshaled by our author in defense not just of *technē* generally but of medicine in particular; moreover, they serve as lenses through which we may gain a more focused view of Greek medicine as it was developing during the period of *de Arte*'s composition. A full account of that development falls outside the current scope, but a brief outline of its broader trends is required to appreciate *de Arte*.[3]

To this point, I have described how the attempt to control nature by cognitive means manifested in Hippocratic medicine as an intention to acquire foreknowledge of a patient's fate, but it had other ramifications as well. On the whole, the Hippocratics moved toward what is often termed a 'rational' view of the world, or at least of medical matters, eschewing healing traditions that relied on religious rituals, relics, and the like. The Hippocratic *Morb. Sacr.*, for example, is foremost a polemic against μάγοι, itinerant magicians who claimed that epilepsy, as a 'sacred' disease brought on by the gods, could be cured only by their ritual therapy. In a set of introductory arguments, the author exposes the magicians' divine mandate as fundamentally impious and questions the validity of their explanations. He then presents his own naturalistic explanation of epilepsy, closing with the assertion that all diseases have a nature and cause and, in addition to this (or perhaps *because* of this), are divine (31.16–32.3 = L. 6.394). The compatibility of the author's alternately religious language and rational attitudes continues to incite controversy, but the interpretive problem may be emblematic of the Greek physician's dilemma: in a culture captivated by magic and myth, he faced the daunting task of promoting a naturalistic approach to medical explanation and intervention without alienating those who might put stock in religious alternatives. That is not to say that rational medicine was always the sworn enemy of the religious.[4] There is ample evidence that the

---

3 Authoritative accounts include, among others, Jouanna 1999, Nutton 2004, and Craik 1998.

4 For a comprehensive study of the compatibility, both culturally and theoretically, of Greek rational and religious medicine, see Wickkiser 2008, especially pp. 22ff.

two approaches coexisted relatively peacefully, and occasionally one finds traces of 'supernaturalism' in the *Corpus*, e.g., in *Prog.* (2.112.5) and the fourth book of *Vict.* (e.g., 218.14 = L. 6.640). Still, as G.E.R. Lloyd has pointed out, the Hippocratic critique of magic distinguishes itself from that encountered in other traditional societies by its denunciation of magicians across the board (1979, 18–19). The Greek medical treatises do not single out magicians who malpractice an otherwise sound profession. Instead, they criticize the assumptions common to all magical practices, thereby effecting what Lloyd and others take to be a profound paradigm shift in the explanation and treatment of disease.

Diseases are not, on the rational view, the consequences of divine disfavor. Generally speaking, they come about when environmental events or dietetic deviations aggravate a person's constitutional weaknesses or disturb the natural balance of his body. This balance consists in a harmony of fluids, often called 'humors' (χυμοί), that permeate the body in various configurations and concentrations. The standard Hippocratic paradigm came to include phlegm, blood, and yellow and black bile (cf. *Nat. Hom.* 172.13–15 = L. 6.40), but other fluid substances may play equally vital roles—*de Arte* is not the only Hippocratic treatise to emphasize the importance of air and ichor, for example (10.3; see further Introduction 4). These are subject to a standard array of primitive physical reactions, perhaps most commonly to heating, cooling, drying, and moistening, as well as to mechanical processes like occlusion, constriction, and dilation.[5] Not surprisingly, treatment proceeds by manipulating these conditions and processes. A doctor might prescribe phlebotomy to rid the patient of excess blood. He might recommend a purgative drug to reestablish ideal levels of yellow bile or feed the patient barley gruel and confine him or her to bed. In some cases he might even cauterize an abscess with a red-hot iron.[6]

Such an approach is laden, whether implicitly or explicitly, with physical and physiological theory, and theoretical ambitions lead some Hippocratics into an alliance with contemporary philosophy.[7] At times, those same ambitions come into conflict with another trend in Greek medicine: empiricism, broadly construed as the conviction that the accumulated observations

[5] Langholf 1990 gives a comprehensive account of Hippocratic medical theory.

[6] For general descriptions of ancient therapeutic approaches, see Jouanna (1999, 112 ff.), Nutton (2004, 87–102).

[7] The literature on the *Corpus* and its philosophical influences is extensive. A good guide to the topic is Longrigg 1989 (including bibliography). See also the edite collection by Wittern and Pellegrin (1996).

of medical phenomena are useful, perhaps even central, to the successful practice of medicine.[8] In works such as the *Epidemics*, for example, empiricism manifests in carefully written case histories that strive to capture potentially salient details about the genesis, progress, and resolution of different diseases. In others, empiricism becomes a philosophical and methodological commitment capable of inspiring genuine passion. So the author of *Nat. Hom.* lambasts material monists on empirical grounds: 'for I say neither that a human being is completely air, nor fire, nor water, nor earth, nor anything else that is not evident as a constituent of a human being' (164.5–7 = L. 6.32). He goes on to levy similar criticism at medical monists (166.12–15 = L. 6.34) and demonstrates the soundness of his own physiological theory by means of an empirical challenge: 'evidence of this [that phlegm is the coldest constituent in the body] is that if you are willing to touch phlegm and bile and blood, you will find phlegm to be the coldest' (182.6–8 = L. 6.46). A similar sentiment informs *VM*, whose author condemns whoever 'attempted to speak or write about medicine, hypothesizing for themselves a hypothesis in their account—hot or cold or wet or dry or whatever else they should wish—reducing the explanatory principle of disease and death in humans, and giving the same principle in all cases, hypothesizing a unity or a duality' (118.1–6 = L. 1.570). Medicine, however, 'does not need any new-fangled hypothesis as do non-evident and puzzling matters, concerning which it is necessary to use a hypothesis, should someone try to say something of significance, e.g., investigations concerning the things in heaven and below the earth. If someone says he has knowledge that these are thus and so, it would not be clear either to him who said it or to his listeners whether these things were true or not' (119.4–10 = L. 1.572).

These trends—a growing preference for reason, knowledge, observation and natural explanation over recourse to myth, magic, and luck—were coherent enough to give medicine a sense of identity but relaxed enough to allow for considerable disagreement between practitioners of the *technē*. It is here that the author of *de Arte* finds himself as he fends off attacks on the healing art, unrepentantly embracing the emerging ideals of rational medicine while confronting the harsh realities of clinical practice.

[8] The classic study is Bourgey 1953. See also Lloyd 1979, 126–169.

## 2. De Arte *as Rhetorical* Epideixis

To the extent that the foregoing remarks leave the impression that *de Arte* is 'merely' a medical treatise, they are misleading. For despite its membership in the *Hippocratic Corpus*, it is both a rhetorical piece of considerable skill and a philosophical tract of some interest. In what follows I will identify and discuss those features of its form and content that lead me to this view, always with an eye to their specific rhetorical, philosophical, and medical contexts.

It is plain that the purpose of *de Arte* is to persuade (see, for example, 13.1), namely, to persuade its audience that certain public criticisms of the *technai* generally (1.1) and of medicine in particular (1.3) are unfounded. This alone does not make it unique in the *Corpus*. Several of the treatises in the *Corpus* are composed with persuasive intent—*Nat. Hom.*, *Flat.*, *VM*, and *Acut.*, just to name a few of the most conspicuous. But *de Arte* stands out among these and other works in key respects. First, the debate into which its author enters is primarily public, that is, the primary audience is the public at large, or, more precisely, an ignorant lay public (1.2). While it is true that other Hippocratic works acknowledge the publicity of the debate in which they are engaged (most notably *Nat. Hom.* 166.2–11 = L. 6.32–34, *VM* 120.12–15 = L. 1.574, and *Acut.* 39.10–12 = L. 2.240; see also Jouanna 1984, 28 ff.), the debates themselves are essentially conflicts between doctors of various convictions and methods. This is not so in the case of *de Arte*, whose author struggles against rhetorical antagonists (I will refer to them usually as 'the critics') from outside the art to win the hearts and minds of laypersons. If doctors are at all the intended audience, it is only indirectly, a point to which I shall return. Second, and related, is the putative subject matter of *de Arte*, which is not the superiority of any one medical theory or method to another, but rather the 'being' and 'power'—what we will for now gloss as the legitimacy and efficacy—of medicine. *De Arte*, in sharp contrast to the intra-disciplinary squabbles typical of the *Corpus*, mounts a defense of doctors *en bloc*.[9]

I do not apply the term 'defense' arbitrarily. Among the many virtues of Gomperz' original study of *de Arte* was his recognition of the treatise's affinity, in both form and content, with surviving examples of ancient forensic rhetoric. Gomperz judged *de Arte* an *apologia*, or legal defense, of the

[9] Mann 2008a.

art of healing. His own map of the work's rhetorical structure illustrated the point (1910, 86):[10]

1. *Prooimion* (cc. 1–3)
    - c. 1: General introduction and articulation of theme (*prothesis*)
    - c. 2: Ontological excursus
    - c. 3: Definition of the main idea and articulation of the simultaneously positive and negative methods of proof (*apodeixis* and *lusis*)
2. *Apodeixis* and *lusis*
    - a. *Technē* versus chance
        - c. 4: General remarks on the relation between *technē* and *tuchē*
        - c. 5: The efficacy of medicine extends beyond the activity of doctors
        - c. 6: Foundation of this thesis in the nature of things
    - b. Limited efficacy of medicine
        - c. 7: Medical failures do not count against the existence of medicine
        - c. 8: Even less so does non-intervention in hopeless cases
    - c. The orientation of medicine with respect to visible and hidden diseases
        - i. Anatomical background
            - c. 9: General distinction between the two species of disease
            - c. 10: Detailed elaboration of this distinction
        - ii. General application
            - c. 11: General remarks on knowledge and the treatment of hidden diseases
            - c. 12: Illustration of the above through comparison with other arts
        - iii. Specific application
            - c. 13: Detailed outline of diagnostic method and the practical application proceeding therefrom
3. *Epilogos*
    - c. 14: Recapitulation (*anakephalaiosis*) and parting remarks from the orator to doctors

[10] Gomperz, following the editorial custom at the time, divided *de Arte* into fourteen chapters by printing section 11.7 as a chapter of its own.

While some, like Jori, have attempted to elaborate or improve that map,[11] the basic points of Gomperz' topography remain intact. In my view, the plan for *de Arte* is best revealed by concentrating on the treatise's formal structures, especially those that are characteristic of Greek forensic rhetoric, as follows.

1. *Prooimion* major (1.1–3.3)
    a. *Prooimion* minor (1.1–3)
        i. *Prothesis* minor (1.3)
    b. *Prokataskeuē* (2.1–3)
    c. *Prothesis* major (3.1–3)
        i. *Diorismos* (3.2)
2. *Pistis* (4.1–8.7)
3. *Diēgēsis* (9.1–12.6)
        i. *Prothesis* minor (9.1)
4. *Epilogos* (13.1)
        i. *Anakephalaiosis*

If we focus for the moment on form at the expense of thematic content, we may better appreciate the basic affinity between *de Arte* and that rhetoric in the forensic style for which Attic orators and logographers were especially known. Not unreasonably, Gomperz divides the treatise into three sections: *prooimion*, or prologue; *apodeixis* and *lusis*, or demonstration and refutation; and *epilogos*, or epilogue. But he and others have overlooked the structural nuances of these sections, e.g., the recursive or 'fractal' pattern of certain elements. The *prooimion* major, which comprises cc. 1–3, closes with a *prothesis*, a statement of the work's purpose, but nested within this *prooimion* is a smaller (c. 1) that closes with its own *prothesis*, which is itself echoed at 9.1.[12] Also striking is our author's preliminary argument, or *prokataskeuē*, which is isolated from the battery of other proofs that begins at 4.1. Such preliminary argumentation is a common feature of Antiphon's forensic speeches (Gagarin 1997, 18), and its presence in *de Arte* suggests a genuine sophistication of style. More importantly, however, the *apodeixis* may be further divided into two distinct sections: one for proof (*pistis*),

[11] Both Gomperz and Jori rely heavily on thematic elements to govern their analyses of structure. This leads Jori to posit an implausibly sharp break between cc. 7 and 8 on the grounds that there our author transitions from a discussion of medicine's being to one of its power (1996, 102).

[12] Jouanna observes that the prologue's length and sophistication set it apart from most other works in the *Corpus* (1984, 34).

which as in Attic forensic rhetoric consists in a series of distinct arguments designed to refute the 'prosecution's' charges; and a second for narrative (*diēgēsis*), a tendentious recounting of events that absolves the defendant of blame. Thus, the formal structure of *de Arte* may be analyzed into the traditional four-part division of a forensic speech with the traditional positions of the narrative and proof reversed.[13]

The content of the proofs themselves is further revealing. Three of them deserve special attention for their 'pragmatism'—that is, their applicability to disagreements that might naturally arise in the course of a doctor's practice—as well as their 'rhetorical' quality. An argument is rhetorical in this sense just in case it is used to commit a person to some proposition, p, without directly demonstrating the truth of p. A rhetorical argument is not necessarily a bad one, as an example from c. 4 shows. There, our author imagines a debate with a patient who denies that the doctor's treatment was responsible for his recovery. The argument proceeds as follows (see further my notes on 4.3):

1. The patient made a voluntary decision to undergo the prescribed therapy.
2. If the patient made a voluntary decision, then he had a reason or set of reasons for making the decision.
3. Thus, he had a reason or set of reasons.
4. This set of reasons either included the expectation that the therapy would benefit him, or it did not.
5. If it did not, then the patient is guilty of recklessness, stupidity, intemperance, *vel sim.*
6. If it did, then he has no grounds for now overturning his previous conviction that the prescribed therapy is beneficial, i.e., causally effective in curing his condition.

This is a perfectly valid argument and may even be sound, depending on the situation. It may even persuade the recalcitrant patient to repent. But it clearly does not demonstrate that the doctor's therapy was causally responsible for the patient's recovery. Moreover, it is utterly irrelevant to the

[13] The basic division may be applied also to quasi-forensic speeches such as Gorgias' *Helen* (which contains a brief narrative of Helen's backstory immediately after the *prooimion* and before the *pisteis*), though one should be cautious about imposing the four-part division on fifth-century rhetoric as though it were an ironclad rule of composition (see Schiappa 1999, 105 ff., and Cole 1991, 170). Jouanna stresses the similarities between *Helen* and both *de Arte* and *Flat.* to bring out their peculiarly rhetorical character (1984, 38 ff.).

general question of medicine's legitimacy or effectiveness, and in this lies its practicality. The argument is meant not to quell any general theoretical revolt against medicine but only to deflect the charge of incompetence leveled against a particular physician.

I find traces of the same pragmatic orientation in arguments made also in chapter 5 (see my notes on 5.5), but perhaps the clearest instances occur in chapters 7 and 8. After having defended at some length the principle that certain diseases may be too powerful for doctors to cure, our author adds that 'my argument is the same on behalf of all other instruments allied with medicine. I claim that if the doctor is unsuccessful with each of all these, he ought to (δεῖν) hold responsible the power of the affliction, not the art' (8.5). This is not a theoretical point about technical limitations; it is an instruction to the doctor who has exhausted his medical resources and yet failed to heal his patient (i.e., it is pragmatic), one that may be useful even to an incompetent physician who has failed to acquire or apply the correct medical knowledge (i.e., it is rhetorical). It should be added that the Hippocratic writers are often didactic, but their instructions usually take the form of medical advice (see the discussion of *Loc. Hom.* in Craik 1998, 18). In *de Arte*, the advice is exclusively rhetorical, as exemplified also by the opening lines of c. 7: 'someone could make such arguments against those who attribute health to chance and discredit the art' (7.1). Our author goes on to give what may be the earliest recorded defense against a malpractice charge. The defense relies on an argument from εἰκός (see notes on 7.1–2, 7.5), 'likelihood,' generally acknowledged to be the calling card of sophistic rhetoric. Aristotle depicts εἰκός as having been devised by Protagoras primarily for defensive legal contexts (*Rh.* 1402a17–29), and at *Theaetetus* 162d–e, Plato provides indirect testimony that εἰκός arguments (or perhaps only a specific kind) were associated especially with Protagoras and rhetoric while shunned by the other arts. But Protagoras had no patent on the εἰκός argument. Mastery of likelihood is attributed also to Tisias and Gorgias at *Phaedrus* 267a–b, and these arguments are indeed found in the extant speeches of Gorgias. Furthermore, εἰκός reasoning is central to the opposed speeches in Thucydides,[14] and Antiphon' tetralogies—especially the first—are rife with it.[15]

---

[14] See further Woodruff 1994.

[15] The role of εἰκός in the first of Antiphon's tetralogies is discussed in Gagarin 2002, 112 ff. With respect to Protagoras, Gagarin cautions that despite Aristotle's remarks we have no extant examples of reverse-probability (or any kind of probability) arguments attributed to the sophist (2002, 29 n. 59).

Indeed, scholars have curiously ignored the striking affinities in strategy and dramatic content between *de Arte* and extant legal speeches, especially those between c. 7 and Antiphon's tetralogies. Our author's basic argument is connected to the second and third tetralogies by a particularly outrageous thread: the defendants in all three cases attempt to shift the blame from themselves onto the victims, who, incidentally, are dead. The third tetralogy, however, has special relevance to *de Arte*'s defense of medicine. There, the defendant stands accused of beating to death an old man, though the old man attacked the defendant first, and the latter struck back only in self-defense. Naturally, the defendant argues that the party who provoked the fight is to blame for its consequences. Worried that the jury will not sympathize with this argument, the defendant drags in a scapegoat: the attending physician.

> But in fact he died many days later, after having been turned over to an incompetent doctor, and he died because of the doctor's incompetence and not from the blows. For other doctors had warned him that, if he underwent this particular form of treatment, he would meet his death. Now, on account of your advice, he is dead, and an unholy charge has been leveled at me. (4.2.4)

In contrast with *de Arte*, the defendant charges that the attending physician's prescription contravened medical orthodoxy. This may of course be merely an invention devised to better support his case—at no point in the remainder of the tetralogy is this evidential fact mentioned again. Neither the prosecution nor the defense is particularly focused on whether or not the doctor is guilty of malpractice; indeed, it is suggested that the law absolves the doctor of responsibility even if he is the cause of death.

> When he claims that the victim died at the hands of the doctor, I'm amazed that he claims also that the victim died by our hand—we who advised him to turn himself over to the doctor. For if we had not turned him over to a doctor, he would claim that the victim died from the lack of treatment. Now even if he died by the doctor's hand (which in fact he did not), still the doctor is not his murderer, since the law grants him immunity. And seeing as we were forced to turn him over to a doctor because of the blows he received from this man, how could anyone be the murderer other than he who forced us to consult a doctor? (4.3.5)

The prosecution offers three distinct arguments here. Interestingly, not one of them relies on or otherwise supports the physician's innocence. While the physician may escape the trial without being charged with murder, the prosecutor's unwillingness to defend him leaves the impression that even he suspects the victim received inadequate medical attention. Legally, the doctor is in the clear, though his honor hobbles out of court in tatters.

Thus, c. 7 of *de Arte* emerges as the perfect complement to Antiphon's third tetralogy. The former serves as a sort of epilogue to the latter, ensuring that all concerned parties receive competent 'legal' representation. The defendant blames the doctor, insinuating thereby the guilt of the prosecution, who hired the doctor to begin with. The prosecution, for its part, argues that even if the doctor killed his patient, those who called in the physician are not to blame. Here in *de Arte*, the physician himself steps forward and denies any responsibility. The patient's own weakness, not the medical prescription, was the cause of death. Anyone who suggests otherwise is blaming the innocent, while letting the guilty go free, and the referent of the definite description is tantalizingly underdetermined.[16] 'The guilty' may be the patients themselves—that is certainly the foreground meaning. On the other hand, they are dead. If they are the culprits, they have also already paid the ultimate (and perhaps legally ordained) price. The physician's argument ought to be (as it is in the second tetralogy, 3.2.8) that the guilty have already been punished. Instead, our author implies that the true criminals are still on the loose, and that could include (metaphorically) the disease itself or the family of the deceased, which at the time did not adequately supervise the patient's convalescence and so now attempts to allay a guilty conscience by unjustly blaming the innocent.

In the tetralogies generally, Antiphon's defendants are wont to intimidate the jury by stoking the fear of wrongful conviction.

> This man, if he is put to death contrary to all that is holy, will bring upon those who kill him a double defilement from the avenging spirits. Fear this, then, and bear in mind your obligation to absolve the guiltless of responsibility. Let time make evident the identity of the defiled person, and leave it to the victim's family to exact a penalty. For thus would you do what is most just and most holy. (4.4.10–11; cf. also 4.2.9)

The defendant reminds the jury how critical their decision is. If they convict an innocent, they will not only have allowed the murder-pollution to persist through failing to punish the real killer, but they will have added more pollution to the mix. If they refuse to convict, they have only the original pollution to worry about. The language of piety and justice is brought to bear in personal and even *ad hominem* attacks of the kind found in c. 7 and elsewhere in *de Arte*. Throughout, the critics are subtly but unmistakably charged with various forms of hubris, the wanton violation of traditional values, boundaries, or institutions so familiar from tragedy. This is apparent

[16] Cf. Antiphon's first tetralogy, 2.4.10.

already in the first chapter, where the critics are accused of waging war on the intellect and of violating the natural distinction between expert and layperson and, implicitly, that between aristocracy and rabble (see notes on 1.2). The patient's failure to credit the art with his recovery is depicted at 4.3–4, in a crafty turn of phrase, as an act of greed, πλεονεξίη, and perhaps even of impiety, ἀνοσιότης, an accusation that probably informs the complaint at 8.6 that 'people who criticize doctors for not handling those who have been overcome are demanding that they touch what is improper no less than what is proper,' which exploits public anxiety about μίασμα, or religious pollution (see comments ad loc.). It is suggested finally that the critics suffer not from ignorance but from some deeper, more spiritual malignancy: μανίη, or madness (8.2). Our author is willing at times to attack even the patient's character. The sick suffer from weakness, ἀκρασίη, specifically weakness of will (7.1–3, with echoes at 11.5), and are guilty, among other things, of ὀλιγωρίη, negligence or neglect of duty (11.6).

The critics' hubris extends also to the intellectual sphere, where, so charges our author, they run roughshod over conventional conceptual oppositions, or antitheses. The binary opposition of words and concepts was of course a common feature of classical Greek thought, one that was heavily exploited by sophists such as Gorgias and Antiphon, among others. Perhaps the most important such antithesis was that between νόμος and φύσις, or 'convention' and 'nature,' and the distinction figures crucially in *de Arte*'s argument regarding language (2.3).[17] Other antitheses on which *de Arte* depends include, but are not limited to,[18] the contrasts between λόγος and ἔργον ('word' and 'deed,' 1.2 and 13.1)[19] and βούλησις and δύναμις ('desire' and 'power,' 1.2–3 and 9.4).[20] But if our author uses and respects these various antitheses, the critics confuse and abuse them, whether intentionally or unintentionally. Their rhetorical displays are the work neither of art nor of artlessness, but of ἱστορίη (1.1), which I translate, with the appropriate irony, as 'skill,' though perhaps 'knack' or 'aptitude' would better express our author's point, which is that the critics have natural talent but inadequate training and so inhabit a *Zwischenwelt* between expert and layperson

---

[17] The νόμος and φύσις antithesis is treated at length in Heinimann 1945. For a more recent discussion, see Ostwald 1992.

[18] Indeed, the list is long, including art and chance (4.1), help and hindrance (1.3), being and non-being (2.2), knowing and seeing (2.2, 11.2), freedom and compulsion (12.3), nature and teaching (9.4), and name and being (6.4).

[19] This was a favorite of Thucydides. See Parry 1981.

[20] For the contrast between desire and power, see Gorgias DK 82 B6 and B8, as well as Antiphon 5.73.

(see further my notes on 1.2). After all, the very purpose of the critics' attack is to obliterate the distinction between expert and layperson altogether by destroying the deeds (ἔργα) of experts through the force of mere words (λόγοι). If successful, *technē* will vanish, *tuchē* will reign (4.1), and there will be no acknowledged difference between correct and incorrect procedure in any domain (τό τε ὀρθὸν καὶ τὸ μὴ ὀρθόν, 5.6).

Against this attack our author mounts an impassioned and highly stylized defense exhibiting an uncommon deftness with language. Jouanna has documented his predilection for certain metrical and euphonic effects, especially parisosis and paromoiosis (172–173; 1984, 37–38). Examples are too numerous to list, but perhaps the most well known comes at the close of the second chapter: τὰ μὲν γὰρ ὀνόματα φύσιος νομοθετήματά ἐστιν, τὰ δὲ εἴδεα οὐ νομοθετήματα, ἀλλὰ βλαστήματα (2.3). Our author's syntactic creativity is evident in his use of chiasmus (τῶν γε μὴ ἐόντων τίνα ἂν τίς οὐσίην, 2.1), hypallage (κακαγγελίῃ μᾶλλον φύσιος, 1.2) and hendiadys (ὁδοῖσί τε προσάντεσι καὶ δρόμοισιν, 12.4; perhaps also μετὰ τοῦ ὀφθῆναι ἐνεργοὶ καὶ τοῖσιν εὐεπανορθώτοισι σώμασι, 11.7). We encounter anacoluthon at least twice, once to relax the tone following a particularly dense and abstruse passage (3.1), and again later to impart a casual feel to the rhetoric (11.7). Pace Jouanna (1988, 171), metaphors are common and developed at length. As with the other effects, I shall not catalog them in detail here—I discuss all rhetorical figures and effects at length in the commentary, especially in the introductory remarks on each chapter—but one extended conceit deserves special attention. At 1.3, the critics are compared to foreign invaders on an unjust crusade against the *polis* of medicine, and the military metaphor continues to dominate the work, though our author molds it to fit his changing rhetorical needs. In the *prooimion* and *epilogos*, the critics are the aggressors, and our author, or *de Arte* itself, is depicted as the defender of medicine (13.1). But sometimes the aggressor is the disease lying hidden in ambush (11.6). Its emissaries are the dietetic elements that run contrary to the doctor's prescription (7.3), and the patient's body is a collaborator whom the doctor turns into an informant through the provocation of signs (12.3).

Among other things, this conceit has the effect of allying *de Arte* and its author with doctors and medicine generally as their friend and defender, which requires that the treatise both praise the *technē* and blame its enemies. This two-fold intent is articulated already from the beginning: 'the present discourse will oppose those who thus march against medicine, emboldened on account of these invaders, whom it blames; well equipped through the art to whose rescue it comes; and powerful through wisdom, in which it has been trained' (1.3). It is reaffirmed in the transition to *pistis*: 'in giving this demonstration (ἀπόδειξις) of the art, I will at the same time refute (ἀναιρεῖν) the arguments of those who think they are demeaning it' (3.3). Accordingly, Gomperz labeled *de Arte* both an *apodeixis*, or demonstration through argument, and a *lusis*, or refutation (86). For Aristotle, the species of oratory designed to praise or blame was *epideictic* (*Rh.* 1358b11–12). This is certainly applicable to *de Arte* insofar as our author is responding to those who have given *epideixeis* denigrating medicine. His response is to praise medicine, repair the damage done by these detractors and return medicine to its rightful place in the pantheon of *technai*. As Aristotle explains, the speech of praise achieves its goal by describing the actions of its subject in a way that reflects well upon his character (1366a23 ff.). In *de Arte*, this is accomplished chiefly through the continuous military imagery. The physician is a hero of war, fighting valiantly to vanquish the diseases that prey upon helpless patients (see especially cc. 7, 11, and 12). The enemy is well hidden and the fight is hard, but the physician-warrior perseveres serenely, with a sound mind and body, eschewing any approach that might be deemed reckless or foolhardy.

While *de Arte* may well have epideictic qualities according to Aristotle, and while our author himself hints that the speech is an *epideixis* (see commentary on 13.1), it is not plain that our author and Aristotle agree on what this means. Two facts give us pause. First, our author writes that an *epideixis* can be given in action as well as in word. Second, an *epideixis* in speech, though it may cast aspersions upon its target, glorifies the speaker himself. This point is made in the opening sentence of *de Arte*, where medicine's detractors are accused of abusing the art simply as a means of giving *epideixeis* of their own knowledge. This is the kind of epideictic grandstanding that is usually attributed to the sophists. Epideictic performers like Hippias and Gorgias reportedly wore purple robes and gave competitive recitations of their compositions at festivals (DK 82 A9). In this way, the sophists associated themselves with the Greek wisdom-tradition by appropriating the trappings of poets and rhapsodes. An epideictic speech was an opportunity to show off one's intellectual and poetic virtues.[21]

His reduction of epideictic to praise and blame notwithstanding, Aristotle does retain in the *Rhetoric* a trace of the older, sophistic notion of *epideixis* as display. As Chase has shown in a short but decisive study of the

[21] For a study of the contrast between the earlier notion of *epideixis* as a performative 'showing off' and Aristotle's later transformation of the term to denote a rhetorical genre, see Schiappa (1999, 198 ff.).

Greek conception of epideictic oratory, the praise-blame dichotomy is not the only characterization Aristotle gives of epideictic speech (1961). When first he marks the distinction between deliberative, forensic and epideictic oratory, he writes that

> The forms of rhetoric are three in number, this being the number of forms the audience for a speech may take. For a speech has three components, the speaker, the subject of the speech, and the audience, and the aim of the speech is geared toward this (the audience, I mean). Necessarily, the audience is either a spectator or a judge, namely, a judge of what has happened or what will happen. A member of the assembly judges what will happen, and a member of the jury judges what has happened, while the spectator judges ability; hence, of necessity there will be three forms of rhetorical speech: deliberative, forensic, and epideictic. (1358a36–b7)

This idea, as Chase recognizes (295–296), harmonizes with the pre-Aristotelian criterion of display, insofar as the audience does not listen with the intent of subsequently passing judgment on the subject under debate. They are interested in the speech for reasons incidental to its thesis, and we shall suppose that these include its innovation in content and style. In short, the forensic and deliberative audiences judge the *issue* addressed in the speech; the epideictic audience judges the *speech* itself and, by extension, the *speaker*.

The centrality of display to the pre-Aristotelian idea of epideictic explains the application of the term *epideixis* to cover demonstrations given by a physician. The physician's *epideixis* presumably did not involve elaborate costumes or poetry, but it does seem, by our author's account, to have been intended as a display of his specialized knowledge. This is the thread common to the *epideixis* of both the sophist and the physician: each is a direct display of some skill or fact, where by 'direct' I mean readily and immediately apprehended. The physician shows us that he can heal sick people by healing a sick person as we watch. The sophist shows us that he can compose an aesthetically appealing speech by giving one in our presence. Likewise, our author has, with *de Arte*, given us a display of his mastery of rhetoric. This kind of proof of the speaker's skill should be kept distinct from the objective of the speech itself, which is to prove that medicine is real. This is done by means of arguments that lead us to a conclusion, that is, by means of what in our author's terms falls under the province of the *apodeixis*, literally, a 'showing at a distance' as opposed to a 'showing in the presence of' (*epideixis*). *De Arte* may be an *epideixis* that proves the reality of medicine, but it is not qua *epideixis* that it does so.

Rhetoric properly conceived, or, as our author calls it, τὸ λέγειν (13.1), blames and praises, attacks and defends. This is to be contrasted with the rhetoric practiced by the critics, who are accused of harboring 'the eagerness to debase the discoveries of others by a *technē* of mean discourse, not suggesting any improvements but instead slandering the discoveries of those who have knowledge in front of those who do not' (1.2). The critics practice a rhetoric that is completely destructive, that only blames and attacks, and which lacks a constructive component—that is what our author means when he refers to it as a *technē* of 'mean discourse' or 'shameful words' (λόγων οὐ καλῶν τέχνη). But he means also that the activity itself is shameful insofar as it works against the realization of the common good. Finally, and perhaps as an implication of the foregoing, their words are aesthetically defective—ugly, if you will. We may describe the rhetoric of *de Arte* by implicit contrast: 1) it will include praise of things that deserve it; 2) it will contribute somehow to the realization of a common good, or as we might put it, it will possess a positive ethical dimension; and 3) it will do so with fine language. The purpose of rhetoric is to produce speeches or arguments (7.1, 13.1) that meet these three conditions, and one expects that the capable orator, in order to support the arts, will 'have rationally considered (λελογισμένων) in relation to what the products of craftsmen are fully finished; in what respect imperfect products are deficient; and further, concerning these deficiencies, which are to be attributed to the craftsmen and which to the things being crafted' (8.7). This suggests that arts such as medicine have need of an external observer who will not only judge accurately their successes and failures (presumably the doctor, too, is capable in virtue of his *technē* of judging that—see my notes on 8.7) but, more importantly, distribute praise and blame accordingly. In principle, nothing prevents the expert in a *technē* from playing this 'rhetorical' role himself—a doctor might well make a good case for medicine, but it will not be *qua* doctor that he does so. In practice, however, it may be difficult (but not impossible) for the expert to take on such a role, since most of his time and energy will be dedicated to the practice of his particular art. Thus, our author remarks in closing that for those knowledgeable in the art, 'it is easier to give a display in action rather than in word, since they have not made a study of speaking' (13.1).

Is there any deeper sense in which the ἔργα of medicine need the λόγοι of rhetoric? The answer will depend, in part, on the meaning of λόγος. The word itself is notoriously protean, but we can distinguish three major domains of application (following Kerferd 1981, 83–84). First, there is the linguistic. We will find λόγος to mean word, speech, discourse, description, or statement, and this at least partly accounts for its occurrence in *de Arte*, where I usually translate it as 'discourse.' The linguistic domain is separable from, but not unrelated to, the epistemic and ontological. A λόγος can be what we would term an explanation, reason, or even the activity of thinking, reasoning or investigating. Accordingly, the author of *de Arte* speaks at 6.3 of an ὀρθὸς λόγος, a correct account or explanation. Often, it is understood that an explanation will be correct just in case it accurately reflects the natural order of reality, and so λόγος at times is applied to the principle of order or structure operating in the world. Heraclitus frequently employs λόγος in this way, and *de Arte* gestures at it when the author contends that a certain thesis is not only ἄλογον—absurd, unthinkable—but ἀδύνατον, flat-out impossible given the actual structure of reality (2.1, 2.3). The boundaries between these three categories are not impermeable. It can be difficult to pinpoint the proper domain for every application of λόγος; what we often translate as 'argument,' especially in sophistic or rhetorical contexts (e.g., at 6.1, ὁ ἐμὸς λόγος), clearly has a foot in both the linguistic and epistemic. Indeed, if the art of τὸ λέγειν is taken to encompass λόγος in a broader sense that includes logic (to say nothing of epistemology and ontology proper), then it is all the more likely that medicine, whose practitioners are described as 'reasoning' (λογίζεσθαι, 7.3) or applying 'reasoning' (λογισμός, 11.3) and 'making inferences' (τεκμαίρεσθαι, 12.2, 12.4), will depend materially on rhetoric for its legitimacy.

For a variety of possible reasons, then, medicine needs rhetoric, and our author pitches *de Arte* as just what the doctor ordered. Availing himself of the principles and precepts of the art, he devises for doctors an apologetic *epideixis* in high-flown forensic style, praising medicine's power and practitioners while blaming and criticizing its enemies. But though it may be first and foremost a piece of rhetoric, *de Arte* is also a work of philosophy and of medical theory, and I turn now to consider each in its own right.

## 3. De Arte *as Philosophical Tract*

Students of the Greek concept of *technē* are familiar with the pivotal role it plays in the philosophy of Plato and Aristotle. In *de Arte*, we can see that the debate over *technē* predated Plato and Aristotle, though we discover also that the terms of that early debate were somewhat different. Certain works in the Hippocratic *Corpus* evince a concern over the charge, evidently in circulation among the Greeks, that medicine 'is not' (*de Arte* 2.1; cf. *VM* 132.18–133.1 = L. 1.596, *Acut.* 39.10–12 = L. 2.240). Both *de Arte* and *Acut.* point to a public display of some sort in which medicine has been slandered, and even Hippocratic writers who do not explicitly mention this particular attack on medicine fret about the art's ability to defend itself in a public setting (*Nat. Hom.* 166.3–11 = L. 6.32–34 and *Morb. I* 6.140.1–2). It is unclear whether these writers had to worry about medicine's ability to attract patients.[22] It is enough that some of them took exception to this affront on intellectual grounds, and it is for this reason that the Hippocratic response is of interest to historians of philosophy.

What does it mean, first and foremost, to say that medicine 'is not' or 'wholly is not'? One might read the expression through the lens of Plato's discussions of *technē* in dialogues such as the *Gorgias*, in which Socrates asks whether rhetoric is a *technē* (465a). This, however, would be a mistake. For Socrates grants that rhetoric 'is' (463a), but he denies that it is a *technē*, terming it instead a knack born of experience (465a). Simply put, to say that something, whether rhetoric or medicine, is not a *technē* does not commit one to denying that it is at all. On the other hand, when the Greeks say of something that it 'is not' (οὐκ ἔστιν), we encounter a syntactically complete occurrence of ἔστι functioning as what Charles Kahn calls an 'existential predicate.'[23] To say that a *technē* is not, for example, would be to say that it cannot be the subject of a sentence with existential import. Thus, if medicine is not, then it is not beneficial, not because medicine is harmful but because it is neither beneficial nor harmful, there being no such thing as medicine in the first place.

Jonathan Barnes has marked the same distinction in Sextus' *Against the professors* (1988, 54, 67–69, 72–73). There, Barnes argues, Sextus engages with two different kinds of global skepticism about *technē*, one 'reformative' and the other 'nihilistic' (my names, not Barnes'). The reformative skeptic will argue that something—rhetoric, for example—is not a *technē* but will not deny that rhetoric is useful for accomplishing certain ends. The nihilistic

---

[22] Lesley Dean-Jones (2003) denies that the attack on medicine had any real public support.

[23] Kahn notes that to speak of an "existential" use is potentially misleading insofar as copulative uses may have existential import (10). But in such cases it is not the existence of the subject term that is in question. So it is in the *Gorgias*, when Socrates calls rhetoric *empeiria*, but also in *VM*'s discussion of the evolution of medicine: "if this [cooking and basic nutrition] is thought not to be a *technē* (μὴ τέχνη αὕτη νομίζεται εἶναι), it is not unreasonable. Where no one is a layperson but all are knowledgeable about something because they are compelled by necessity to use it, it is not appropriate for anyone to be called a *technitēs*." (123.9–12 = L. 1.578). Cooking is (that is, there is such a thing as cooking), though it is not a *technē*.

skeptic, by contrast, will argue that rhetoric 'is not,' by which he means that there is no such thing at all. What is conventionally called rhetoric is utter nonsense. These two varieties of skepticism are easily transposed into a modern idiom. One might deny that political science is indeed a science without questioning its utility, much less its existence. The same person might easily deny that there is any such thing as astrology. In Greek terms, astrology 'is not.' In order to refute this charge, the defender of astrology must demonstrate not only that there is a causally coherent natural phenomenon to be studied (e.g., a determinate causal relationship between the stellar configuration at the time of one's birth and one's mature psychological dispositions), but also that self-described experts indeed have been relatively successful at understanding the phenomenon and applying that understanding in practice. Our author is fully aware that both conditions must be met, and arguing that they have been met in the case of medicine is his primary objective in cc. 4–6, which culminates in the declaration that 'medicine evidently has and always will have being, both in virtue of things that come to be 'because of something' and in virtue of things known in advance' (6.4).

We must take care to distinguish these intellectual concerns about the foundations of medicine from moral concerns about the physician's character that become salient to Hellenistic writers whose works are also among those included in the *Corpus*, notably *Jusj.*, *Decent.*, and *Praec.* The earlier authors have little to say about a physician's personal appearance or bedside manner. Instead, they focus on refuting or deflecting the accusation that medicine's apparent successes are the work of mere chance (*de Arte*, *VM*, and perhaps *Morb.* I) or that physicians cannot know anything about the internal processes of the body since they are not open to inspection (*de Arte*, *VM*, and perhaps *Nat. Hom.*). These are the main problems that occupy the author of *de Arte*, and I discuss them at some length in my commentary. The second of these is especially interesting in the history of philosophy, for the proper role of unobservable entities in scientific theories is a perennial question in the philosophy of science. It was a major point of contention between the Sceptics and their philosophical opponents, and the issue saw a revival in the twentieth century at the hands of the logical positivists.[24]

Comparison of the critics of medicine with the logical positivists is especially apt in that both groups seem to have launched their attack from the

---

[24] See Carnap, Hahn, and Neurath 1929 for the classic statement of the logical positivists' anti-realist program.

same point of origin: the positive epistemological thesis that, in order to count as knowledge, beliefs about matters of fact must be justified, usually directly verified, by perceptual experience. Thus, alleged knowledge of unobservable entities is no knowledge at all. But while they share a severe empiricism, the ancient critics and the logical positivists part ways in their conclusions about where this critique leaves science. The logical positivists sought to reform science by purging it of its 'metaphysical' tendencies; the ancient critics, from what we read in the Hippocratic *Corpus*, were happy to fiddle as *technē* burned.

Viewed in this light, *de Arte* emerges as perhaps the earliest defense of scientific realism in the history of philosophy. So what precisely is its defense? Understandably few historians of philosophy or medicine have dared to wade into its murky waters. Its highly compressed and high-toned arguments do not invite friendly analysis. Nonetheless, I believe *de Arte* is greater than the sum of these parts. When we take an aerial view of our author's philosophical positions, we may be surprised to find that they fit comfortably together. For him, one of the tasks of the medical *technē* is to discover ἀνάγκαι, or necessary connections, in nature (12.3). This amounts to discovering the observable εἴδεα, or forms, of nature, which is to say natural kinds and their characteristic configurations of causal powers, or δύναμεις (2.2, 4.4). Not surprisingly, he embraces a theory of names that recognizes the constraints that the real structure of natural kinds places upon the terms conventionally applied to the world (2.3).

It is revealing that modern defenses of scientific realism tend to cluster around these same ideas. If natural kinds have real essences, so the reasoning goes, and if natural kind terms rigidly designate natural kinds, then we may hold out the hope of fitting our language to the world so as to make induction possible (Boyd 1999; Putnam 1972). And induction is crucial to any attempt to make inferences about (and therefore acquire knowledge of) the unobservable. If the juxtaposition of these ideas with the doctrines of *de Arte* seems anachronistic, I hasten to clarify that my claim is not that we encounter here a fully worked-out philosophy of science. Rather, it is that *de Arte* bears a prima facie family resemblance to these realist accounts, and this raises the interesting question as to whether its author is reacting to primitive versions of skepticism that anticipate those that motivate modern anti-realists. Indeed, many have tried to put faces on these early skeptics, principally by comparing passages from c. 2 to fragments of various pre-Socratic philosophers. Let us review the chapter in full. (For the sake of clarity and precision, I add lower-case Roman numerals as subsection headers.)

> 1 (i) It seems quite clear to me that, on the whole, there is no art that is not, (ii) since it's just absurd to believe that one of the things-that-are is not. (iii) For what being could anyone observe of the things-that-are-not and report that they are? (iv) For if indeed it is possible to see the things-that-are-not, just as it is to see the things-that-are, I don't know how anyone could believe of those things that it were possible both to see with his eyes and to know with his mind that they are, that they are not. 2 (v) Isn't it rather more like the following? (vi) Whereas the things-that-are always are in every case seen and known, the things-that-are-not are neither seen nor known. (vii) Accordingly, the arts are known only once they have been taught, and there is no art that is not seen as an outgrowth of some form. 3 (viii) In my opinion, they acquire their names, too, because of their forms. (ix) For it's absurd—not to mention impossible—to think that forms grow out of names: (x) names for nature are conventions imposed by and upon nature, whereas forms are not conventions but outgrowths.

> 1 (i) Δοκεῖ δή μοι τὸ μὲν σύμπαν τέχνη εἶναι οὐδεμία οὐκ ἐοῦσα · (ii) καὶ γὰρ ἄλογον τῶν ἐόντων τι ἡγεῖσθαι μὴ ἐνεόν · (iii) ἐπεὶ τῶν γε μὴ ἐόντων τίνα ἂν τίς οὐσίην θεησάμενος ἀπαγγείλειεν ὡς ἔστιν; (iv) Εἰ γὰρ δὴ ἔστι γε ἰδεῖν τὰ μὴ ἐόντα ὥσπερ τὰ ἔοντα, οὐκ οἶδ' ὅπως ἄν τις αὐτὰ νομίσειε μὴ ἐόντα ἅ γε εἴη καὶ ὀφθαλμοῖσιν ἰδεῖν καὶ γνώμῃ νοῆσαι ὡς ἔστιν. 2 (v) Ἀλλ' ὅπως μὴ οὐκ ᾖ τοῦτο τοιοῦτον · (vi) ἀλλὰ τὰ μὲν ἐόντα αἰεὶ ὁρᾶταί τε καὶ γινώσκεται, τὰ δὲ μὴ ἐόντα οὔτε ὁρᾶται οὔτε γινώσκεται. (vii) Γινώσκεται τοίνυν δεδιδαγμένων ἤδη τῶν τεχνέων καὶ οὐδεμία ἐστὶν ἥ γε ἔκ τινος εἴδεος οὐχ ὁρᾶται. 3 (viii) Οἶμαι δ' ἔγωγε καὶ τὰ ὀνόματα αὐτὰς διὰ τὰ εἴδεα λαβεῖν · (ix) ἄλογον γὰρ ἀπὸ τῶν ὀνομάτων ἡγεῖσθαι τὰ εἴδεα βλαστάνειν καὶ ἀδύνατον · (x) τὰ μὲν γὰρ ὀνόματα φύσιος νομοθετήματά ἐστιν, τὰ δὲ εἴδεα οὐ νομοθετήματα, ἀλλὰ βλαστήματα.

These passages are discussed at length in the commentary, and I am hesitant to duplicate the points made there. However, it will be helpful to reproduce the relevant fragments of the various pre-Socratics thought to be lurking in the background. The language and style of the argument is perhaps most often dubbed 'Eleatic' or 'Parmenidean,'[25] and I would concur, with qualification, on the basis of the following fragments.

> For never can this be victorious, that the things-that-are-not are (εἶναι μὴ ἐόντα),
> but you, block your thought from this path of inquiry,
> and do not let habit, derived from much experience, force you down this much-experienced path[26]

---

[25] E.g., by Taylor (1911, 225), Jouanna (1988, 175), and Hankinson (1998, 77).

[26] The Greek is ἔθος πολύπειρον ὁδοῦ, and I take the adjective to modify both nouns, which I think is consistent with the poetic genre and yields a richer sense. Conveniently, it also mirrors my construal of αἰεί in 2.2.

to guide your sightless eye (ἄσκοπον ὄμμα) and clanging ear
and tongue, but judge by reason (κρῖναι δὲ λόγωι) the much-contested
refutation
uttered by me. (DK 28 B7)

For neither could you know what-is-not, for this can't be done,
nor could you say it.

οὔτε γὰρ ἂν γνοίης τό γε μὴ ἐὸν (οὐ γὰρ ἀνυστόν)
οὔτε φράσαις. (DK 28 B2, ll. 7–8)

The syntax of DK 28 B2 is echoed at (vi), while its sense is captured in (vi) and (iii). But that is not to say that our author is a devout disciple of Parmenides. While he may, like many pre-Socratics, accept that what-is-not cannot be known, he diverges from the doctrine articulated in DK 28 B7 by insisting in (vi) that the-things-that-are are present to the senses. Likewise, while he seems to agree with Melissus that what is is always (ἔστιν ἀεί, DK 30 B3), some have detected in (vi) a rebuke of a Melissan argument.

> For if there is earth and water and air and fire and iron and gold, and the living as opposed to the dead, and black and white, and everything else that human beings claim are true, if indeed these are, and we see and hear correctly (εἰ δὴ ταῦτα ἔστι, καὶ ἡμεῖς ὀρθῶς ὁρῶμεν καὶ ἀκούομεν), each must be such as we first thought, and must not change or become different, but each must be always the sort of thing it is. But as it stands now, we claim to see and hear and understand correctly (νῦν δέ φαμεν ὀρθῶς ὁρᾶν καὶ ἀκούειν καὶ συνιέναι). We think that what is hot becomes cold and what is cold, hot, and what is hard becomes soft, and the soft, hard, and what is alive dies and comes to be from what is not alive, and all these things become different, and that what was and what is now are not at all alike, but iron, though it is hard, is worn down by a finger, as is gold and stone and everything else that seems to be strong; and earth and stone come to be from water. So that it turns out that we neither see nor know the things that are (ὥστε συμβαίνει μήτε ὁρᾶν μήτε τὰ ὄντα γινώσκειν). (DK 30 B8)

No doubt the language of (vi) would appear to echo that in the above fragment, though the echo becomes far fainter if Barnes is correct that the final clause, ὥστε συμβαίνει μήτε ὁρᾶν μήτε τὰ ὄντα γινώσκειν, ought to be secluded.[27] In any case, the sentiment expressed in *de Arte* seems directly opposed to that voiced by Melissus, though it is difficult to say more than this, since (vi) is a programmatic statement lacking direct support in

[27] Jonathan Barnes (1982a, 298 n. 3) argues that συμβαίνειν is not pre-Socratic Greek and that γινώσκειν does not have the requisite sense to mirror συνιέναι. While it strikes me as possible that the clause stood in Melissus' original, it does stick out rather awkwardly from the surrounding text, and Barnes may be right that this is a gloss in a later hand.

argument and thus cannot be coordinated with the substantive remarks in the fragment. We encounter the same problem when considering a fragment from Antiphon's *Truth*.

> If you have understood these things, you will know that for him (?) is nothing any one thing, neither of the things that he who sees most deeply sees with his vision, nor the one that knows most deeply knows with his mind (οὔτε ὧν ὄψει ὁρᾶι ⟨ὁ ὁρῶν⟩ μακρότατα οὔτε ὧν γνώμηι γιγνώσκει ὁ μακρότατα γιγνώσκων).[28]
> (DK 87 B1)

The text and meaning of the fragment is deeply problematic. It may be an empirical argument against monism, but that is at best a conjecture. Again, there is not enough argumentative content for fruitful comparative analysis with *de Arte*. At best we may observe the similarity of language between Antiphon and (iv–vi).

*De Arte* could be 'Eleatic' in its concern for the thinkability and eternity of what-is, but its author departs from the Eleatic path in his insistence that being is a plurality ('the things-that-are') and that it is somehow accessible by perception. These commitments push *de Arte* in the direction of Protagoras, whose *homo mensura* was explicated by Plato with the argument that

> it is possible to think neither what-is-not nor anything other than what one experiences, and these latter are true in every case. (167a)
>
> οὔτε γὰρ τὰ μὴ ὄντα δυνατὸν δοξάσαι, οὔτε ἄλλα παρ' ἃ ἂν πάσχῃ, ταῦτα δὲ ἀεὶ ἀληθῆ.

The language of Plato's gloss is reminiscent of (vi), to be sure, and the meaning may match our author's claim in (iv) that what is seen and known (i.e., thought) must be thought to exist. Indeed, Gomperz held that (vi) and the *homo mensura* expressed the same doctrine (1910, 22) and further suggested that *de Arte* was written either by Protagoras or by a disciple of his (1910, 22–35). Much of Gomperz' discussion relies on an idiosyncratic and outdated interpretation of the *homo mensura*. Our best evidence is that Protagoras was a radical empiricist who attacked the arts, some (e.g., geometry) on the grounds that their principles were non-evident, or ἄδηλον (see further Mann 2008b). That would make Protagoras more likely to have been one of the critics whom our author targets in *de Arte*, not its immediate author or inspiration (see section 5 below).[29] For while there are strains of

---

[28] DK 87 B1 = Pendrick F1. The reading and its interpretation are much disputed, and I am confident neither in Pendrick's version nor in Morrison's (1976, 525).

[29] The idea that the *homo mensura* is in direct opposition to the philosophical commitments voiced in *de Arte* was first suggested by Bourgey (1953, 119 n. 4).

empiricism in *de Arte*, our author is adamant that the epistemic obstacles posed by non-evidence (τὰ ἄδηλα) can be overcome (11.1). In this, his views mirror the more measured empiricism of Xenophanes, who, while denying that no one could have genuine knowledge of the non-evident (DK 21 B34), was optimistic about the possibility of making discoveries over time (DK 21 B18). Our author is more sanguine yet, maintaining that the non-evident indeed can be known, even if, as Xenophanes would have agreed, it requires greater time and effort (11.2).

Our author distills the essence of his epistemology into a vivid dictum: 'what eludes the sight of the eyes is captured by the sight of the mind (τῇ τῆς γνώμης ὄψει)' (11.2). The metaphor of cognitive faculties as a kind of sight is not unique. It is present, at least obliquely, in the famous fragment of Anaxagoras, who certainly shared the view that the non-evident is nonetheless knowable: 'the phenomena are a sight of the non-evident (ὄψις ἀδήλων τὰ φαινόμενα, DK 59 B21a).'[30] Gorgias illustrates the power of speech using as an example the natural philosophers of his day, who 'by removing and producing one opinion in exchange for another make the incredible (τὰ ἄπιστα) and non-evident (τὰ ἄδηλα) appear to the eyes of opinion (τοῖς τῆς δόξης ὄμμασιν)' (DK 82 B11 § 13). His remark is especially relevant because he restricts the layperson's views on the non-evident to the province of 'opinion,' mirroring our author's reliance on mind to apprehend the non-evident, but with an important difference: Gorgias' treatment is probably pejorative. Speech is so powerful it can cause people to subscribe to fantastic ideas about matter of which they have no personal experience.

Generally speaking, though, Greek thinkers (including our author) helped themselves to the 'mind's eye' metaphor in celebration of reason's triumph over the limits on knowledge imposed by the senses. So Plato: 'the sight of reason (ἡ ... τῆς διανοίας ὄψις) sharpens as the sight of the eyes (ἡ τῶν ὀμμάτων *sc.* ὄψις)' (*Symposium* 219a). Socrates is making reference first and foremost to the wisdom one acquires as he ages, and so his words do not carry the technical epistemological weight that they do in *de Arte*. Less poetic but more relevant is a fragment of Democritus.

> Whenever the obscure faculty (γνώμη) is no longer able to see or hear or smell or taste or perceive by touch the infinitesimal, though more subtle matters [must be investigated, then the genuine faculty takes over, since it possesses a more subtle tool for thought.][31] (DK 68 B11)

[30] For the significance of Anaxagoras' dictum in its intellectual-historical context, including brief remarks on *de Arte*, see Diller (1932, 21).

[31] The bracketed material is supplied by Diels, but there is little question that the gist is right.

As in *de Arte*, reason picks up where the senses leave off. For Democritus, of course, it is not so much a matter of the senses 'leaving off' as it is of their abject failure to apprehend reality. Our author's language, too, might be construed as somewhat critical—the eyes 'let the criminal get away'—but his overall tone is decidedly more neutral, and we should not ignore his reversal of the Democritean phrasing. For Democritus, perception and reason are kinds of γνώμη, but for our author γνώμη is a kind of sight. This is not just a difference in metaphor. *De Arte*, as we shall see, upholds the validity, even the superiority, of perception over reason as a mode of knowledge acquisition (12.1), and indeed the image of 'the sight of the mind' suggests that our author holds reason to an epistemological standard set by perception.

So our author contends that, in cases of non-evident disease, 'as it is impossible to achieve perfect clarity (τὴν ἀναμάρτητον σαφήνειαν) by listening to these reports, the doctor must look to something else' (11.4). This he calls λογισμός, 'reasoning' (11.3), or, more specifically, τεκμαίρεσθαι, 'making inferences' (12.2, 12.4), and the terminology recalls a well known fragment of the physician-philosopher Alcmaeon of Croton: 'concerning the non-evident (περὶ τῶν ἀφανέων) and the mortal, gods have clear knowledge (σαφήνειαν), but we, insofar as we are human beings, are left to make inferences (τεκμαίρεσθαι)' (DK 24 B1). The fragment resonates deeply with *de Arte*. In both, perceptual clarity is highly esteemed (it is characterized as worthy of the divine and is obviously preferred by Alcmaeon), but, when it comes to non-evident matters, such perceptual clarity is unavailable to human beings. That is not to say that humans are without recourse; they can make inferences, and there is no denial that sound inferences conduce to knowledge. Still, inference is a second-best, something to which humans resort when they cannot directly perceive the truth.

If some diseases are non-evident, there arise serious questions as to how we should understand our author's declaration in (vi) that 'the things-that-are always are in every case seen and known, the things-that-are-not are neither seen nor known.'[32] In what sense are non-evident diseases seen? On the most literal interpretation, a disease that is not seen would not qualify as one of the 'things that are.' But assuming that our author would not concede such a point to the critics of medicine, we should seek more creative ways of taking his meaning here. Two main avenues appear open

[32] In any case, I cannot agree with commentators like Bourgey who see here little more than half-hearted pass at resolving certain problems of knowledge that plague the *Corpus* (1953, 67).

to us. Either we may read the phrase 'seen and known' more figuratively, or we may assign to the phrase 'the things-that-are (always)' a more technical function. In the first case, it is certainly possible that 'seen' refers broadly to any cognitive procedure that depends in some way on empirical knowledge and not merely to direct perceptual acquaintance with a fact or object. Thus, we may 'see' something indirectly by using empirical knowledge as the basis for further inference, as our author recommends in his discussion of signs in c. 12. But though later chapters are consistent with, perhaps even suggestive of, this interpretation, it strikes me as too metaphorical for the immediate context of (vi). For (vi) is presented in part as a justification of the claims made in (iii) and (iv), and these seem to require that 'seen' imply direct perceptual acquaintance.

Alternatively, we might suppose that the phrase 'the things-that-are always' does not include the particular diseases to which the doctor has no immediate perceptual access. After all, post-Parmenidean philosophers, most notably Anaxagoras and Empedocles, recognized that particulars are continuously perishing and coming to be, concluding that such transient beings could not be identified with 'real' being (cf. DK 59 B17; DK 31 B8). Certainly, such particulars do not exist 'always,' i.e., eternally. However, their finite lives are transcended by their character, structure, or form, which may be realized in multiple particulars. This, I submit, explains in part our author's transition to a discussion of εἴδεα, 'forms' or 'kinds,' which, he insists in (vii), are visible, perhaps in the sense that the characteristic structure or form is thought to be present in each particular (see further the discussion in my commentary on 2.2–3). Accordingly, a particular non-evident disease will be 'seen' just in case it can be known, and it will be known in virtue of the fact that it has a certain natural form, the constitutive causal powers of which are open to observation. As it is put in *de Arte*, diseases are 'the sorts of things they are through the presence or absence of each of these [sc. 'powers,' i.e., hot, cold, and perhaps solidity and liquidity]' (9.3), and, since we know the nature of hot and cold through observation, we know something about the diseases in which such causal factors play a role, whether or not they are immediately accessible by perception. Even if it is not at the moment actually seen, a particular case of non-evident disease is an instance of a natural kind that is, in an important sense, evident.

In fact, it is the 'formal' structure of reality that makes the correct use of language (and, ultimately, knowledge and teaching) possible. There have been many attempts to understand our author's brief excursus on language in (viii) through (x); my own attempt is found in the commentary on 2.3. Whatever the specific differences between the going scholarly views, however, a general consensus has emerged that *de Arte* recognizes the constraints that the natural order of the world places on language while acknowledging also the conventional or social aspect of language. As some have pointed out (Vegetti 1964, 68; Jori 1996, 380), this anticipates Plato's picture of language in the *Cratylus*, which emphasizes the functional role of language in distinguishing between forms in nature (386c–388c) while conceding that names are in certain respects the products of legislation (388e; cf. *de Arte* 2.3). In this and perhaps other ways, *de Arte* serves as a bridge between the clumsy but original treatment of forms in Empedocles, to which the discussion in c. 2 owes a substantial debt (see my notes ad loc.), and the more sophisticated theories of Plato and Aristotle. This, I would argue, is partly responsible for the treatise's philosophical appeal. Highly eclectic yet complete and coherent, *de Arte* affords us a glimpse of a vibrant, progressive pre-Platonic tradition that honors its origins and anticipates its intellectual heirs.

## 4. De Arte *as Medical Treatise*

Perhaps because its form is 'sophistic' and its content so philosophical, scholars sometimes ignore the more medical aspects of *de Arte*, by which I mean the basic theoretical commitments in the areas of anatomy, physiology, and nosology that justify or ground a doctor's therapeutic approach. Even if Lloyd is correct that 'the actual medical knowledge [our author] displays is none too impressive' (1991, 254), this is easily accounted for by the treatise's rhetorical and philosophical objectives, which require that its author expend his energies elsewhere. But it is possible, too, that the medical background to the philosophical and rhetorical arguments in *de Arte* is more complex than is usually allowed. Of the major studies of *de Arte* to date, only Vegetti's makes a serious effort to investigate such questions. His conclusion is that *de Arte* is thoroughly 'Coan' and, thus, 'Hippocratic' (1964, 320), and while I will not wade into the dark waters surrounding such designations, some of the evidence cited by Vegetti in defense of his thesis deserves attention. The conclusion is based largely (but not completely) on *de Arte*'s alleged affinity with three treatises, namely, *VM*, *Acut.*, and *Prog.* Vegetti cites *de Arte* 5.4 in connection with the first two.

> For it was by fasting or by overeating (ἀσιτίῃ ἢ πολυφαγίῃ), by drinking much fluid or by abstaining from it, by bathing or by not bathing, by vigorous exercise or by rest, by sleep or by wakefulness, or by using some combination of these that they recovered.

This is to be compared, Vegetti asserts, with chapters in *VM* that identify κένωσις and πλήρωσις (deficiency and repletion of food) as the principal factors that cause disease (e.g., 128.7–9 = L. 1.588). The comparison appears less apt, however, once we recognize that *de Arte* is listing therapeutic measures that *cure* disease, not giving a general aetiology of disease. In *VM*, deficiency and repletion are essentially harmful, and the author does not recommend them as cures. Much closer to *de Arte* would be *Acut.*, which, as Vegetti points out, addresses the therapeutic value of fasting (e.g., 57.9–11 = L. 2.330), drinking (e.g., 44.16–19 = L. 2.266), bathing (e.g., 65.4–67.18 = L. 2.364–374), rest (e.g., 55.17–18 = L. 2.318), and sleep (57.16–18 = L. 2.330).

Vegetti is probably correct that *de Arte* at times appears to share with *VM* and *Acut.* a basic model of health as the product of dietetic, and probably even humoral, balance (see, for example, 7.1–3 and my comments). Our author, no less than the authors of *VM* and *Acut.*, is adamant that regimen is an indispensible component of medicine (6.1–3). However, he shows no apprehension about the practice of cautery (8.4), and his examples of sign-provocation depend largely on pharmaceutical effects (12.4–5). Moreover, there is no obvious agreement between *de Arte* and the other two treatises on the underlying principles or processes that figure in the dietetic balance. In *VM*, for example, this balance is explicitly described as a tempering (κρῆσις) of powers (δύναμεις) in the body, one which is achieved, at least in part, through a process of coction (πέψις) (143.3–6 = L. 1.616, 145.12–16 = L. 1.620). But while δύναμις, or power, is something of a technical term in *de Arte*, it does not denote the basic phenomenal-chemical humor that serves as a fundamental *explanans* of disease in *VM* (149.1–3 = L. 1.626). Likewise, the axiom of dietetic theory laid down in *Acut.*, i.e., that 'great changes in conditions related to our natures and constitutions are most productive of disease' (50.9–11 = L. 2.296), is nowhere to be found in *de Arte*. Nevertheless, the case for affinity between *de Arte* and the two dietetic treatises is bolstered by certain overlaps in anatomical and physiological theory. Vegetti perhaps overstates the general similarity between c. 10 of *de Arte* and the twenty-second chapter of *VM* (149.1–152.17 = L. 1.626–634), but he is right to remark on the mutual interest on the porosity and hollowness of the abdominal and thoracic cavities and their organs. Both use the technical term θώρηξ (*de Arte* 10.4, *VM* 151.8–9 = L. 1.630); *de Arte* says it is empty (κενόν), while *VM* calls it hollow (κοῖλον). In the case of *Acut.*, a discussion of oxymel's acidic properties, especially its value for bringing up sputum (61.14–62.1 = L. 2.348–350), resonates with a textually difficult passage in *de Arte* on the role of acrid food and drinks (σιτίων δριμύτητι καὶ πωμάτων) in dispersing phlegm (12.4).

Comparison of *de Arte* with *Prog.* produces similarly mixed results. Our author's conviction that the art uses signs (σημεῖα) to form a diagnosis of non-evident diseases, 'including what has already been suffered and what it is possible yet to suffer' (12.2), recalls the famous proclamation in *Prog.* that 'if [the doctor] prognosticates and predicts in the presence of his patients what *is* happening, what *has* happened, and what *will* happen (to the extent that any of these things were left out of the patient's original account), the more he will be believed to know his patients' real situations, so that people will dare to place themselves in the doctor's hands' (2.110.2–9). And Vegetti is correct in noting that *Prog.* discusses the importance of many of the signs mentioned in c. 12 of *de Arte*: respiration (2.122.11–17; in relation to abscesses specifically, 2.152.13–158.2), urine (2.138.15–142.15), expectoration (2.144.9–146.15), and sweats (2.122.18–124.12). This is hardly surprising, since the objective in *Prog.* is to connect observable symptoms of a patient to his outcome. To that end, the author supplies the reader with rules to be used in concert with observations of particular cases to yield an accurate prognosis.

> One must also observe the parts of the eyes that are visible during sleep. For if some part of the white shows when the lids are shut (unless this arises from diarrhea or purgative drugs or the patient usually sleeps like this), this is a bad—in fact, an extremely deadly—sign. (2.116.11–118.3)

At first, *Prog.* seems to employ a straightforwardly syllogistic model of sign-inference that anticipates the Stoic definition of a sign as the antecedent of a true conditional (see Appendix 4). The doctor is advised to observe the totality of the particular patient's symptoms, and *Prog.* provides the doctor with general conditionals that allow him to determine in any particular case what the outcome will be. For example:

1. If patients' eyeballs show during sleep, then they will die.
2. This patient's eyeball is showing during sleep.
3. Therefore, this patient will die.

But not all sign-inferences in *Prog.* can be analyzed as *modus ponens* syllogisms. Sometimes the consequent of a conditional contains the semiotic information. 'If a sore happens to have developed either before or during the course of the disease, examine it closely. For if the sick patient is about to die, before he dies it will be livid and dry or pale and hard' (2.122.1–4). The sign-inference available to the student of *Prog.* will not be deductively valid in this case.

1. If patients with sores are about to die, then they will have sores of such and such a character.

2. This patient has a sore of such and such a character.
3. Therefore, this patient will die.

The physician will not be able to say with absolute certainty that a patient with this kind of sore is about to die, but he is right to be concerned, since the appearance of such a sore is consistent with the patient's death.

There is little evidence that the author of *Prog.* is concerned with absolute certainty at all. Instead, his language suggests that his objective is to provide his readers with the resources to calculate the relative probabilities of different outcomes based on the competing signs they observe in the patient.

> The following are good [signs]: to endure the disease easily; to breathe well; to be free of pain; to bring up expectorate easily; for the body to be uniformly warm and soft and not be thirsty; for the urine and stool and sleep and sweat to exhibit the good qualities described earlier. For the person will not die if all these signs are present. But if some of these things are present, but not others, he will die after having survived for fourteen days or more. The bad signs are the opposite of these: enduring the disease with difficulty; heavy, deep breathing; no relief from pain; expectorate brought up with difficulty; extreme thirst; the body having an uneven fever, the stomach and the lungs being extremely hot; cold forehead, hands and feet; for the urine and stool and sleep and sweat to exhibit the bad qualities described earlier—if any of these occurs along with expectoration, the person will die within a fortnight, either on the ninth or eleventh day. Thus, one must make these inferences (συμβάλλειν), insofar as this expectorate is especially deadly and, if it does not recede, the patient will not reach the fourteenth day. A person must make his predictions on the basis of the good and bad signs he has included in his calculation. For in this way you would most likely speak the truth.
>
> (2.148.9–150.15)

The kind of sign-inference recommended here defies any attempt to reduce medical reasoning from signs to a set of simple syllogisms, whether deductively valid or not. What the author needs is a statistical model that would offer some way of weighting the various observations so as to arrive at the probabilities of various outcomes, not unlike what the Hellenistic Empirics would later implement (see Appendix 4). Probability is a much looser standard than the author of *de Arte* would likely accept, however. Though he never gives a complete concrete example of a typical sign-inference, his epistemic standard is the certainty afforded by direct observation (11.2, 11.4, 12.1). Moreover, a probabilistic model would mean that the source of some failures would be in some sense internal to the *technē*, a conclusion that our author strenuously rejects (see Appendix 3).

Of further (and related) interest is the ultimate subject matter of sign-inferences in *de Arte*. In the Appendix (section 4), I review Sextus Empiricus' account of the Stoic distinction between commemorative and indicative signs. Indeed, he takes Stoics and Epicureans to task for employing indicative signs; they erroneously believe that they can make inferences about what is unperceivable based on what they can perceive. This mirrors a debate in the Hellenistic medical community between Empirics and Rationalists, who argued over whether the task of medicine was to ferret out the underlying (and unperceivable) causes of disease (the Rationalist view), or whether medicine should restrict itself to making inferences about things of which it had direct experience (the view of the Empirics).[33] In comparing *Prog.* and *de Arte*, we find the early seeds of this eventual disagreement. Each depicts medicine as a certain kind of enterprise. The author of *Prog.* sees it as do the Empirics. Physicians observe closely what combinations of symptoms and treatments precede recovery or death. (Empirics, however, will deny that they use such observations to make inferences, properly speaking.) There is no effort to discover the internal causes of the disease. In fact, there is no explicit acknowledgement that such causes exist. In *de Arte*, by contrast, our author not only assumes that there are such causes, but also that discerning these is the principal task of the physician. His concern is not with the patient's future condition as such—there is no discernible interest, for example, in predicting the crises of fevers, as in *Prog.* and many other Hippocratic texts. Rather, the doctor in *de Arte* is determined to diagnose the patient's present internal state, from which inferences can be made regarding the future, especially regarding 'what should be done' (12.3).

All in all, there is some basis for endorsing, with qualification, Vegetti's view that *de Arte* bears a sort of family resemblance to these 'Coan' treatises. But it bears resemblance to other Hippocratic 'families,' as well. More recent work by Elizabeth Craik has uncovered affinities between *de Arte* and the pair of treatises *Loc. Hom.* and *Gland.* In the commentary, I flag some striking parallels, including the view of chance articulated at *de Arte* 4.2, which echoes *Loc. Hom.* 85.25–35 (= L. 6.342), and the description of the synovial joints at 10.5, which closely mirrors a description at *Loc. Hom.* 46.17–27 (= L. 6.290). But there are others. Indeed, there is significant overlap between *de Arte* and the two other treatises in the areas of anatomy and physiology. *De Arte* describes both φλέβες (vessels) and νεῦρα (cords) as 'stretched out

[33] I omit, for the sake of simplicity, the Methodist view. For a concise account of the differences between the Hellenistic medical schools, see further Hankinson (1998, 306–322). For a more detailed treatment, see Nutton (2004, 128–247).

along the bones (πρὸς τοῖσιν ὀστέοισι προστεταμένα);' in *Loc. Hom.*, both vessels and cords are said to be located 'along the bone' (38.25 = L. 6.280, 42.4 = L. 6.284). As Craik points out, there is an implicit general division in *Gland.* between the cavities of the body and the joints (2009, 15; see *Gland.* 68.1–6 = L. 8.556–558), while in *de Arte* non-evident diseases are 'those affecting the bones and the bodily cavity' (10.1), and the ensuing discussion devotes special attention to the contents of the cranial, thoracic, and abdominal cavities as well as to the synovial joints (cf. Craik 2009, 19–20).

According to *Gland.*, the physiological process primarily responsible for disease is the aberrant flow of moisture (66.11–12 = L. 8.556), and this is consistent with the general pathology given in *Loc. Hom.*: 'fluxes happen when the flesh is over-chilled or over-heated, or has an excess or a deficiency of phlegm' (46.30–31 = L. 6.290–292; trans. Craik). The author regularly associates phlegm with moisture, and 'phlegm-moisture-growth' as a theoretical axiom is taken to be broadly explanatory of health and disease (Craik 1998, 15). At the most basic physical level, two qualitative axes are operative: the hot-cold and the dry-moist:

> Pain occurs because of cold and because of heat and because of excess and because of deficiency. Pain occurs in parts of the body which have been chilled naturally, parts on the outside of the body towards the skin, by what heats too much, and in parts which are naturally hot by the cold; and in naturally dry parts by being moistened, and in naturally moist parts by being dried. (78.13–17 = L. 6.334; trans. Craik)

While, as in *de Arte*, drugs are said either to purge or bind (Craik 1998, 234; cf. *Loc. Hom.* 84.1–6 = L. 6.340), often drugs are identified by their natural heating or cooling properties (e.g., 52.1–12 = L. 6.296). Among the pathological conditions to which the underlying theory is applied are abscess, fever, and skin sores. Abscesses in the lung are indicated by various signs, including breathlessness and hoarseness of voice (58.28 = L. 6.308). The general approach to treating abscesses includes administering purgatives and inducing expectoration by 'harsh wine' (62.1–7 = L. 6.310), which, the author divulges a few lines later, is heating (62.9–12 = L. 6.312). Fevers, he writes, are caused by an excess of phlegm, and 'when fatigue and fever and excess affect [the patient], you must give copious baths and anoint with liquids and warm the patient as far as possible so that, the body being laid open, the feverish heat may escape through sweat' (66.15–20 = L. 6.318). Excessive phlegm is responsible also for chronic sores on the skin. By swelling the surrounding flesh, the phlegm invites the accumulation of ichor, the peccant, serous fluid that plays an unspecified pathological role also in *de Arte* (10.3; cf. Craik 1998, 233) and *Gland.* (72.16 = L. 8.562).

The few remarks in *de Arte* on pathology and therapeutics conform well to the picture presented in *Loc. Hom.* Diseases are classified as either evident or non-evident, and the former are exemplified by skin eruptions, obvious from their irregular color or swelling (9.3). The doctor may 'perceive their solidity and liquidity (or moistness, ὑγρότης) by our senses of sight and touch, as well as which of them are hot and cold, these diseases being the sorts of things they are through the presence or absence of each of these' (9.3). Non-evident disease generally is linked to the presence of ichor in the cavities (10.3), though later abscess (12.1) and fever (12.4–5) are treated as paradigms of non-evident disease, and there ichor is not mentioned. (However, it may be that abscesses and skin eruptions are both viewed as kinds of suppuration, in which case the relevance of ichor could be assumed. See also my notes on 12.1.) As in *Loc. Hom.*, signs of abscess may include rapidity of breath and scratchiness of voice (12.2), while fever is connected, at least in some cases, to 'congealed phlegm' (cf. *Loc. Hom.* 50.28–29 = L. 6.296), the expectoration of which may be induced by 'acrid food and drink' (12.4, though the passage is textually uncertain; see my notes ad loc.). Heat-producing pathogens in the body are melted by means of 'hot' food and drink, and the general approach to diagnosing non-evident diseases is based on heating processes such as exercise and vapor baths, which are designed to induce sweating (12.5).

Thus, the affinities between *de Arte* and the two treatises *Gland.* and *Loc. Hom.* are just as strong, and perhaps stronger, than those between *de Arte* and *VM*, *Acut.*, and *Prog.* Not every medical peculiarity in *de Arte* can be accounted for by these affinities, however. Our author's claim that any healthy cavity 'is full of breath,' for example, finds no parallel in the treatises examined by Vegetti and Craik but is more consistent with 'pneumatic' treatises like *Flat.* and *Morb. Sacr.* Moreover, certain phrases and ideas in *de Arte* correspond to passages from other treatises, most notably from *Vict.* and *Alim.* These two works, like *Gland.* and *Loc. Hom.*, espouse elements of a phlegm-moisture-growth theory of health and disease (*Vict.* 126.5–19 = L. 6.472–474; *Alim.* 140.2–4 = L. 9.98, 147.17 = L. 9.120), but their ambitions, or at least their approaches, are as much philosophical as medical. Both contain echoes in content and style of Heraclitus (*Vict.* 130.1–2 = L. 6.478; *Alim.* 146.14 = L. 9.116) as well as the post-Parmenidean pluralists Anaxagoras (*Vict.* 126.27–28 = L. 6.474; *Alim.* 143.2–3 = L. 9.106) and Empedocles (*Vict.* 126.25–26 = L. 6.474; *Alim.* 140.16–17 = L. 9.100). It is the last of these who ties *Alim.* perhaps most closely to *de Arte*. Alluding to Empedocles' remarks on the subject of forms and growth (e.g., Inwood 26 9–10 = DK 31 B21, Inwood 27 5–6 = DK 31 B23), the author of *Alim.* writes that '[nutriment] sends forth shoots of its own form' (τὴν μὲν ἰδίην ἰδέην ἐξεβλάστησε; 140.16 = L. 9.100; see *de Arte* 2.2–3 and my notes). To this may be added the similarity of remarks on spontaneity (*de Arte* 6.4; *Alim.* 141.20–22 = L. 9.102), names (*de Arte* 6.4; *Alim.* 142.20–22 = L. 9.104–106), the natural limits of medicine's power (*de Arte* 8.2; *Alim.* 141.22–23 = L.9.102), and the nature-education antithesis (*de Arte* 9.4; *Alim.* 145.12 = L. 9.112), not to mention a shared concern for non-evident diseases and their causes (*de Arte* 11.1ff.; *Alim.* 141.22–23 = L. 9.102, 142.6 = L. 9.104). The two treatises have more specific medical content in common, as well. When the author of *Alim.* lists the bodily secretions important to medicine (142.7–13 = L. 9.104), he includes some, like urine and sweat, that are singled out in *de Arte* (12.5; cf. also *Alim.* 143.16 = L. 9.106, which mentions sediment in the urine), and he ends the section with a sophistic declaration of relativity like the one that concludes *de Arte*'s discussion of secretions and their semiotic value (*Alim.* 142.11–13 = L. 9.104; *de Arte* 12.6; see my notes ad loc.).

The treatise *Vict.*, on the other hand, says little about signs; its subject is dietetic theory and practice, and the dietetic components with which the author is primarily concerned include food, drink, exercise, sleep, bathing, sex, and purging (see especially 194.17 = L. 6.594ff.), a list that overlaps substantially with that presented at *de Arte* 5.4. Further, *Vict.* features an extended analysis of foods and drinks in terms of their heating powers (162.9 = L. 6.534ff.; cf. *de Arte* 12.4), and the author frequently touts the dietetic virtues of running, with special attention to the kinds of courses that are to be run (e.g., *Vict.* 186.6–19 = L. 6.578–580; cf. *de Arte* 12.5). Indeed, the affinity between *de Arte* and *Vict.* is felt already in their respective *prooimia*, both of which denounce the pettiness of criticizing the mistakes and incomplete discoveries of predecessors while recommending that they be corrected discreetly (*Vict.* 122.3–21 = L. 6.466; *de Arte* 1.1–3). Later, the author of *Vict.* indulges in a digression that compares 'the nature of man' (by which he means medicine) to various *technai*, including prophecy, smithing, cobblery, carpentry, and others. Prophecy is like the nature of man in that it 'acquires knowledge of the non-evident (τὰ ἀφανέα) by means of the evident' (136.6–8 = L. 6.488); smithing in that it reduces iron with fire and nourishes it with water (136.16–17 = L. 6.488); cobblery in that it divides wholes into parts and makes parts whole (136.24–25 = L. 6.490); and carpentry in that it 'makes more by making less' (138.4–5 = L. 6.490). It is difficult not to be reminded of the argument at *de Arte* 11.7, which assimilates medicine to the other handicrafts (especially 'those that work with wood, or with leather, or the numerous others that work with bronze or iron or similar metals') insofar as all must come to a halt when their materials are missing. Finally, in *Vict.* we find a theory of mind that postulates certain physical constraints on intelligence: as in the case of physical health, mental health or intelligence (φρόνησις) depends on achieving the proper balance of material constituents (150.29 = L. 6.512 ff.), an idea perhaps hinted at—but only hinted at—in *de Arte* (7.1–3; see my notes ad loc.). Those with excessively watery souls are referred to as ἄφρονας ('senseless,' 154.8 L. 6.518; cf. *de Arte* 8.7) and their condition as μανίη ('madness,' 154.9 = L. 6.518; cf. *de Arte* 8.2).

There are a great number of affinities, then, between *de Arte* and diverse works in the Hippocratic *Corpus*. Clearly, our author embraces a medical eclecticism to rival his philosophical eclecticism; his ability to combine so many disparate ideas while avoiding contradiction is impressive in its own right. Less clear, however, is the explanation for this eclecticism. It is possible that in his attempt to defend the *technē* of medicine without qualification, he constructs a sort of composite image of that *technē*. This would explain also his surprising silence on the first principles (ἀρχαί) of health and disease; his surrender of medical detail to 'to those who care about these matters' (10.2); as well as his reticence about the specific content of specific medical diagnoses or prescriptions (see my notes on 12.4). In short, the 'theoretical void' at the center of *de Arte* may be calculated to avoid the appearance of theoretical prejudice. Alternatively, the void may be no void at all. Our author might well have developed a systematic theory to underpin his statements about medicine, but he may have chosen to obscure it for other reasons, possibly reasons of a rhetorical nature. After all, the treatise appears to be geared toward non-specialists, and the oversimplified presentation of medical ideas may simply reflect his audience.

The major obstacle to this last explanation is the almost complete lack of medical innovation or originality in *de Arte*; our author's ideas and methods are derivative. The sole exception is his suggestion that signs be actively provoked in cases where they are not forthcoming, a practice which, to my knowledge, is reported nowhere else in the *Corpus*, with the possible exception of *VC*, where the writer recommends that 'a dark drug' be applied to make evident suspected skull fractures and contusions (3.238–242; cf. Hirschberg 1913, 173), but even this example is only tenuously analogous. Indeed, our author might have anticipated resistance to the suggestion on grounds that it was gratuitously invasive—witness his paradoxical description of the procedure as 'harmless violence,' i.e., a temporary discomfort without lasting effects (12.3). But it could also be significant that the sign-provocations subsequently described correspond to many of the cures and treatments found in the Hippocratic treatises canvassed above. Supposing the administration of a purgative or diuretic by a doctor failed to cure the patient, what is the doctor's best defense? Perhaps that the prescription was issued not just to cure, but, failing that, also to coax further information about the disease from the patient's body. Thus, the apparent innovation may be a mere *ex post facto* contrivance, in which case *de Arte* would reveal itself once again as more rhetorical than medical in its mission.

## 5. *The Text and Its Questions*

Even in antiquity, *de Arte* does not appear to have been appreciated for its medical content as such. It was known to Erotian (and, before him, to Heraclides of Tarentium), who counted it not among the 'semiotic' or 'aetiological' works of Hippocrates, but rather as one of the 'therapeutic' works, and only then on something of a technicality. Erotian declined to classify it as a surgical or dietetic treatise, but included it in a special subset of treatises 'relating to the art,' which comprised also *Jusj.*, *Lex.*, and *VM* (Nachmanson, 9). Galen was aware of *de Arte*, but his only reference to it is in his glossary, where he is concerned not with a special medical term but with the exotic compound κακαγγελίη in 1.2 (Kühn 19, 107.8; see Jouanna 1988, 205–206). *De Arte* is directly quoted in two pseudo-Galenic works (*Introductio sive medicus* Kühn 14, 687.3–8; *Def. Med.* Kühn 19, 350.11–17). Both are concerned exclusively with the definition of medicine given at 3.2. The relative lack of interest on the part of ancient commentators has meant that editions of *de Arte* have had to rely almost exclusively on the surviving manuscripts. Jouanna gives a full account and reconstruction of the manuscript tradition (1988, 194–203), and I will not attempt in vain to improve on it. For present purposes, it suffices to say that there are two main lines of transmission, one represented by *Marcianus gr.* 269 (coll. 533) (= M), and another represented by *Parisinius gr.* 2253 (= A).

These two manuscripts, A and M, descend directly from the original *de Arte*, generally thought to have been written sometime in the late fifth-century BCE, after the rise of sophistic rhetoric but before the floruits of Plato and Aristotle.[34] Gomperz' commentary established this period as the literary and philosophical context for the work, and subsequent commentators have for the most part concurred. Heinimann argues (1961, 112 n. 32) that

[34] For a discussion of the reasons for assigning *de Arte* to the fifth century, as opposed to the fourth, including an admirably thorough review of the literature and refutation of dissident views, see Jori 1985, 245.

our author's use of words like ἀγγεῖα ('receptacles,' 10.4) demonstrates no awareness of the technical meanings they would take on in fourth-century treatises ('vessel'). Jouanna adds that adjectival forms ending in -ώδης and -ικός, ubiquitous in medical prose of the fourth century, are conspicuously absent from *de Arte* (1988, 191). The few attempts at dissent have not garnered scholarly sympathy. Diller, for example, believes (1975, 86–87) the occurrence of terms such as οὐσία and εἶδος to indicate that our author is familiar with Attic philosophy, but a closer analysis of their use does not support the hypothesis (see my comments on 2.1–3 and 6.4).

Though there is widespread agreement as to *when* our author composed *de Arte*, there is less agreement as to *why* it was written, or, more to the point, *for whom*. The most obvious answer, and in some ways the least interesting, is that it was written for a lay public (see Introduction 2 above).[35] But *de Arte* was written also in response to unnamed sophists and in defense of doctors. There is a very real sense, then, in which the critics targeted by our author, as well as the doctors he defends, constitute parts of the intended audience. This becomes still clearer when we consider the likely identity of our author's main opponent: Protagoras of Abdera. The identification is made with help from an exchange in Plato's *Sophist*.

> STRANGER: And what about the laws and all other civic matters? Don't [sophists] promise to make people capable of debating about them?
> THEAETETUS: In a word, *nobody* would talk to them if they didn't promise this.
> STRANGER: Indeed, the points one ought to raise in a debate against each craftsman himself, concerning all *technai* in general and each *technē* specifically, have been put down in writing and published somewhere for the benefit of anyone who wants to learn.
> THEAETETUS: You appear to me to be talking about the works by Protagoras on wrestling and the other *technai*.
> STRANGER: And on many other subjects, too, my good man.[36] (232d–e)

There are four important points to take away from the Platonic testimony. First, the Protagorean work was a kind of *logograph*; it laid out arguments that were to be recited by laypersons in the presence, and no doubt to the dismay, of a craftsman. Second, the work was designed to undermine the *technai* in two ways, namely, by disputing the *technai* generally, presumably

[35] This seemingly obvious thesis is questioned, however, in Demand 1996, where it is argued that the lack of philosophical influence upon the few discussions of medicine in the extant works of the Attic orators indicates a lack of public interest in philosophical medicine.

[36] For a discussion of the common misinterpretations of this passage, see Mann 2008b, 106–107.

calling into question the very notion of *technē*, and by disputing the claims made by experts in the particular *technai*. Third, Protagoras' ambition seems to have been to smear as many of the *technai* as he could; there is no indication that his attack was limited to a subset of the known *technai*. Fourth, and finally, the work—whatever its title—was well known to the public.

These four points make it plausible, even probable, that Protagoras' work attacked medicine, and that *de Arte* is written at least in part as a response to this attack.[37] Its logographic intent would explain what appear to be *de Arte*'s didactic asides to the beleaguered doctor (e.g., 7.1, 8.5). The plan to attack *technē* generally and then each *technē* in particular explains *de Arte*'s peculiar structure, i.e., our author's detour into the obscure territory of c. 2 before returning to the subject of medicine in c. 3. Further, given the ambitious scope of the Protagorean attack on the *technai*, it is difficult to imagine that such a prominent *technē* as medicine was spared. Finally, the public nature of Protagoras' criticism fits our author's description of those 'slandering the discoveries of those who have knowledge in front of those who do not' (1.2). Indeed, elsewhere Plato depicts Protagoras engaged in just such slander, ridiculing sophists who include the *technai* in their curricula on the grounds that they are irrelevant to a liberal man's political and personal success (*Protagoras* 318d–319a). Medicine is not listed among the *technai* scorned by Protagoras, but geometry is, and Aristotle reconstructs part of Protagoras' refutation of the geometers at *Metaph.* 997b–998a4.

The Protagorean critique seems to have been the most well known in antiquity, and I think it a reasonable assumption that our author would have striven for the greatest possible acclaim by opposing the most prominent of any *technē*-critics. Still, it is possible that our author has in mind other critics, as well. In the *Memorabilia*, for example, Xenophon reports that Socrates cautioned against studying arts, or any parts thereof, that either were not useful (4.7.2–5) or whose subject matter he deemed undiscoverable (4.7.6), going so far as to attempt a refutation of Anaxagoras' physical theories (4.7.7). With respect to medicine, he urged his companions to regulate their health through close attention to regimen, adding that, for a person who followed this advice, 'it would be a difficult task to find a doctor who knew more about what conduced to his health' (4.7.9). Xenophon cannot, of course, be taken as gospel, and in any case the Socratic

---

[37] This thesis was first put forward by Heinimann (1961, 111). It is accepted in some form by Vegetti (1964, 335), Jouanna (1988, 174), and Jori (1996, 346–357). The nature and impact of the Protagorean attack is addressed at some length in Mann 2008b.

reservations fall far short of the charge that medicine 'is not,' but the notions that obscure matters are beyond human ken and that the layperson may be better at maintaining his health than the doctor resonate with our author's responses to the problems of non-evident diseases (cc. 11–12) and success *sans médecin* (c. 5), respectively.

According to Sextus Empiricus, Anacharsis of Scythia (one of the so-called 'seven wise men') challenged the arts by questioning whether disputes between experts over the quality of technical products could ever be satisfactorily adjudicated. Anacharsis allegedly argued that laypersons are not qualified to judge such disputes, since they are ignorant of the rules and procedures of the art; nor can experts settle them, since they will necessarily disagree with one of the experts involved in the dispute, and the original problem will recur (M 7.55–59). Both Vegetti (1964, 337–338) and Jori (1996, 352–355) read *de Arte* 8.7 as our author's solution to the dilemma.

> Those experienced in this craft have no need for criticism or praise that is so senseless. Instead, they need people who have rationally considered in relation to what the products of craftsmen are fully finished; in what respect imperfect products are deficient; and further, concerning these deficiencies, which are to be attributed to the craftsmen and which to the things being crafted.

Jori takes the idea to be that judgments about the quality of technical products will be referred not to laypersons or experts in the particular *technē* but to the 'scientific community' at large (1996, 354), by which he means presumably the set of all technical experts, irrespective of specialization. Our author's reversion to the generic label 'craftsmen' is construed as a signal that the judges in question have reflected on the nature of *technē* generally and so are qualified to evaluate (objectively and neutrally) the success or failure of experts in any particular *technē*. But, as I say in my notes on the above passage, the point seems rather that a competent judge would need little more than a clear conception of the art's *telos* and the full use of his rational faculties; human reason provides the necessary objectivity and neutrality for an authoritative judgment. In any case, it is far from obvious that our author's remarks are directed against Anacharsis. It is still less obvious that we should follow both Vegetti and Jori in accepting the conjecture, first proposed by Untersteiner (1948a, 37–44), that the 'dilemma of judgment' did not originate with the historical Anacharsis, but rather that the Scythian figured as a character in the fourth book of Protagoras' *Antilogy*. The attribution rests on a tenuous equation of the argument in *Against the professors* (7.55–59) with one in the *Outlines* (3.264), and then a still more dubitable connection between that argument and Protagoras' famous discussion of virtue and teaching in Plato's *Protagoras* (326e–328b). There may well be reason to doubt Sextus' attribution of the dilemma to the historical Anacharsis (Untersteiner 1948a, 43–44), but subsequent scholarship on the sophists has not incorporated the attribution to Protagoras, and I remain unconvinced.

Gorgias, too, is sometimes cited as an antagonist of the *technai*.[38] According to Plato, Gorgias held that his art was superior to all others, and Socrates in the *Gorgias* imagines a dispute between Gorgias, a doctor, a trainer, and a businessman (452a–d). Whose art brings about the greatest good for humankind? Gorgias argues that it is rhetoric, since it produces persuasion, which is the source of human freedom generally and, for individual persons, the key to wielding power over others (452d). Moreover, all other arts are subordinate to rhetoric (*Gorgias* 456–b), and here Gorgias adduces as proof two examples. First, he claims, it is common for his brother, a doctor, to fail to convince a patient to undergo the prescribed therapy, while Gorgias, through his art, manages to persuade him (456b). Second, if an orator were to contest with a doctor over appointment as city physician, the orator would win, since the orator is able to speak more persuasively about all crafts than even the craftsmen themselves (456b–c).

But while this might qualify in some sense as 'speaking poorly of the arts' (τὰς τέχνας αἰσχροεπεῖν, 1.1), Gorgias comes nowhere close to posing the sort of existential threat to the arts, either collectively or individually, that is of central concern in *de Arte*. Gorgias never questions that the doctor is a better healer than the orator, and in fact his first example portrays rhetoric as an aid to medicine. Later in the dialogue, Plato has Gorgias condemn the misuse of oratory to denigrate the *technai*:

> For the orator has the power to argue against anyone about anything, and as a result he is more apt to persuade the masses about—well, in short, about whatever he wants. But, even though he has the power to do so, he ought not diminish the reputation of doctors or any other craftsman, but rather use rhetoric justly. (457a–b)

Indeed, in the *Helen*, Gorgias likens the art of speaking to medicine. Speech offers control over the soul just as medicine offers control over the body. Neither medicine nor *technē* as such is explicitly attacked, though some, like Vegetti (1964, 340), have read two passages as potentially hostile. As an example of the fact that persuasion, when added to words, has the power

[38] Jori argues heroically that Gorgias could be one of our author's adversaries (1996, 335–346), though some of his argument depends on an outdated interpretation of *On not being* (335–338).

to affect the soul in accordance with the speaker's desire, Gorgias cites "the words of those who study the heavens (τοὺς τῶν μετεωρολόγων λόγους), who by removing and producing one opinion in exchange for another make the incredible (τὰ ἄπιστα) and non-evident (τὰ ἄδηλα) appear to the eyes of opinion (τοῖς τῆς δόξης ὄμμασιν)" (DK 82 B11 §13). As I note above (Introduction 3), the language is reminiscent of the mind's eye metaphor in *de Arte* (11.2), and the reference to non-evident matters (τὰ ἄδηλα) reminds us of our author's preoccupation with non-evident diseases (e.g., 11.1ff.). But it is not clear that Gorgias is taking a position contrary to that articulated in *de Arte*. Again, his aim is to praise the power of persuasion, and his observation about the μετεωρολόγοι is designed to show that they require persuasive speech in order to propagate their theories. Gorgias does not question whether they themselves have knowledge of the matters they investigate, though he does say that 'as it stands, it is not easy (εὐπόρον) for [human beings] to remember the past, observe the present, or divine (μαντεύεσθαι) the future' (DK 82 B11 §11).[39] That it is difficult to have such knowledge does not entail that it is impossible, and the sentiment is in line with *de Arte*, whose author assures us that the art is not 'unequipped' (ἀπορεῖν) to deal with less evident diseases (10.1), though 'they are known with no less time and with even greater effort than they would have been if seen with the eyes' (11.2). Moreover, our author would agree with Gorgias that rhetoric ought to be used justly for the benefit of all (1.2–3), and perhaps even that arts like medicine were dependent on or subordinate to the art of speaking (see Introduction 2 above).

Thus, it is more plausible that Gorgias was an inspiration to the author of *de Arte* and not an antagonist. That Gorgias himself might be the author is not, I suppose, impossible, but it is unlikely (cf. Jori 1985, 259). Gomperz has shown convincingly that the style and language of *de Arte* is continuous with Attic oratory in the manner of Antiphon, and though there are 'Gorgianic' effects in the piece (antithesis, paromoiosis, isocolon), *de Arte* is more fluid and less formulaic than Gorgias' standard fare. Who, then, is the author? The question has captivated the attention of scholars since Gomperz' original

[39] The allusion to prophecy leads Vegetti (1964, 340) to wonder whether it is Gorgias' *Helen* that the author of *Acut.* has in mind when he complains that 'if in acute diseases practitioners differ from each other to such an extent that whatever one doctor thinks best to apply are considered bad by another, it is likely to be said in such cases that the *technē* is similar to divination (μαντικῄ)' (39.12–17 = L. 2.240–242). This is an interesting possibility, though Gorgias does not himself make the comparison. Further, the Hippocratic writer is worried about disagreement between doctors and diviners, a concern that Gorgias does not address.

study, and much ink—too much ink, I think—has been spilled without yielding consensus. An exhaustive study of the question and its history has been made by Jori (1985), who concludes that 1) our author was a sophist, not a practicing physician (252–253), and 2) he was likely Hippias of Elis (266). In what follows, I will briefly make the case for qualifying both claims.

I agree, as have most (but not all) scholars, that *de Arte* was in all likelihood composed by a sophist whose clinical experience was not extensive (see Jori 1985, 246ff.). Our author's facility with speech is plain, his facility with medicine less so. He avoids discussion of complicated anatomical and physiological detail (10.2). He neither describes the results of a diagnosis nor prescribes a single course of treatment (12.3). His remarks on the nature and causes of disease are vague and non-committal (9.3; 10.3). He is overconfident where he ought to be cautious (e.g., 9.4; see Hirschberg 1913, 171). But the affinities between *de Arte* and other works in the *Corpus*, traced above (Introduction 4), complicate the picture, and the lack of evidence of clinical experience should never be confused with evidence for the lack of clinical experience, the former of which could be explained in various ways. We might imagine, for example, that *de Arte*'s clinical vacuity is a clever rhetorical calculation. Writing in defense of medicine as a whole and for a lay audience, our author might have opted to simplify his material and suppress potentially controversial elements of his theory (see further Mann 2008a).

Nonetheless, the most plausible candidates for authorship are two figures who would be recognized primarily as sophists, Hippias of Elis and Antiphon of Rhamnus.[40] Hippias was suggested first by Diels (1914, 379). The attribution was argued for at greater length by Dupréel in a comprehensive study of the sophists (1948), and revived again by Jori (1985). The positive case for Hippias rests largely on external evidence that he was a polymath and champion of the *technai*. In the two Platonic dialogues named for him, Hippias boasts of his skill in various arts, including mathematics, astronomy, poetry, music, history, mnemotechnics, metalworking, tailoring, and cobblery (*Hippias major* 285b–d; *Hippias minor* 368b–c). Elsewhere Plato hints at friction between Hippias and Protagoras; the former apparently

[40] Gomperz' attribution to Protagoras or a Protagorean (1910, 21ff.) was undercut by the correct construal of *Sophist* 232d (Diels 1914, 378); nor has Ducatillon's more recent ascription of *de Arte* to the gymnastic physician Herodicus of Selymbria gained favor among scholars (1977b).

held that lectures on the *technai* were integral to education, while the latter, consistent with his attack on the *technai* documented at *Sophist* 232d–e, denied their value (*Protagoras* 318d–e). Lacking is evidence that Hippias took an interest in medicine or that the content of his theoretical views could have informed *de Arte*.[41] Jori compensates for this lack by linking *de Arte* to Hippias through the Greek doctor Eryximachus, son of Acumenus. At *Protagoras* 315c, Plato portrays him as a pupil of Hippias, and Jori recommends that in the *Symposium* his character be understood as a stand-in for the sophist (1985, 264). The speech of Eryximachus, with its emphasis on the medicine-gymnastics-farming triad (*Symposium* 187a), is paired with a theory of nature and convention described in the *Laws* (889c–e) as evocative of the sort of naturalistic bent that Hippias probably exhibited (265). (Jori confesses surreptitiously in a footnote (1985, 265 n. 120) that Untersteiner credits Antiphon, not Hippias, with the theory.) The medical views of Eryximachus are then mined for affinities with *de Arte*, and a jewel is discovered (265): Eryximachus' (or, rather, Hippias') distinction between a 'good love' manifested in health and a 'bad love' manifested in disease (*Symposium* 186b) is, in Jori's words, 'singularly analogous' to *de Arte*'s description of diseased patients 'consenting at last to admit those things that promote disease rather than those that promote health' (7.3).

It is nothing of the sort, of course. Our author goes on to add that patients succumb to the disease 'not because they desire death, but because they are powerless to endure' (7.3). That is, the patient's desire itself is not inherently bad or destructive (see my comments ad loc.). If the attribution to Hippias rests on this alleged affinity, then the positive evidence for it remains weak. The case for Antiphon is somewhat the inverse. While there is no record of his views on the subject of *technē* generally, much less of his involvement in a public conflict over the matter, there is ample evidence of overlap between the philosophical views of Antiphon and those laid out in *de Arte*. As I contend in my commentary on 2.2–3, some of the more obscure points cannot be made sense of without the advantage of Antiphon's fragments, and in places Antiphon confers real benefit upon our reconstruction of the text (e.g., 11.6). That Antiphon could have been the author of *de Arte* was first intimated by Untersteiner (1948b, 237) and later entertained also by

[41] Dupréel points to the apparent similarity of Hippias' position on nature and convention at *Protagoras* 337d, but Cherniss neutralizes the significance of the parallel by comparing Antiphon F44(a) II.10–20 (202).

Cherniss (201–203), whose advancement of the thesis served as a satirical ploy to expose the absurdity of Dupréel's attribution to Hippias (202 n. 10). In addition to the similarities in thought and expression I discuss above (Introduction 2, 3)[42] and in the commentary (esp. 2.2–3 and 11.6), Cherniss notes some extraordinary coincidences in diction that come down to us in bits of commentary on Antiphon's language.

> Antiphon: ἐπιθύμημα (object of desire). (DK 87 B110;[43] cf. *de Arte* 1.2: ἐπιθύμημά τε καὶ ἔργον)
>
> ὀδμή (scent) and εὐοδμία (fragrance) seem to many to be fine names, but they are poetic, confined to Ionic and Aeolic prose. Only in Antiphon would you find ὀδμάς and εὐοδμίαν. (F8; cf. *de Arte* 12.2: τὰ μὲν ὀδμῇσι τὰ δὲ χροιῇσι τὰ δὲ λεπτότητι καὶ παχύτητι)

Cherniss concludes, inexplicably, that 'all of this and more too would not constitute evidence that Antiphon wrote the *de Arte*, which he certainly did not' (202 n. 10). The source of Cherniss' pessimistic certainty is a mystery; perhaps he assumed that *de Arte* must be the work of a doctor. Jori, too, dismisses the attribution, but he does so less casually, citing the following testimony from Plutarch.

> [Antiphon] is said to have composed tragedies, both by himself and together with Dionysus the tyrant. While he was still working on poetry, he contrived a *technē* of alleviating distress, just like the therapy that doctors provide the sick. In Corinth he set up a workshop next to the marketplace and put out a sign saying that he was able to provide therapy, through words, to those who were distressed. And he comforted the troubled, asking after the causes. But thinking the *technē* beneath him, he turned to rhetoric. (T6(a))

Jori sees here an application and amplification of the Gorgianic pharmaco-linguistic analogy, according to which all knowledge is subordinate to rhetoric (1985, 261). This interpretation is transparently tendentious. Antiphon's invention of a 'talking cure' does not require Gorgias' analogy; nor does the sentiment that such work was 'beneath' him imply that it is subordinate to rhetoric in the sense Jori suggests. Yet even if it did, I have argued above (Introduction 2, 5) that our author's attitude toward rhetoric may be closer to Gorgias' than is usually allowed.

---

[42] I proceed on the assumption that there was one Antiphon responsible for the tetralogies, the fragments, and the court speeches, though even if this is not granted, the attribution remains plausible since it is based in the main on the fragments. For different views on the controversy surrounding the unity of Antiphon's corpus, see Gagarin (2002, 37–62), Pendrick (2002, 1–25), and Woodruff (2004, 323–336).

[43] The fragment is omitted by Pendrick.

More importantly, Plutarch tells us that Antiphon had clinical experience in a quasi-medical setting. To this we may add the fact that in his magnum opus, *Truth*, Antiphon propounded his own medical theories, fragments of which are preserved in the Arabic translation of Galen's *On medical names*.

> If you ask me for evidence from the utterances of the rhetors to serve as proof, so that you may know that these too meant by the word 'fever' fiery, unnatural heat, then listen to the utterance of Antiphon where he says: 'these, as I told you, are things that were caused by bile, because it was present in the hands and feet; whereas the bile which advanced to the flesh produced chronic fevers, when its mass was great. For when it advances to the flesh, there arises through it a corruption in the flesh's very substance and it swells up. The unnatural warmth therefore will come from this place; and if it lasts and becomes engrained, that will result from the bile, when it is present in abundance in the flesh and does not quickly disperse and subside, but remains, by persisting alongside the unnatural warmth.' You find, therefore, that in these words of his Antiphon does not restrict himself to calling unnatural warmth by the name by which all Greek speakers of the dialect known as Attic call it, i.e., *thermē*, so as to say that in the case of all who suffer from fever there is a warmth, which is known by this name. But he also informs you how this heat will arise, and traces the cause of its genesis to varieties of bile. Again in this same second book of his discourse, *Truth*, he makes another remark in which he traces the cause of the genesis of fever to varieties of gall, by saying: 'any one of them that advances to the flesh produces strong, long-lasting fevers.' Thereafter, when going into it a little further, he will use for the warmth that arises in an unnatural way in connection with arthritis (gout) a designation other than that used by all his colleagues, namely, *phlegmonē* and fever, two names which in this context point to burning. We can show that the ancients used to call everything resembling inflammation *phlegmonē* from the exegesis of what they said; for it has been explained by more than a few commentators. And that they also used to call it fever, you can show from the following remark, which I reproduce for you from the text of Antiphon: 'thus when more gets into the vessels than they can bear, they open up, and because of this there arises through it *phlegmonē*. And when *phlegmonē* arises through them and starts to cause pain for the one afflicted by it, and this takes root, then one calls this disease arthritis (gout). (F29A)

The views expressed by Antiphon offer no decisive parallels to *de Arte*, nor do they contradict it. The basic medical model is humoral, though the fragments stress the role of bile, a humor not mentioned in *de Arte*. Disease arises through the pathological accumulation of humors (cf. *de Arte* 10.3–4), and Antiphon exhibits a special concern with fever (cf. *de Arte* 12.4–5) and diseases of the joints (cf. *de Arte* 10.5). None of this is definitive proof that Antiphon was the author of *de Arte*, though it is at the very least evidence that he could have been. So might Hippias, too, but the argument in favor is considerably weaker. That is probably as close as we will come to achieving certainty on the question. As our anonymous author would be the first to admit, it is difficult to achieve perfect clarity about non-evident matters.

# ΠΕΡΙ ΤΕΧΝΗΣ

1 1 Εἰσίν τινες οἳ τέχνην πεποίηνται τὸ τὰς τέχνας αἰσχροεπεῖν, ὡς μὲν οἴονται, οὐ τοῦτο διαπρησσόμενοι ὃ ἐγὼ λέγω, ἀλλ' ἱστορίης οἰκείης ἐπίδειξιν ποιεύμενοι. 2 Ἐμοὶ δὲ τὸ μέν τι τῶν μὴ εὑρημένων ἐξευρίσκειν, ὅ τι καὶ εὑρεθὲν κρέσσον ἢ ἀνεξεύρετον, συνέσιος δοκεῖ ἐπιθύμημά τε καὶ ἔργον εἶναι, καὶ τὸ τὰ ἡμίεργα ἐς τέλος ἐξεργάζεσθαι ὡσαύτως · τὸ δὲ λόγων οὐ καλῶν τέχνῃ τὰ τοῖσιν ἄλλοισιν εὑρημένα αἰσχύνειν προθυμεῖσθαι, ἐπανορθοῦντα μὲν μηδέν, διαβάλλοντα δὲ τὰ τῶν εἰδότων πρὸς τοὺς μὴ εἰδότας ἐξευρήματα, οὐκέτι συνέσιος δοκεῖ ἐπιθύμημά τε καὶ ἔργον εἶναι, ἀλλὰ κακαγγελίη μᾶλλον φύσιος ἢ ἀτεχνίη. Μούνοισι γὰρ δὴ τοῖσιν ἀτέχνοισιν ἡ ἐργασίη αὕτη ἁρμόζει, φιλοτιμεομένων μὲν οὐδαμὰ δὲ δυναμένων κακίῃ ὑπουργεῖν ἐς τὸ τὰ τῶν πέλας ἔργα ἢ ὀρθὰ ἐόντα διαβάλλειν ἢ οὐκ ὀρθὰ μωμεῖσθαι. 3 Τοὺς μὲν οὖν ἐς τὰς ἄλλας τέχνας τούτῳ τῷ τρόπῳ ἐμπίπτοντας, οἷσι μέλει τε καὶ ὧν μέλει, οἱ δυνάμενοι κωλυόντων · ὁ δὲ παρεὼν λόγος τοῖσιν ἐς ἰητρικὴν οὕτως ἐπιπορευομένοισιν ἐναντιώσεται, θρασυνόμενος μὲν διὰ τούτους οὓς ψέγει, εὐπορέων δὲ διὰ τὴν τέχνην ᾗ βοηθεῖ, δυνάμενος δὲ διὰ σοφίην ᾗ πεπαίδευται.

2 1 Δοκεῖ δή μοι τὸ μὲν σύμπαν τέχνη εἶναι οὐδεμία οὐκ ἐοῦσα · καὶ γὰρ ἄλογον τῶν ἐόντων τι ἡγεῖσθαι μὴ ἐνεόν · ἐπεὶ τῶν γε μὴ ἐόντων τίνα ἄν τίς οὐσίην θεησάμενος ἀπαγγείλειεν ὡς ἔστιν; Εἰ γὰρ δὴ ἔστι γε ἰδεῖν τὰ μὴ ἐόντα ὥσπερ τὰ ἐόντα, οὐκ οἶδ' ὅπως ἄν τις αὐτὰ νομίσειε μὴ ἐόντα ἅ γε εἴη καὶ ὀφθαλμοῖσιν ἰδεῖν καὶ γνώμῃ νοῆσαι ὡς ἔστιν. 2 Ἀλλ' ὅπως μὴ οὐκ ᾖ τοῦτο τοιοῦτον · ἀλλὰ τὰ μὲν ἐόντα αἰεὶ ὁρᾶταί τε καὶ γινώσκεται, τὰ δὲ μὴ ἐόντα οὔτε ὁρᾶται οὔτε γινώσκεται. Γινώσκεται τοίνυν δεδιδαγμένων ἤδη τῶν τεχνέων καὶ οὐδεμία ἐστὶν ἥ γε ἔκ τινος εἴδεος οὐχ ὁρᾶται. 3 Οἶμαι δ' ἔγωγε καὶ τὰ ὀνόματα αὐτὰς διὰ τὰ εἴδεα λαβεῖν · ἄλογον γὰρ ἀπὸ τῶν ὀνομάτων ἡγεῖσθαι τὰ εἴδεα βλαστάνειν καὶ ἀδύνατον · τὰ μὲν γὰρ ὀνόματα φύσιος νομοθετήματά ἐστιν, τὰ δὲ εἴδεα οὐ νομοθετήματα, ἀλλὰ βλαστήματα.

3 1 Περὶ μὲν οὖν τούτων εἴ γέ τις μὴ ἱκανῶς ἐκ τῶν εἰρημένων συνίησιν, ἐν ἄλλοισιν ἂν λόγοισιν σαφέστερον διδαχθείη · περὶ δὲ ἰητρικῆς—ἐς ταύτην γὰρ ὁ λόγος—, ταύτης οὖν τὴν ἀπόδειξιν ποιήσομαι. 2 Καὶ πρῶτόν γε διοριεῦμαι ὃ νομίζω ἰητρικὴν εἶναι · τὸ δὴ πάμπαν ἀπαλλάσσειν τῶν νοσεόντων τοὺς καμάτους καὶ τῶν νοσημάτων τὰς σφοδρότητας ἀμβλύνειν, καὶ τὸ μὴ ἐγχειρεῖν τοῖσι κεκρατημένοισιν ὑπὸ τῶν νοσημάτων, εἰδότας ὅτι πάντα ταῦτα δύναται ἰητρική.

3 Ὡς οὖν ποιεῖ τε ταῦτα καὶ οἵη τέ ἐστιν διὰ παντὸς ποιεῖν, περὶ τούτου μοι ὁ λοιπὸς λόγος ἤδη ἔσται. Ἐν δὲ τῇ τῆς τέχνης ἀποδείξει ἅμα καὶ τοὺς λόγους τῶν αἰσχύνειν αὐτὴν οἰομένων ἀναιρήσω, ᾗ ἂν ἕκαστος αὐτῶν πρήσσειν τι οἰόμενος τυγχάνῃ.

4 1 Ἔστι μὲν οὖν μοι ἀρχὴ τοῦ λόγου, ἥ καὶ ὁμολογήσεται παρὰ πᾶσιν · ὅτι γὰρ ἔνιοι ἐξυγιαίνονται τῶν θεραπευομένων ὑπὸ ἰητρικῆς ὁμολογεῖται. Ὅτι δ' οὐ πάντες, ἐν τούτῳ ἤδη ψέγεται ἡ τέχνη, καί φασιν οἱ τὰ χείρω λέγοντες διὰ τοὺς ἁλισκομένους ὑπὸ τῶν νοσημάτων τοὺς ἀποφεύγοντας αὐτὰ τύχῃ ἀποφεύγειν καὶ οὐ διὰ τὴν τέχνην. 2 Ἐγὼ δὲ οὐκ ἀποστερέω μὲν οὐδ' αυτὸς τὴν τύχην ἔργου οὐδενός, ἡγεῦμαι δὲ τοῖσι μὲν κακῶς θεραπευομένοισι νοσήμασι τὰ πολλὰ τὴν ἀτυχίην ἕπεσθαι, τοῖσι δὲ εὖ τὴν εὐτυχίην. 3 Ἔπειτα δὲ καὶ πῶς οἷόν τ' ἐστὶ τοῖσιν ἐξυγιανθεῖσιν ἄλλο τι αἰτιήσασθαι ἢ τὴν τέχνην εἴπερ χρεώμενοι αὐτῇ καὶ ὑπουργέοντες ὑγιάνθησαν; Τὸ μὲν γὰρ τῆς τύχης εἶδος ψιλὸν οὐκ ἐβουλήθησαν θεήσασθαι ἐν ᾧ τῇ τέχνῃ ἐπέτρεψαν σφᾶς αὐτούς · 4 ὥστε τῆς μὲν ἐς τὴν τύχην ἀναφορῆς ἀπηλλαγμένοι εἰσί, τῆς μέντοι ἐς τὴν τέχνην οὐκ ἀπηλλαγμένοι · ἐν ᾧ γὰρ ἐπέτρεψαν αὐτῇ σφᾶς καὶ ἐπίστευσαν, ἐν τούτῳ αὐτῆς καὶ τὸ εἶδος ἐσκέψαντο καὶ τὴν δύναμιν περανθέντος τοῦ ἔργου ἔγνωσαν.

5 1 Ἐρεῖ δὴ ὁ τἀναντία λέγων ὅτι πολλοὶ ἤδη καὶ οὐ χρησάμενοι ἰητρῷ νοσέοντες ὑγιάνθησαν · καὶ ἐγὼ τῷ λόγῳ οὐκ ἀπιστέω. 2 Δοκεῖ δέ μοι οἷόν τε εἶναι καὶ ἰητρῷ μὴ χρεωμένους ἰητρικῇ περιτυχεῖν, οὐ μὴν ὥστε εἰδέναι ὅ το ὀρθὸν ἐν αὐτῇ ἔνι ἢ ὅ τι μὴ ὀρθόν, ἀλλ' ὥστε ἐπιτυχεῖν τοιαῦτα θεραπεύσαντες ἑωυτοὺς ὁποῖάπερ ἂν ἐθεραπεύθησαν εἰ καὶ ἰητροῖσιν ἐχρέωντο. 3 Καὶ τοῦτό γε τεκμήριον μέγα τῇ οὐσίῃ τῆς τέχνης ὅτι ἐοῦσά τέ ἐστι καὶ μεγάλη, ὅπου γε φαίνονται καὶ οἱ μὴ νομίζοντες αὐτὴν εἶναι σῳζόμενοι δι' αὐτήν. 4 Πολλὴ γὰρ ἀνάγκη καὶ τοὺς μὴ χρεωμένους ἰητροῖσι, νοσήσαντας δὲ καὶ ὑγιασθέντας, εἰδέναι ὅτι ἢ δρῶντές τι ἢ μὴ δρῶντες ὑγιάνθησαν · ἢ γὰρ ἀσιτίῃ ἢ πολυφαγίῃ, ἢ ποτῷ πλέονι ἢ δίψῃ, ἢ λουτροῖσιν ἢ ἀλουσίῃ, ἢ πόνοισιν ἢ ἡσυχίῃ, ἢ ὕπνοισιν ἢ ἀγρυπνίῃ, ἢ τῇ ἁπάντων τούτων ταραχῇ χρεώμενοι ὑγιάνθησαν. 5 Καὶ τῷ ὠφελῆσθαι πολλὴ ἀνάγκη αὐτούς ἐστιν ἐγνωκέναι ὅ τι ἦν τὸ ὠφελῆσαν, καὶ εἴ τί γ' ἐβλάβησαν, τῷ βλαβῆναι, ὅ τι ἦν τὸ βλάψαν. Τὰ γὰρ τῷ ὠφελῆσθαι καὶ τὰ τῷ βαβλάφθαι ὡρισμένα, οὐ πᾶς ἱκανὸς γνῶναι; Εἰ τοίνυν ἐπιστήσεται ἢ ἐπαινεῖν ἢ ψέγειν ὁ νοσήσας τῶν διαιτημάτων τι οἷσιν ὑγιάνθη, πάντα ταῦτα τῆς ἰητρικῆς ἐστι. Καὶ ἔστιν οὐδὲν ἧσσον τὰ ἁμαρτηθέντα τῶν ὠφελησάντων μαρτύρια τῇ τέχνῃ ἐς τὸ εἶναι. Τὰ μὲν γὰρ ὠφελήσαντα τῷ ὀρθῶς προσενεχθῆναι ὠφέλησε, τὰ δὲ βλάψαντα τῷ μηκέτι ὀρθῶς προσενεχθῆναι ἔβλαψε. 6 Καίτοι ὅπου τό τε ὀρθὸν καὶ τὸ μὴ ὀρθὸν ὅρον ἔχει ἑκάτερον, πῶς τοῦτο οὐκ ἂν τέχνη εἴη; Τοῦτο γὰρ ἔγωγέ φημι ατεχνίην εἶναι ὅπου μήτε ὀρθὸν ἔνι μηδὲν μήτε οὐκ ὀρθόν · ὅπου δὲ τούτων ἔνεστιν ἑκάτερον, οὐκέτι ἂν τοῦτο ἔργον ἀτεχνίης εἴη.

6 1 Ἔτι τοίνυν εἰ μὲν ὑπὸ φαρμάκων τῶν τε καθαιρόντων καὶ τῶν ἱστάντων ἡ ἴησις τῇ τε ἰητρικῇ καὶ τοῖσιν ἰητροῖσιν μοῦνον ἐγίνετο, ἀσθενὴς ἦν ἂν ὁ ἐμὸς λόγος. 2 Νῦν δὲ φαίνονται τῶν ἰητρῶν οἱ μάλιστα ἐπαινεόμενοι καὶ διαιτήμασιν ἰώμενοι καὶ ἄλλοισί τε εἴδεσιν ἃ οὐκ ἄν τις φαίη, μὴ ὅτι ἰητρός, ἀλλ' οὐδὲ ἰδιώτης ἀνεπιστήμων ἀκούσας, μὴ οὐ τῆς τέχνης εἶναι. 3 Ὅπου οὖν οὐδὲν οὔτ' ἐν τοῖσιν ἀγαθοῖσι τῶν ἰητρῶν οὔτ' ἐν τῇ ἰητρικῇ αὐτῇ ἀχρεῖόν ἐστιν, ἀλλ' ἐν τοῖσι πλείστοισι τῶν τε φυομένων καὶ τῶν ποιευμένων ἔνεστιν τὰ εἴδεα τῶν θεραπειῶν καὶ τῶν φαρμάκων, οὐκ ἔστιν ἔτι οὐδενὶ τῶν ἄνευ ἰητροῦ ὑγιαζομένων τὸ αὐτόματον αἰτιήσασθαι ὀρθῷ λόγῳ. 4 Τὸ μὲν γὰρ αὐτόματον οὐδὲν φαίνεται ἐὸν ἐλεγχόμενον · πᾶν γαρ τὸ γινόμενον διά τι εὑρίσκοιτ' ἂν γινόμενον, καὶ ἐν τῷ διά τι τὸ αὐτόματον οὐ φαίνεται οὐσίην ἔχον οὐδεμίαν ἀλλ' ἢ ὄνομα · ἡ δὲ ἰητρικὴ καὶ ἐν τοῖσι διά τι καὶ ἐν τοῖσι προνοευμένοισι φαίνεταί τε καὶ φανεῖται αἰεὶ οὐσίην ἔχουσα.

7 1 Τοῖσι μὲν οὖν τῇ τύχῃ τὴν ὑγιείην προστιθεῖσι, τὴν δὲ τέχνην ἀφαιρέουσι, τοιαῦτ' ἄν τις λέγοι · τοὺς δ' ἐν τῇσι τῶν ἀποθνησκόντων συμφορῇσι τὴν τέχνην ἀφανίζοντας θαυμάζω ὁτέῳ ἐπαιρόμενοι ἀξιόχρεῳ λόγῳ τὴν μὲν τῶν ἀποθνησκόντων ἀκρασίην ἀναιτίην καθιστᾶσι, τὴν δὲ τῶν τὴν ἰητρικὴν μελετησάντων σύνεσιν αἰτίην, ὡς τοῖσι μὲν ἰητροῖσιν ἔνεστι τὰ μὴ δέοντα ἐπιτάξαι, τοῖσι δὲ νοσέουσιν οὐκ ἔστι τὰ προσταχθέντα παραβῆναι. 2 Καὶ μὴν πολύ γε εὐλογώτερον τοῖσι κάμνουσιν ἀδυνατεῖν τὰ προστασσόμενα ὑπουργεῖν ἢ τοῖσιν ἰητροῖσι τὰ μὴ δέοντα ἐπιτάσσειν. 3 Οἱ μὲν γὰρ ὑγιαινούσῃ γνώμῃ μεθ' ὑγιαίνοντος σώματος ἐγχειρέουσι, λογισάμενοι τά τε παρεόντα τῶν τε παροιχομένων τὰ ὁμοίως διατεθέντα τοῖσι παρεοῦσιν ὥστε ποτὲ θεραπευθέντα εἰπεῖν ὡς ἀπήλλαξαν, οἱ δ' οὔτε ἃ κάμνουσιν οὔτε δι' ἃ κάμνουσιν, οὐδ' ὅ τι ἐκ τῶν παρεόντων ἔσται οὐδ' ὅ τι ἐκ τῶν τούτοισιν ὁμοίων γίνεται εἰδότες ἐπιτάσσονται, ἀλγέοντες μὲν ἐν τῷ παρεόντι, φοβεύμενοι δὲ τὸ μέλλον καὶ πλήρεις μὲν τῆς νούσου, κενεοὶ δὲ σιτίων, ἐθέλοντες δὲ τὰ πρὸς τὴν νοῦσον ἤδη μᾶλλον ἢ τὰ πρὸς τὴν ὑγιείην προσδέχεσθαι, οὐκ ἀποθανεῖν ἐρῶντες ἀλλὰ καρτερεῖν ἀδυνατέοντες. 4 Οὕτω δὲ διακειμένους πότερον εἰκὸς τούτους τὰ ὑπὸ τῶν ἰητρῶν ἐπιτασσόμενα ποιεῖν ἢ ἄλλα ποιεῖν ἢ ἃ ἐπετάχθησαν; ἢ τοὺς ἰητροὺς τοὺς ἐκείνως διακειμέ νους ὡς ὁ πρόσθεν λόγος ἡρμήνευσεν ἐπιτάσσειν τὰ μὴ δέοντα; 5 Ἆρ' οὐ πολὺ μᾶλλον τοὺς μὲν δεόντως ἐπιτάσσειν, τοὺς δὲ εἰκότως ἀδυνατεῖν πείθεσθαι, μὴ πειθομένους δὲ περιπίμπτειν τοῖσι θανάτοισιν, ὧν οἱ μὴ ὀρθῶς λογιζόμενοι τὰς αἰτίας τοῖσιν οὐδὲν αἰτίοισιν ἀνατιθεῖσι, τοὺς αἰτίους ἐλευθεροῦντες;

8 1 Εἰσὶ δέ τινες, οἳ καὶ διὰ τοὺς μὴ θέλοντας ἐγχειρεῖν τοῖσι κεκρατημένοισιν ὑπὸ τῶν νοσημάτων μέμφονται τὴν ἰητρικήν, λέγοντες ὡς ταῦτα μὲν καὶ αὐτὰ ὑφ' ἑωυτῶν ἂν ἐξυγιάζοιτο ἃ ἐγχειρέουσιν ἰᾶσθαι, ἃ δ' ἐπικουρίης δεῖται μεγάλης οὐχ ἅπτονται · δεῖν δέ, εἴπερ ἦν ἡ τέχνη, πάνθ' ὁμοίως ἰᾶσθαι. 2 Οἱ μὲν ταῦτα λέγοντες, εἰ ἐμέμφοντο τοῖσιν ἰητροῖσιν ὅτι αὐτῶν τοιαῦτα λεγόντων οὐκ ἐπιμέλονται ὡς

παραφρονεύντων, εἰκότως ἂν ἐμέμφοντο μᾶλλον ἢ κεῖνα μεμφόμενοι· εἰ γάρ τις ἢ τέχνην, ἐς ἃ μὴ τέχνη, ἢ φύσιν, ἐς ἃ μὴ φύσις πέφυκεν, ἀξιώσειε δύνασθαι, ἀγνοεῖ μανίῃ ἁρμόζουσαν ἄγνοιαν μᾶλλον ἢ ἀμαθίῃ· **3** ὧν γάρ ἔστιν ἡμῖν τοῖσί τε τῶν φυσίων τοῖσι τε τῶν τεχνέων ὀργάνοισιν επικρατεῖν, τούτων ἔστιν ἡμῖν δημιουργοῖς εἶναι, ἄλλων δὲ οὐκ ἔστιν. ὅταν οὖν τι πάθῃ ὥνθρωπος κακὸν ὃ κρέσσον ἐστὶν τῶν ἐν ἰητρικῇ ὀργάνων, οὐδὲ προσδοκᾶσθαι τοῦτό που δεῖ ὑπὸ ἰητρικῆς κρατηθῆναι ἄν. **4** Αὐτίκα γὰρ τῶν ἐν ἰητρικῇ καιόντων τὸ πῦρ ἐσχάτως καίει, τούτου δὲ ἡσσόνως ἄλλα πολλά. Τῶν μὲν οὖν ἡσσόνων τὰ κρέσσω οὔπω δῆλον ὅτι ἀνίητα, τῶν δὲ κρατίστων τὰ κρέσσω πῶς οὐ δῆλον ὅτι ἀνίητα; Ἃ γὰρ πῦρ οὐ δημιουργεῖ, πῶς οὐ τὰ τούτῳ μὴ ἁλισκόμενα δηλοῖ ὅτι ἄλλης τέχνης δεῖται καὶ οὐ ταύτης ἐν ᾗ τὸ πῦρ ὄργανον; **5** Ωὑτὸς δέ μοι λόγος καὶ ὑπὲρ τῶν ἄλλων, ὅσα τῇ ἰητρικῇ συνεργεῖ. Ὧν ἁπάντων φημὶ δεῖν ἑκάστου οὐ κατατυχόντα τὸν ἰητρὸν τὴν δύναμιν αἰτιᾶσθαι τοῦ πάθεος, ἀλλὰ μὴ τὴν τέχνην. **6** Οἱ μὲν οὖν μεμφόμενοι τοὺς τοῖσι κεκρατημένοισι μὴ ἐγχειρέοντας παρακελεύονται καὶ ὧν μὴ προσήκει ἅπτεσθαι οὐδὲν ἧσσον ἢ ὧν προσήκει, παρακελευόμενοι δὲ ταῦτα ὑπὸ μὲν τῶν ὀνόματι ἰητρῶν θαυμάζονται, ὑπὸ δὲ τῶν καὶ τέχνῃ καταγελῶνται. **7** Οὐ μὴν οὕτως ἀφρόνων οἱ ταύτης τῆς δημιουργίης ἔμπειροι οὔτε μωμητέων οὔτ' αἰνετέων δέονται, ἀλλὰ λελογισμένων πρὸς ὅ τι αἱ ἐργασίαι τῶν δημιουργῶν τελευτώμεναι πλήρεις εἰσί, καὶ ὅτευ ὑπολειπόμεναι ἐνδεεῖς, ἔτι τε τῶν ἐνδειῶν ἅς τε τοῖσι δημιουργεῦσιν ἀναθετέον, ἅς τε τοῖσι δημιουργεομένοισι.

**9** **1** Τὰ μὲν οὖν κατὰ τὰς ἄλλας τέχνας ἄλλος χρόνος μετ' ἄλλου λόγου δείξει· τὰ δὲ κατὰ τὴν ἰητρικὴν οἷά τέ ἐστιν ὥς τε κριτέα, τὰ μὲν ὁ παροιχόμενος, τὰ δὲ ὁ παρεὼν διδάξει λόγος. **2** Ἔστι γὰρ τοῖσι ταύτην τὴν τέχνην ἱκανῶς εἰδόσι τὰ μὲν τῶν νοσημάτων οὐκ ἐν δυσόπτῳ κείμενα, καὶ οὐ πολλά, τὰ δὲ οὐκ ἐν εὐδήλῳ, καὶ πολλά. **3** Ἔστιν δὲ τὰ μὲν ἐξανθεῦντα ἐς τὴν χροιὴν ἢ χροιῇ ἢ οἰδήμασιν ἐν εὐδήλῳ· παρέχει γὰρ ἑωυτῶν τῇ τε ὄψει τῷ τε ψαῦσαι τὴν στερεότητα καὶ τὴν ὑγρότητα αἰσθάνεσθαι, καὶ ἅ τε αὐτῶν θερμὰ ἅ τε ψυχρά, ὧν τε ἑκάστου ἢ παρουσίῃ ἢ ἀπουσίῃ τοιαῦτ' ἐστίν. **4** Τῶν μὲν οὖν τοιούτων πάντων ἐν πᾶσι τὰς ἀκέσιας ἀναμαρτήτους δεῖ εἶναι, οὐχ ὡς ῥηϊδίας, ἀλλ' ὅτι ἐξεύρηνται· ἐξεύρηνταί γε μὴν οὐ τοῖσι βουληθεῖσιν, ἀλλὰ τούτων τοῖσι δυνηθεῖσιν· δύνανται δὲ οἷσι τά τε τῆς παιδείης μὴ ἐκποδών, τά τε τῆς φύσιος μὴ ἀταλαίπωρα.

**10** **1** Πρὸς μὲν οὖν τὰ φανερὰ τῶν νοσημάτων οὕτω δεῖ εὐπορεῖν τὴν τέχνην· δεῖ γε μὴν αὐτὴν οὐδὲ πρὸς τὰ ἧσσον φανερὰ ἀπορεῖν. Ἔστιν δὲ ταῦτα ἃ πρός τε τὰ ὀστέα τέτραπται καὶ τὴν νηδύν. **2** Ἔχει δὲ τὸ σῶμα οὐ μίαν ἀλλὰ πλείους· δύο μὲν γὰρ αἱ τὸ σιτίον δεχόμεναί τε καὶ ἀφιεῖσαι, ἄλλαι δὲ τούτων πλείους, ἃς ἴσασιν οἷσι τούτων ἐμέλησεν· **3** ὅσα γὰρ τῶν μελέων ἔχει σάρκα περιφερέα, ἣν μῦν καλέουσιν, πάντα νηδὺν ἔχει· πᾶν γὰρ τὸ ἀσύμφυτον, ἤν τε δέρματι ἤν τε σαρκὶ καλύπτηται, κοῖλόν ἐστι, πληροῦται τε ὑγιαῖνον μὲν πνεύματος, ἀσθενῆσαν δὲ ἰχῶρος. Ἔχουσι μὲν τοίνυν οἱ βραχίονες σάρκα τοιαύτην, ἔχουσι δ' οἱ μηροί, ἔχουσι δ' αἱ κνῆμαι. 4 Ἔτι δὲ καὶ ἐν τοῖσιν ἀσάρκοισιν τοιαύτη ἔνεστιν οἵη καὶ ἐν τοῖσιν εὐσάρκοισιν ἐνεῖναι δέδεκται · ὅ τε γὰρ θώρηξ καλεόμενος, ἐν ᾧ το ἧπαρ στεγάζεται ὅ τε τῆς κεφαλῆς κύκλος, ἐν ᾧ ὁ ἐγκέφαλος, τό τε νῶτον πρὸς ᾧ ὁ πλεύμων, τούτων οὐδὲν ὅ τι οὐ καὶ αὐτὸ κενόν ἐστιν, πολλῶν διαφυσίων μεστόν · ἔστι δ' οἷσιν οὐδὲν ἀπέχει πολλῶν ἀγγεῖα εἶναι τῶν μέν τι βλαπτόντων τὸν κεκτημένον, τῶν δὲ καὶ ὠφελεύντων. 5 Ἔτι δὲ καὶ πρὸς τούτοισι φλέβες πολλαὶ καὶ νεῦρα οὐκ ἐν τῇ σαρκὶ μετέωρα ἀλλὰ πρὸς τοῖσιν ὀστέοισι προστεταμένα ⟨ἃ⟩ σύνδεσμός ἐστι τῶν ἄρθρων, καὶ αὐτὰ τὰ ἄρθρα ἐν οἷσιν αἱ συμβολαὶ τῶν κινεομένων ὀστέων ἐγκυκλέονται, καὶ τούτων οὐδὲν ὅ τι οὐχ ὕπαφρόν ἐστι καὶ ἔχον περὶ αὐτὸ θαλάμας ἃς καταγγέλλει ὁ ἰχώρ, ὅς, ἐκδιοιγομένων αὐτέων, πολλός τε καὶ πολλὰ λυπήσας ἐξέρχεται.

11 1 Οὐ γὰρ δὴ ὀφθαλμοῖσί γ' ἰδόντι τούτων τῶν εἰρημένων οὐδενὶ οὐδὲν ἔστιν εἰδέναι. Διὸ καὶ ἄδηλα ἐμοί τε ὠνόμασται καὶ τῇ τέχνῃ κέκριται εἶναι · οὐ μὴν ὅτι ἄδηλα κεκράτηκεν ἀλλ' ᾗ δυνατὸν κεκράτηται · δυνατὸν δὲ ὡς αἵ τε τῶν νοσεόντων φύσιες ἐς τὸ σκεφθῆναι παρέχουσιν, αἵ τε τῶν ἐρευνησόντων ἐς τὴν ἔρευναν πεφύκασιν. 2 Μετὰ πλείονος μὲν γὰρ πόνου καὶ οὐ μετ' ἐλάσσονος χρόνου ἢ εἰ τοῖσιν ὀφθαλμοῖσιν ἑωρᾶτο, γινώσκεται. Ὅσα γὰρ τὴν τῶν ὀμμάτων ὄψιν ἐκφεύγει, ταῦτα τῇ τῆς γνώμης ὄψει κεκράτηται. 3 Καὶ ὅσα δ' ἐν τῷ μὴ ταχὺ ὀφθῆναι οἱ νοσέοντες πάσχουσιν, οὐχ οἱ θεραπεύοντες αὐτοὺς αἴτιοι, ἀλλ' ἡ φύσις ἥ τε τοῦ νοσέοντος ἥ τε τοῦ νοσήματος. Ὁ μὲν γὰρ ἐπεὶ οὐκ ἦν αὐτῷ ὄψει ἰδεῖν τὸ μοχθέον οὐδ' ἀκοῇ πυθέσθαι, λογισμῷ μετῄει. 4 Καὶ γὰρ δή, καὶ ἃ πειρῶνται οἱ τὰ ἀφανέα νοσέοντες ἀπαγγέλλειν περὶ τῶν νοσημάτων τοῖσι θεραπεύουσι, δοξάζοντες μᾶλλον ἢ εἰδότες ἀπαγγέλλουσιν · εἰ γὰρ ἠπίσταντο, οὐκ ἂν περιέπιπτον αὐτοῖσι · τῆς γὰρ αὐτῆς συνέσιός ἐστιν ἧσπερ τὸ εἰδέναι τῶν νούσων τὰ αἴτια, καὶ τὸ θεραπεύειν αὐτὰς ἐπίστασθαι πάσῃσι τῇσι θεραπείῃσιν αἳ κωλύουσι τὰ νοσήματα μεγαλύνεσθαι. Ὅτε οὖν οὐδ' ἐκ τῶν ἀπαγγελλομένων ἔστι τὴν ἀναμάρτητον σαφήνειαν ἀκοῦσαι, προσοπτέον τι καὶ ἄλλο τῷ θεραπεύοντι. 5 Ταύτης οὖν τῆς βραδυτῆτος οὐχ ἡ τέχνη, ἀλλ' ἡ φύσις αἰτίη ἡ τῶν σωμάτων. Ἡ μὲν γὰρ αἰσθομένη ἀξιοῖ θεραπεύειν καὶ σκοπεῦσα ὅπως μὴ τόλμῃ μᾶλλον ἢ γνώμῃ καὶ ῥᾳστώνῃ μᾶλλον ἢ βίῃ θεραπεύῃ, ἡ δ' ἢν μὲν διεξαρκέσῃ ἐς τὸ ὀφθῆναι, ἐξαρκέσει καὶ ἐς τὸ ὑγιανθῆναι, ἢν δ' ἐν ᾧ τοῦτο ὁρᾶται κρατηθῇ διὰ τὸ βραδέως αὐτὸν ἐπὶ τὸν θεραπεύσοντα ἐλθεῖν ἢ διὰ τὸ τοῦ νοσήματος τάχος, οἰχήσεται. 6 Ἐξ ἴσου μὲν γὰρ ὁρμώμενον τῇ θεραπείῃ οὐκ ἔστι θᾶσσον, προλαβὸν δὲ θᾶσσον. Προλαμβάνει δὲ διά τε τὴν τῶν σωμάτων στεγνότητα ἐν ᾗ οὐκ ἐν εὐόπτῳ οἰκέουσιν αἱ νοῦσοι διά τε τὴν τῶν καμνόντων ὀλιγωρίην ⟨ἣν⟩ ἐπιτίθενται · οὐ λαμβανόμενοι γὰρ ἀλλ' εἰλημμένοι ὑπὸ τῶν νοσημάτων ἐθέλουσι θεραπεύεσθαι. 7 Εἶτα τῆς γε τέχνης τὴν δύναμιν ὁπόταν τινὰ τῶν τὰ ἄδηλα νοσεύντων ἀναστήσῃ θαυμάζειν ἀξιώτερον ἢ ὁπόταν μὴ ἐγχειρήσῃ τοῖσιν ἀδυνάτοισιν; Οὔκουν ἐν ἄλλῃ γε δημιουργίῃ τῶν ἤδη εὑρημένων οὐδεμιῇ ἔνεστιν οὐδὲν τοιοῦτον · ἀλλ' αὐτέων ὅσαι πυρὶ δημιουργεῦνται, τούτου

μὴ παρεόντος, ἀεργοί εἰσι· καὶ ὅσαι μετὰ τοῦ ὀφθῆναι ἐνεργοὶ καὶ τοῖσιν εὐεπανορθώτοισι σώμασι δημιουργεῦνται, αἱ μὲν μετὰ ξύλων, αἱ δὲ μετὰ σκυτέων, αἱ δὲ [γραφῇ] χαλκῷ τε καὶ σιδήρῳ καὶ τοῖσι τούτων ὁμοίοισι χύμασιν αἱ πλεῖσται, τὰ δ' ἐκ τούτων καὶ μετὰ τούτων δημιουργεύμενα, καὶ εὐεπανόρθωτα, ὅμως οὐ τῷ τάχει μᾶλλον ἢ ὡς δεῖ δημιουργεῖται, οὐδ' ὑπερβατῶς, ἀλλ', ἢν ἀπῇ τι τῶν ὀργάνων, ἐλινύει· καίτοι κἀκείνῃσι τὸ βραδὺ πρὸς τὸ λυσιτελέον ἀσύμφορον· ἀλλ' ὅμως προτιμᾶται.

12 1 Ἰητρικὴ δέ, τοῦτο μὲν τῶν ἐμπύων, τοῦτο δὲ τῶν τὸ ἧπαρ ἢ τοὺς νεφροὺς, τοῦτο δὲ τῶν συμπάντων τῶν ἐν τῇ νηδύι νοσεύντων ἀπεστερημένη τι ἰδεῖν ὄψει ᾗ τὰ πάντα πάντες ἱκανωτάτως ὁρῶσιν, ὅμως ἄλλας εὐπορίας συνεργοὺς εὗρε· 2 φωνῆς τε γὰρ λαμπρότητι καὶ τρηχύτητι καὶ πνεύματος ταχυτῆτι καὶ βραδυτῆτι, καὶ ῥευμάτων ἃ διαρρεῖν εἴωθεν ἑκάστοισι δι' ὧν ἔξοδοι δέδονται ὧν τὰ μὲν ὀδμῇσι τὰ δὲ χροιῇσι τὰ δὲ λεπτότητι καὶ παχύτητι διασταθμωμένη τεκμαίρεται ὧν τὰ σημεῖα ταῦτα ἅ τε πεπονθότων ἅ τε παθεῖν δυναμένων. 3 Ὅταν δὲ ταῦτα τὰ μηνύοντα μηδ' αὐτὴ ἡ φύσις ἑκοῦσα ἀφιῇ, ἀνάγκας εὕρηκεν ᾗσιν ἡ φύσις ἀζήμιος βιασθεῖσα μεθίησιν· ἀνεθεῖσα δὲ δηλοῖ τοῖσι τὰ τῆς τέχνης εἰδόσιν ἃ ποιητέα. 4 Βιάζεται δὲ τοῦτο μὲν πῦρ τὸ σύντροφον φλέγμα διαχεῖν σιτίων δριμύτητι καὶ πωμάτων ὅπως τεκμαρεῖταί τι ὀφθὲν περὶ ἐκείνων ὧν αὐτῇ ἐν ἀμηχάνῳ τὸ ὀφθῆναι ἦν· τό τ' αὖ πνεῦμα, ὧν κατήγορον, ὁδοῖσί τε προσάντεσι καὶ δρόμοισιν ἐκβιᾶται κατηγορεῖν· ἱδρῶτάς τε τούτοισιν τοῖσι προειρημένοισιν ἄγουσα ⟨καὶ⟩ ὑδάτων θερμῶν ἀποπνοίῃσι, τεκμαίρεται. 5 Ἔστι δὲ ἃ καὶ διὰ τῆς κύστιος διελθόντα ἱκανώτερα δηλῶσαι τὴν νοῦσόν ἐστιν ἢ διὰ τῆς σαρκὸς ἐξιόντα· ἐξεύρηκεν οὖν καὶ τοιαῦτα πώματα καὶ βρώματα ἃ τῶν θερμαινόντων θερμότερα γινόμενα τήκει τε ἐκεῖνα καὶ διαρρεῖν ποιεῖ, ᾗ οὐκ ἂν διερρύη μὴ τοῦτο παθόντα. 6 Ἕτερα μὲν οὖν πρὸς ἑτέρων καὶ ἄλλα δι' ἄλλων ἐστὶ τά τε διιόντα τά τ' ἐξαγγέλλοντα, ὥστε οὐ θαυμάσιον αὐτῶν τάς τε πίστιας χρονιωτέρας γίνεσθαι τάς τ' ἐγχειρήσιας βραχυτέρας, οὕτω δι' ἀλλοτρίων ἑρμηνειῶν πρὸς τὴν θεραπεύουσαν σύνεσιν ἑρμηνευομένων.

13 1 Ὅτι μὲν οὖν καὶ λόγους ἐν ἑωυτῇ εὐπόρους ἐς τὰς ἐπικουρίας ἔχει ἡ ἰητρικὴ καὶ οὐκ εὐδιορθώτοισι δικαίως οὐκ ἂν ἐγχειρέοι τῇσι νούσοισιν ἢ ἐγχειρευμένας ἀναμαρτήτους ἂν παρέχοι, οἵ τε νῦν λεγόμενοι λόγοι δηλοῦσιν αἵ τε τῶν εἰδότων τὴν τέχνην ἐπιδείξιες, ἃς ἐκ τῶν ἔργων ἥδιον ἢ ἐκ τῶν λόγων ἐπιδεικνύουσιν, οὐ τὸ λέγειν καταμελετήσαντες, ἀλλὰ τὴν πίστιν τῷ πλήθει, ἐξ ὧν ἂν ἴδωσιν, οἰκειοτέρην ἡγεύμενοι ἢ ἐξ ὧν ἂν ἀκούσωσιν.

# ON THE ART OF MEDICINE

1 1 There are some who make an art of demeaning the arts, so they think, not achieving the result I just mentioned, but rather making a display of their special 'skill.' 2 But it seems to me that to discover fully something that has not yet been discovered and which, once it has been discovered, is better than if it had not been fully discovered, is an object and occupation of the intellect, as is likewise to accomplish fully what has been accomplished only in part. In contrast, the eagerness to debase the discoveries of others by an art of mean discourse, not suggesting any improvements but instead slandering the discoveries of those who have knowledge in front of those who do not—this no longer seems to be an object or occupation of the intellect, but rather an indication of a mediocre nature or a lack of art. For indeed, such business is fit for the artless alone, namely, serving the mediocrity of those with ambition but utterly without power in slandering their fellows' achievements when they are right or criticizing them when they are not. 3 As for those who attack the other arts in this way, let those who are able deter such attacks when and where they care to. The present discourse will oppose those who thus march against medicine, emboldened on account of these invaders, whom it blames; well equipped through the art to whose rescue it comes; and powerful through wisdom, in which it has been trained.

2 1 It seems quite clear to me that, on the whole, there is no art that is not, since it's just absurd to believe that one of the things-that-are is not. For what being could anyone observe of the things-that-are-not and report that they are? For if indeed it is possible to see the things-that-are-not, just as it is to see the things-that-are, I do not know how anyone could believe of those things that it were possible both to see with his eyes and to know with his mind that they are, that they are not. 2 Is it not rather more like the following? Whereas the things-that-are always are in every case seen and known, the things-that-are-not are neither seen nor known. Accordingly, the arts are known only once they have been taught, and there is no art that is not seen as an outgrowth of some form. 3 In my opinion, they acquire their names, too, because of their forms. For it's absurd—not to mention impossible—to think that forms grow out of names: names for nature are conventions imposed by and upon nature, whereas forms are not conventions but outgrowths.

3 1 Concerning these matters, then, should anyone not have reached a sufficient understanding from what has been said, clearer instruction may be given in other discourses. Concerning medicine—as this is the subject of the discourse—about this, then, I will now give a demonstration. 2 First, I will define what I think medicine is, namely, totally removing the sufferings of the sick or alleviating the violent effects of their diseases, as well as not handling the sick who have been overwhelmed by their diseases, knowing that all these things are in medicine's power. 3 That it does these things and always is able to do so will be the focus of my discourse from this point forward. In giving this demonstration of the art, I will at the same time refute the arguments of those who think they are demeaning it, and on the very points where any one of them happens to think they are accomplishing something substantial.

4 1 Now my discourse starts from the following premise, which will be accepted by all. That some of those who have been treated by medicine fully recover is generally accepted. But, in light of the fact that not all recover, the art is now criticized, and those who speak more meanly of it on account of those defeated by their diseases claim that those who escape them do so by chance and not because of art. 2 I myself do not deprive chance of its accomplishment; however, I do believe that for the most part misfortune follows upon the poor treatment of a disease, while good fortune follows upon good treatment. 3 How, then, could those who fully recovered hold something other than the art responsible for this, if indeed they did so while using and submitting to it? For in turning themselves over to the art, they did not wish to observe the form of pure chance, 4 and as a result they are freed from their reliance on chance, though their debt to the art is not discharged. For they turned themselves over to the art and put their faith in it; in this, they observed its form and, once the work was accomplished, they came to know its power.

5 1 Now he who makes the opposite argument will say that many who were sick have recovered even without consulting a physician, and I do not doubt the claim. 2 It seems to me, however, that it is possible even for those who do not consult a doctor to chance upon medicine. This does not, of course, actually result in their knowing what is correct in it and what is not, but rather in their hitting upon by chance the very treatments that would have been applied had they consulted a doctor. 3 And this is powerful evidence of medicine's being—evidence that it both is and is powerful—that even those who do not believe that it is are evidently saved by it. 4 Even those who

did not consult a doctor but recovered after falling sick surely must know that they recovered by doing or not doing something. For it was by fasting or by overeating, by drinking much fluid or by abstaining from it, by bathing or by not bathing, by vigorous exercise or by rest, by sleep or by wakefulness, or by using some combination of these that they recovered. 5 In virtue of having been benefited, they surely must have known what it was that benefited them; and likewise, if they were harmed somehow, then, in virtue of being harmed, what it was that harmed them. For is not everyone capable of knowing the things determined through his benefit or harm? So if the sick person knows how to praise or blame any of the components of regimen by which he recovered, then all these belong to medicine. The mistakes of medicine, too, no less than the benefits, are testimonies to its being. For what is beneficial brings benefit through correct application, while what is harmful causes harm through incorrect application. 6 And where the correct and incorrect each has its own determination, how could this not be art? There is artlessness, I claim, where there is neither correctness nor incorrectness; but where each of these is present, the work of artlessness would be absent.

6 1 Still, if doctors and their art brought about cures only by means of purgative and binding drugs, my argument would be weak. 2 But in fact it is evident that the most highly praised doctors heal by regimen and other forms of treatment that nobody, neither doctor nor unknowledgeable layperson (provided the latter had even heard of them), would claim did not belong to the art. 3 So nothing is useless for good doctors or for medicine itself; rather, forms of treatments and drugs are present in most things, both natural and synthetic. Hence, by a correct account, not a single person who has recovered without a doctor can still give the credit to spontaneity. 4 For, upon examination, it is evident that spontaneity is nothing at all since everything that comes to be would be discovered to do so because of something, and it is in virtue of this 'because of something' that spontaneity evidently has no being other than a name. But medicine evidently has and always will have being, both in virtue of things that come to be 'because of something' and in virtue of things known in advance.

7 1 Someone could make such arguments against those who attribute health to chance and discredit the art. I am further surprised at those who base their denial of the art on the misfortunes of those who died. By what sufficient argument are they moved to exculpate the weakness of those who died while holding responsible the intellect of medical practitioners, as though

it were possible for doctors to give the wrong orders but impossible for the sick to deviate from the orders they are given? 2 In actual fact, it is far more probable that the sick are powerless to follow the orders they are given than it is that doctors give the wrong orders. 3 For the latter handle the situation with healthy mind and body, reasoning about the present condition as well as conditions in the past similar to those in the present, so that they can tell how they were cured once they were treated. The former, however, while knowing neither what they suffer nor because of what they suffer, nor what will come of their present condition, nor what comes of similar conditions, are given orders. Pained in the present and fearing for the future, they are full of disease but empty of food, consenting at last to admit those things that promote disease rather than those that promote health, not because they desire death, but because they are powerless to endure. 4 Which is more likely—that people in such a state do what their doctors ordered, or that they do things that were not ordered? Or is it likely that doctors, in the state mentioned earlier, give the wrong orders? 5 Is it not much more likely that doctors give the right orders, but that in all probability the sick are powerless to obey them, and by not obeying them meet their deaths? And also that those who reason incorrectly attribute responsibility for these deaths to those who are not responsible, thereby setting the guilty free?

**8** 1 There are some, too, who criticize medicine on account of those who do not consent to handle people who have been overcome by their diseases: they say that doctors make an attempt to heal diseases that would resolve themselves on their own but do not touch those in great need of help. But if indeed medicine is, it ought to try to heal all alike. 2 Now if such people criticized doctors for ignoring them because they were out of their heads, then their criticism would be more plausible than it is. For if a person expects art to have power in matters where art is not, or expects nature to have power in matters where it is not present, then he is ignorant of an ignorance more in tune with madness than with lack of learning. 3 For of those things that we can master using the instruments of art and nature, we can be craftsmen. Of other things, we cannot. Thus, whenever a person suffers some evil that is stronger than the instruments of medicine, he should not expect medicine to be able somehow to overcome this. 4 For example, fire burns the most intensely of all the caustics used in medicine, but there are many others that burn less so. Clearly, then, things that are stronger than the lesser caustics are by no means untreatable. But is it not clear, too, that things stronger than the most powerful caustics are untreatable? As for the things that fire does not work on, is it not clear that if undefeated by it they require an art other than the one of which fire is an instrument? 5 My argument is the same on behalf of all other instruments allied with medicine. I claim that if the doctor is unsuccessful with each of all these, he ought to hold responsible the power of the affliction, not the art. 6 So people who criticize doctors for not handling those who have been overcome are demanding that they touch what is improper no less than what is proper. And while in making these demands they gain the admiration of those who are doctors in name, they are ridiculed by those who are doctors also in virtue of their art. 7 Those experienced in this craft have no need for criticism or praise that is so senseless. Instead, they need people who have rationally considered in relation to what the products of craftsmen are fully finished; in what respect imperfect products are deficient; and further, concerning these deficiencies, which are to be attributed to the craftsmen and which to the things being crafted.

9 1 Demonstrations concerning the other arts will take place at another time and with another discourse. But concerning medicine—that is, what sorts of things it involves and how they are to be judged—the first half of this discourse has elucidated in part, and from here forward it will address the remaining issues. 2 According to those with sufficient knowledge of this art, some diseases are located where they are not hard to see—though these are few—while others are located where they are not easy to see, and these are many. 3 Things that erupt on the skin are evident by their color or swelling. They offer us the opportunity to perceive their solidity and liquidity by our senses of sight and touch, as well as which of them are hot and cold, these diseases being the sorts of things they are through the presence or absence of each of these. 4 In all cases, then, the treatments for diseases of this sort ought to be free from error, not because they are easy, but rather because they are fully discovered, such discoveries being made not by those who have merely the desire, but by those who have also the power. And power is available to those whose training is not lacking and whose natures are not indolent.

10 1 With respect to evident diseases, then, the art ought to be thus well equipped. But neither ought it be unequipped with respect to less evident diseases, namely, those affecting the bones and the bodily cavity. 2 Actually, the body does not have just one cavity, but many. There are two that take in and expel food, for example, and there are many others that are known to those who care about these matters. 3 For all of the limbs surrounded by flesh (so-called 'muscle') have a cavity. For everything that is not grown together, whether covered by skin or flesh, is hollow, and when healthy is

full of breath; when weak, of fluid. Accordingly, the arms have this kind of flesh, as do the upper and lower parts of the legs. 4 Moreover, the sort of cavity shown to exist in the flesh-covered parts is found also where there is no flesh. For the so-called trunk encases the liver and the round part of the head contains the brain; next to the back are the lungs. None of these is not itself empty, each being full of natural fissures, and in these cases nothing prevents the presence of receptacles for many things, some of which are harmful to their possessor, and some of which are beneficial. 5 In addition, there are numerous vessels, as well as sinews that are not on the surface of the flesh but rather are stretched out along the bones and form a bond for the joints, and also the joints themselves, in which the balls of the moving bones circle round. None of these does not have a viscous quality, each being surrounded by chambers that are indicated by fluid, which issues forth copiously when the cells are completely ruptured, causing a great deal of pain.

11 1 Of course, it is impossible for a person who sees only with his eyes to know any of the things just mentioned. For this reason, I have given them the name 'non-evident,' and so they have been judged by the art. However, they have not prevailed just because they are non-evident; rather, they have been prevailed over where possible. And it is possible insofar as the natures of the sick submit to examination and the natures of those searching for the non-evident are well suited to the role. 2 For they are known with no less time and with even greater effort than they would have been if seen with the eyes. For what eludes the sight of the eyes is captured by the sight of the mind. 3 And if the sick suffer from a lack of speed in being seen, it is not those providing treatment who are responsible, but rather nature, specifically, the nature of the sick person as well as the nature of the disease. For the former, since it was possible neither to see the problem with his sight nor to learn about it by hearing, tried to pursue it using reason. 4 After all, even the reports that those who are sick with non-evident diseases attempt to give to their doctors are based on opinion rather than on knowledge. For if they had knowledge, they would not have run afoul of those diseases, since knowing the causes of diseases and knowing how to treat them by all the means that hinder their progress belong to the same intellect. Now as it is impossible to achieve perfect clarity by listening to these reports, the doctor must look to something else. 5 Thus, it is not the art that is responsible for slowness, but rather the nature of human bodies. For the art sees fit to provide treatment only after it has perceived the problem, taking care that its treatments are applied not rashly, but, rather, thoughtfully, and gently

rather than violently, while the nature of the human body, if it can hold out until it is seen, will hold out long enough to be healed, as well. But if, in the time it takes for this to be seen, the sick person is overcome, whether on account of his slowness in going to the doctor or the speed of the disease, he will be lost. **6** For if it starts the race from the same mark as treatment, disease is not the swifter, though it will be swifter if given a head start. And it gets a head start both from the impenetrability of human bodies, which diseases occupy without being seen, and from the negligence of the sick, which they impose upon themselves. For they consent to treatment only once their diseases have taken hold, and not before. **7** So then the power of the art is worthier of admiration when it restores those sick with non-evident diseases than when it does not handle impossible cases? Surely such is not the case in any of the other crafts that have been discovered up to now. Instead, those that work with fire cannot function when it is not present, and those that work with materials that are visible and malleable—for example, those that work with wood, or with leather, or the numerous others that work with bronze or iron or similar metals—as I was saying, though the things crafted from and with these materials are easy to work with, all the same they are crafted not with mere speed in mind, but with regard for what is required and without skipping any steps, and if ever one of the tools is missing, all work ceases. And though even in these crafts slowness is an obstacle to turning a profit, nonetheless it is paid greater respect.

**12 1** But medicine, though deprived of seeing any of the abscesses, whether of the liver or the kidneys, or indeed any of all those diseases located in the bodily cavity, with the eyesight—by which all people see all things most adequately—nonetheless discovered other resources to work with. **2** From the clarity or scratchiness of voice, from the speed or slowness of breath, and from each of the fluids regularly discharged through the orifices (gauging some on the basis of their smell, others by their color and still others by their thinness and thickness), it makes an inference to the conditions of which these things are signs, including what has already been suffered and what it is possible yet to suffer. **3** And whenever nature herself does not willingly relinquish these informants, medicine has discovered devices of compulsion by which nature is forced—without injury—to surrender them. She is released once she has made it evident to those knowledgeable in the art what should be done. **4** For example, using acrid food and drink the art forces fever to melt the congealed phlegm in order to draw an inference about what it was unable to see based on what has been seen. In turn, by running up steep roads the art forces breath to bring a charge against those things of which it is the accuser. Inducing sweats by the aforementioned means and by the vapors of hot water, the art makes an inference. **5** There are things that, in passing also through the bladder, are better suited for making the disease evident than when they pass out through the flesh. Accordingly, medicine has discovered food and drink that become hotter than the sources of heat, melting them and causing them to pass from the body along a route by which they never would have passed had they not been subjected to this. **6** Thus, the things that escape the body and betray its secrets differ with respect to the different routes they take and the different information they carry, so that it is no surprise that the time spent coming to some conviction about them exceeds that left for action, especially since their interpretation must pass through foreign translators on its way to the intellect that provides treatment.

**13** **1** The discourse given here makes it evident that medicine has well equipped arguments of its own to help in its fight. It rightly does not handle diseases that cannot be remedied, and, when it does handle a disease, it does so without making mistakes. This is made evident also by the displays of those knowledgeable in the art, for whom it is easier to give a display in action rather than in word, since they have not made a study of speaking. Instead, they hold that the majority of people are more apt to be convinced by what they see rather than by what they hear.

# COMMENTARY

## 1

In this, the first part of the *prooimion*, which I regard as the '*prooimion* minor' (see Introduction 2), our author sets the tone for the work as he playfully mocks the critics of the arts. The critics, as we shall see, have attacked medicine primarily for its lack of practical success, though our author insists that it they themselves, not medicine, who have failed. Thus, their own practice does not deserve to be called a *technē*; instead it is labeled an 'art of mean discourse' and a (mere) 'skill.' Our author is not above the injurious epithet or personal insult, and indeed he uses the *prooimion* to establish the foundations of an ad hominem attack on the critics that will frame the speech. His opponents are, first and foremost, uneducated hacks. Further, they are slaves to the jealous, talentless masses, who use them in their bid to overthrow the intellectual elite. The essential charge, familiar from tragic contexts, is hubris, the irreverence that inevitably results in the violation of boundaries—political, social, religious, epistemological, etc.—set by nature or convention (see Introduction 2). The charge resurfaces in various forms throughout *de Arte*, but here in c. 1 it is pitched most vividly in terms that construct an elaborate conceit. The experts in the *technai*, the aristocrats of the intellect, face rebellion from the useless democratic rabble, who have called for outside reinforcements in the form of unscrupulous argument-mongers (perhaps an allusion to the traveling sophist Protagoras, among others). In turn, *de Arte* joins the fray on the side of the experts, and of experts in medicine in particular, to restore moral, political, and cognitive order.

Our author's introduction defies expectations in at least two ways. First, his *prothesis*, or precise statement of purpose, is slipped in at the end of the chapter, almost as an afterthought. Second, he eschews the usual plea of inexperience, preferring instead to burnish his credentials. He is bold, he is well equipped, and he is powerful—trained in wisdom, no less! From start to finish, c. 1 is a show of force. The weapons at our author's disposal are ample, and not least among them is a stylistic creativity and daring that rivals that of any surviving sophistic text. Metrical and conceptual balance (e.g., φιλοτιμεομένων μὲν οὐδαμὰ δὲ δυναμένων), euphony (e.g., the alliteration of τοὺς μὲν οὖν ἐς τὰς ἄλλας τέχνας τούτῳ τῷ τρόπῳ ἐμπίπτοντας), syntactic effects (e.g., the hypallage κακαγγελίη φύσιος ἢ ἀτεχνίη), complex metaphor and dramatic imagery make *de Arte* a striking reminder of the classical Greek love of language.

**1.1** εἰσίν τινες οἳ τέχνην πεποίηνται τὸ τὰς τέχνας αἰσχροεπεῖν, ὡς μὲν οἴονται, οὐ τοῦτο διαπρησσόμενοι ὃ ἐγὼ λέγω, 'there are some who make an art of demeaning the arts, so they think, not achieving the result I just mentioned': oft-cited rhetorical parallels include the opening lines of Isocrates' *Helen* (εἰσί τινες οἳ μέγα φρονοῦσι, κτλ.; 10.1) and *Nicocles* (εἰσί τινες οἳ δυσκόλως ἔχουσι, κτλ.; 3.1) as well as the beginning of *Flat.* (εἰσί τινες τῶν τεχνέων, αἳ, κτλ.; 102.1 = L. 6.90). I would add to the list Antiphon's *On Concord*: εἰσί τινες οἳ τὸν παρόντα μὲν βίον οὐ ζῶσιν, κτλ. (F53a). *De Arte*'s similarity in diction and syntax to these works establishes its rhetorical resemblance to eminent members of the sophistic family. The subject of these lines—public verbal dispute—further confirms the author's preoccupation with the practices and concerns of classical sophistry. Indeed, the verbal verve characteristic of sophists such as Gorgias is already evident in his play on the word αἰσχροεπεῖν, which brings against the critics a three-fold charge. First (and most obviously), the author charges that the critics' speech attempts to demean the arts. Second, he charges that such an attempt is in itself shameful. Third, he charges that the critics' discourse, that is, the array of arguments marshaled against the arts, is of poor quality. The full range of associations is difficult to convey in translation, though they are key to understanding the opening chapter and, indeed, the treatise as a whole. We see, then, that our author's opening reaction to the critics is subtly layered, and we can begin to discern his own aims by implicit contrast with his opponents. They demean the arts, whereas he will support them generally, with special attention to medicine. But their speech is poor; his will serve as a shining example of the finest rhetorical form. And while their behavior is shameful, he will show himself to be right and honorable.

The phrase ὡς μὲν οἴονται has struck most editors as problematic, driving some to extremes of emendation, as in the case of Diels' change to ὃ μὲν οἴονται οὐ τοῦτο διαπρησσόμενοι, ὡς ἐγὼ λέγω ('which they don't think they're doing, as I claim they are;' 1914, 380). It is difficult to take ὡς as introducing indirect discourse, primarily because the expected order is οἴονται μὲν ὡς. Secondly, indirect discourse employing ὡς and a participle is an unusual and improbable (though not impossible) construction found nowhere else in the treatise. Instead, some have taken ὡς as a relative adverb introducing a dependent clause with οἴονται as the main verb and διαπρησσόμενοι as the auxiliary. Thus, Gomperz renders ὡς as 'wobei;' Jones 'though;' and

Jouanna 'alors que,' though the standard meanings and functions of ὡς do not support these translations.[1] Further, this approach has the consequence of attributing to the critics a lack of either intent or self-awareness that is both curious in itself and inconsistent with 3.3, where in strikingly similar language the author promises to refute the critics on those points where each happens to think he has achieved something (ᾗ ἂν ἕκαστος αὐτῶν πρήσσειν τι οἰόμενος τυγχάνῃ). The better option is to put ὡς μὲν οἴονται in the same family with stock phrases such as ὡς δ' ἐμοὶ δοκεῖ, that is, to treat it as an adverbial clause with a parenthetical function, dependent not on the clause that follows but on that which precedes it, as Jori has argued convincingly (1996, 364 n. 20). It seems to the critics that they have succeeded in artfully demeaning the arts, while this strikes our author (ἐμοὶ δὲ ... δοκεῖ) as nonsense. Instead of practicing a proper art, they merely show off their peculiar ἱστορίην (see note below).

The primary referent of τοῦτο is τὸ τὰς τέχνας αἰσχροεπεῖν. The critics' arguments fail to discredit the arts. This failure has implications for the auxiliary referent, πεποίηνται. Insofar as their case against the arts has fallen short, the critics have failed to demonstrate their mastery of art-denigration. Further, our author may mean to underscore the futility of using art to question the very notion of art: if the critics succeed in making their argument, they thereby refute its conclusion.

**1.1** ἱστορίης οἰκείης, 'special 'skill'': if, in virtue of their bad arguments, the critics fail at the art of art-denigration, they must ground any claim to artistry in something extrinsic to the immediate logical content of their attacks. It is questionable, for example, whether pieces such as Gorgias' *Helen*, or even his *On not being*, were intended to prove the unconventional theses put forward so much as to draw attention to other aspects of the discourse (see further Gagarin 2001). Likewise, the verbal assaults launched by the critics might fail to destroy the arts while still demonstrating some unique facility with another aspect of language. This ἱστορίη is special, οἰκείη, not only because it is the critics' own—in contrast to someone else's—but also because it is uncommon.

Does our author concede, then, that the critics possess some measure of art? In a sense, yes. Gomperz suggests that the author is contrasting the mere ἱστορίη of his opponents with his own σοφία (to which he refers at the close of this chapter) and cites in support a fragment of Heraclitus (DK 22

[1] Jori studiously catalogs the long history of mistranslations (1996, 364 n. 20).

B129) disparaging the ἱστορίη of Pythagoras (87). The implication would be that, while the critics might have a store of rote facts or procedures at the ready, they lack the genuine insight that comes with wisdom and, one might add, technical mastery. On the other hand, ἱστορίη need not carry any pejorative connotation. In Homer, the noun ἵστωρ signifies a person with technical skill or prowess (*h. Hom.* 32.2), and ἱστορίη and its adjectival and adverbial forms continue in philosophical discourse to retain connections to technical precision and knowledge (Aristotle, *de An.* 402a4, *GA* 757b35; Plato, *Sophist* 267e). This is the way in which our author employs it, albeit ironically. Just as their supposed 'art' of art-denigration was a sham, so too the critics' ἱστορίη will, upon further scrutiny, turn out to be nothing more than the ability to slander and criticize. This ability, however loathsome, is real, but it is not an art (see also notes on 1.2 below).

**1.1** ἐπίδειξιν ποιεύμενοι, 'making a display': the author uses this phrase to distinguish between what the critics hope to demonstrate *directly* and what they hope to demonstrate *in argument*. An audience is immediately aware of their facility with words insofar as it is directly evident from the expositions themselves, which are instances of this facility in action, as it were. Again, this is to be considered separately from the particular theses for which these critics argue, which need not bear any strong connection to the aims of the *epideixis*. Our author will refer to the demonstration of a thesis through argument as an *apodeixis*, and he will apply this term to his own project (3.1), though, given its meticulous construction, he surely regards it as an *epideixis* of rhetorical artistry, as well (see also Introduction 2, as well as notes on 3.1 and 13.1).

**1.2** τὸ μέν τι τῶν μὴ εὑρημένων ἐξευρίσκειν ... καὶ τὸ τὰ ἡμίεργα ἐς τέλος ἐξεργάζεσθαι ὡσαύτως, 'to discover fully something that has not yet been discovered ... [and] likewise to accomplish fully what has been accomplished only in part': the completive significance of the prefix ἐξ- is important to establishing the parallel construction of the sentence. As intelligence aims at the full discovery (τὸ ἐξευρίσκειν) of what has not been discovered (τι τῶν μὴ εὑρημένων), so too is its function the full completion (τὸ ἐξεργάζεσθαι) of what is half-done (τὰ ἡμίεργα). The adverb 'likewise' (ὡσαύτως) plays a central role as an indicator of this parallel, which sets the stage for an implied contrast between the author, who uses his intelligence to further the arts, and the critics, who abuse the arts and, in so doing, their own intelligence.

The Greek cognates ἐξευρίσκειν and εὑρίσκειν were the watchwords of the anthropological theory of human progress that gained traction in the fifth century, especially within sophistic circles. It was against the traditional mythology (sanctioned by Hesiod) of human decline from an original state of easy happiness that the 'new anthropology' posited an original 'state of nature' in which human beings lived in a manner akin to that of animals and from which they gradually extricated themselves through the discovery of language, civil law, and the arts. The idea of progress may have come down from Xenophanes, who hints at the possibility of epistemic progress in a surviving fragment (DK 21B18). But our best exemplars come from tragedy and the so-called Great Speech of Protagoras in Plato's dialogue of the same name (320dff.), which is generally thought to be a reasonably faithful reconstruction of Protagoras' περὶ τῆς ἀρχῇ καταστάσεως, 'On the original state.'[2] Protagoras' seems to have been the first sustained theoretical treatment of the subject, and, given the evidence that our author was familiar with sophistic thought—indeed, was perhaps an active participant in the movement—he may have Protagoras in mind when he alludes to human progress here, though perhaps his diction reflects a debt to the tragic poets as well. In Euripides' *Suppliants*, progress is said to have been made possible through human σύνεσις (203); in Aeschylus' *Prometheus Bound*, humans have 'fully discovered' (ἐξευρίσκειν) the arts once and for all (460, 469, 503), and one of the chief arts extolled is medicine (476–483).[3]

However, our author's reference to incompleteness may signal a departure from the 'Aeschylean' view that the arts have been discovered in full. If so, there remains the further question of medicine's completeness. The *Corpus* itself offers no uniform answer. The author of *VM* concedes that medicine has yet to attain perfect precision in all areas of inquiry falling within its purview (132.10–133.6 = L. 1.596–598), while in *Loc. Hom.* the art is said to be complete (84.17 = L. 342). Craik (1998, 233) suggests that *de Arte* takes the Aeschylean view, though no text is cited as evidence, and indeed I have found none that definitively rules out the possibility of its incompleteness.

1.2 συνέσιος ... ἐπιθύμημά τε καὶ ἔργον, 'object and occupation of the intellect': our author conceives of intellect as that faculty of the mind responsible for knowing (7.1, 11.4, 12.6) and making discoveries—I translate as 'occupation'

[2] This was, however, a point of contention among some past scholars. See Guthrie 1971, 64 n. 1 for the relevant bibliography and summary of the arguments involved.

[3] Dodds 1973 is still the most comprehensive study of this idea, though Edelstein 1967 remains valuable, especially for its discussion of the medical corpus. For a more recent, focused account of the anthropology of progress as developed in *VM*, see Rosen 2008.

the Greek noun ἔργον in order to sharpen the author's point that intellect has this characteristic job or function. (This sense predates Aristotle and is found already at Thucydides 2.89 and Plato, *Republic* 335d. However, we must be mindful of ἔργον in its sense of deed or accomplishment. Not only does intellect—metaphorically, of course—desire to make discoveries, but, in keeping with the theme of progress, it also achieves its goal.) Insofar as the arts, on the Greek view, are distinctively human (i.e., in contrast to natural or animal; see Introduction 1), and since they require such knowledge and discovery, it stands to reason that the intellect is a distinctively human faculty. To use it in accordance with its natural function, as our author does by championing the arts, is thus to work in harmony with human nature. As to whether our author holds a comprehensive view about the natural functions of human beings and their parts, see introductory notes to c. 10.

**1.2** λόγων οὐ καλῶν τέχνῃ, 'by an art of mean discourse': with the predicative formula οὐ καλῶν, our author continues to exploit the play on words introduced earlier with the verb αἰσχροεπεῖν. The critics' discourses are 'not fine' insofar as 1) their specific content asserts that the arts are worthless, but they are also 'not fine' in that they are 2) morally shameful and 3) technical products of poor quality—they do not succeed in proving the arts are worthless. This last sense yields an oxymoron (i.e., 'an art of bad arguments') that echoes the paradox and irony of 1.1. There is also an implicit antithetical contrast between the mere words (λόγοι) of the critics and the real accomplishments (ἔργα) of those who practice a *technē*. (On the λόγος-ἔργον antithesis the various senses of λόγος at play in *de Arte*, see also Introduction 2.)

**1.2** κακαγγελίῃ μᾶλλον φύσιος ἢ ἀτεχνίῃ, 'an indication of a mediocre nature or a lack of art': the MSS. diverge here with respect to κακαγγελίῃ (A), which the usually more reliable M has as καταγγελίῃ. The former is likely correct, as it yields a better sense and is attested in Galen. We are left with a striking hypallage, the adjective κακός (properly belonging to φύσις) being transferred to and compounded with ἀγγελίῃ.[4] A more logical and precise expression would have demanded ἀγγελίῃ μᾶλλον κακῆς φύσιος ἢ ἀτεχνίῃ, which reveals the extent to which our author prefers poetic sensibility to

[4] Our author is generally fond of the verb ἀγγέλλειν and its cognate compounds, which take on a technical semiotic significance—see especially 12.6. Gomperz notes that κακαγγελίη and its immediate cognates are, with the exception of *de Arte*, confined almost exclusively to tragedy (91).

semantic precision. In this regard, note also the symmetry between ἐπιθύμημά τε καὶ ἔργον (both neuter singular) and κακαγγελίη ... ἢ ἀτεχνίη (both feminine singular), and, again, the alliteration of the first pair against the homoioteleuton of the second.

There is some question as to whether κακαγγελίη ... ἢ ἀτεχνίη indicates a comparison or disjunction. Traditionally, it has been construed as the latter, but Jouanna has broken with tradition in arguing for a comparison (1988, 244 n. 1), an approach followed uncritically by Jori (1996, 69). Jouanna rationalizes the construal in part by differentiating, quite sensibly, between three classes: those who are technically adept, those who have a bad nature, and those who lack art (1988, 244 n. 1). With the phrase μούνοισι γὰρ δὴ τοῖσιν ἀτέχνοισιν, our author contrasts the bad-natured, who desire to demean the arts, with the artless, who take their marching orders from the ambitious former.[5]

There is reason to resist this last claim on linguistic grounds alone. First, if μούνοισι γὰρ δὴ τοῖσιν ἀτέχνοισιν is intended to contrast the artless with the bad-natured, we might expect a contrastive particle (perhaps μέντοι) instead of the staunchly confirmatory γὰρ δὴ. Moreover, γὰρ δὴ bears a logical load; we should expect our author to give us a reason for assenting to the preceding thought. Neither Jouanna nor Jori account for this in their respective interpretations, and in fact Jori omits altogether the causal element from his translation.

Second, the approach requires that ἡ ἐργασίη αὕτη point forward to ὑπουργεῖν and set it apart from the action (τὸ προθυμεῖσθαι) described at 1.3. As a point of grammar, αὕτη naturally points back to an object or clause already mentioned, and ἥδε is conventionally used to point forward (Smyth 1245), though αὕτη may on occasion do so, as well (Smyth 1247). But it seems to me that what αὕτη cannot do is set the two actions apart in this case. That is, with actions in the clauses immediately preceding and succeeding ἡ ἐργασίη αὕτη, both of which are potential referents, it would be counter-intuitive to use αὕτη in an exclusively forward-looking way, since in cases

[5] In arguing the comparative case, Jouanna points out that our author uses the formula μᾶλλον ἢ elsewhere in the treatise (cf. 7.3, 8.2 (*bis*), 11.4, 11.5 (*bis*), 11.7), always to introduce a comparison. I agree, though it seems to me rather clear that the contrast in this case is between κακαγγελίη and ἐπιθύμημά τε καὶ ἔργον. Our author might easily have written μᾶλλον κακαγγελίη φύσιος ἢ ἀτεχνίη ἢ συνέσιος ἐπιθύμημά τε καὶ ἔργον, but instead he has reversed the normal syntax, and this reversal is the source of what I take to be Jouanna's and Jori's confusion. Incidentally, the grammatical question is logically separable from the tripartite schemas discussed below. That is, any one of the schemas—Jouanna's, Jori's, or mine—is *prima facie* compatible with either construal of κακαγγελίη μᾶλλον φύσιος ἢ ἀτεχνίη.

where successive thoughts or objects are distinguished from one another, its distinctive function is always to point backward while ἥδε points forward. Had our author wished to firmly distinguish ὑπουργεῖν from τὸ προθυμεῖσθαι, he would have used ἥδε, not αὕτη. Linguistic considerations, then, favor the traditional construal, which assigns to αὕτη its natural role of pointing backward to the preceding sentence. The appositive infinitive construction redescribes and elaborates the same idea, and, as Jori rightly observes (1996, 367 n. 29), the subjective genitive construction φιλοτιμεομένων μὲν οὐδαμὰ δὲ δυναμένων κακίῃ reaches back through κακαγγελίῃ ... φύσιος to refer to the bad-natured.

But what is it to have a bad nature in precisely the sense our author intends? The text appears to maintain a distinction between those with bad natures, those with art, and those without it. The bad-natured, according to Jouanna, are those who lack both moral fiber and technical competence, while the artless lack merely technical competence (1988, 244 n. 1). These latter incompetents of decent character will not demean the arts of their own accord, though they will do so upon command of the bad-natured. Putting aside the fundamental implausibility of the proposed psychology, there remain at least two obstacles to Jouanna's interpretation. First, the distinction between the bad-natured and the merely artless rests on Jouanna's subtly misleading translation of the phrase μούνοισι γὰρ δὴ τοῖσιν ἀτέχνοισιν as 'à ceux qui sont *seulement* ignorants de l'art' where the Greek demands '*seulement* à ceux qui sont ignorants de l'art' (224; emphases mine).

Secondly, and more decisively, the logic of the argument gains nothing from the introduction of this second class of good-natured, obsequious incompetents, since, by Jouanna's own admission, they are not 'the adversaries envisioned here' (1988, 245). The real adversaries—those who have 'made an art of demeaning the arts'—are the bad-natured incompetents, according to Jouanna, and it is easy to see why he is compelled to take this position. If κακαγγελίῃ μᾶλλον φύσιος ἢ ἀτεχνίῃ is comparative, then τὸ δὲ λόγων οὐ καλῶν τέχνῃ τὰ τοῖσιν ἄλλοισιν εὑρημένα αἰσχύνειν προθυμεῖσθαι, κτλ. must describe the activities of the bad-natured. Further, it is most likely that the author with this description intends to contrast the critics with technical adepts (including himself). Thus, the critics must be identical to the bad-natured.

Jori, who also favors a comparative construal as well as a tripartite classificatory schema, does not equate the critics with the bad-natured; indeed, he seems unaware that it is an inevitable consequence of his view. Still, certain elements of his interpretation deserve consideration. Whereas Jouanna does not support his interpretation by citing sympathetic passages from elsewhere in *de Arte*, Jori looks hard at 8.6–7 for clues: 'and while in making these demands they (i.e., those who criticize doctors for not dealing with those overcome by their diseases) gain the admiration of those who are doctors in name, (ὑπὸ μὲν τῶν ὀνόματι ἰητρῶν), they are ridiculed by those who are doctors also in virtue of their art. (ὑπὸ δὲ τῶν καὶ τέχνῃ). Those experienced in this craft have no need for criticism or praise that is so senseless (οὕτως ἀφρόνων ... οὔτε μωμητέων οὔτ' αἰνετέων).' From this, Jori distills a detailed typology comprising 1) the real doctor, 2) the quack (the 'physician in name'), and 3) the critic of medicine. The so-called quack desires to be a real doctor but is hopelessly inept. Resentful of the real doctor, he thoughtlessly praises the critic, embracing the critic's arguments and using them against the real doctor. Translating this specific typology into the more general terms of 1.2, Jori depicts the critics of the arts (those who lack art) as putting their arguments in the service of the ineptitude (Jori's rendering of κακίη) of so-called experts in an attempt to undermine the technically adept in front of the ignorant masses (1996, 367 n. 29).

Jori's account of the functional relationship between the artless and the bad-natured has real merit. Furthermore, he is quite right to draw our attention to the structural analogy between the character types of 1.2 and 8.6–7, though I would caution against reading too much of the latter into the former. If familiarity with the more specific features of the doctor-quack-critic typology is required to decode the tripartite scheme of the opening lines, then surely our author deserves reproach for putting the cart before the horse. But in fact, the specific features of the doctor-quack-critic typology do not so neatly translate. While it is true that in c. 8 the quack concedes the validity of a particular criticism, we might reasonably ask whether he would endorse a purely destructive attack against his art as a whole or the arts generally. Presumably he would not, as the success of such an attack would defeat his larger purpose (namely, to appear expert). There is difficulty, too, in grafting the typology in c. 8 onto the categories outlined in c. 1. Is the quack bad-natured or artless? Certainly he lacks genuine art, though Jori reserves ἀτεχνίη for the critics. In what sense, then, might he be bad-natured? Jori contends that κακίη means simply ineptitude, but surely the artless are also inept, a conclusion with which he is curiously comfortable: 'in the judgment of our author, in fact, the characters of κακίη and of ἀτεχνίη will be attributed to both' (sc. categories, namely those of critic and quack; 1996, 370 n. 29).

So while Jouanna interprets 1.2 by concentrating on its immediate context to the exclusion of other potentially illuminating passages in *de Arte*, Jori views it largely through the lens of related passages, in the course of which he loses sight of the immediate context. Clearly, the text requires a more balanced approach that preserves the insights of both while avoiding their excesses. The central task is to discover more completely how and why our author employs the categories of the bad-natured and the artless. Two passages from elsewhere in the treatise provide the relevant background. First, there is the author's remark at 9.4, where one detects distinct echoes of the passage under discussion: 'and power (δυνᾶσθαι; sc. to make discoveries, ἐξευρίσκειν) is available to those whose training (παιδεία) is not lacking and whose natures (φύσις) are not indolent.' Here the author presents two necessary conditions for the development of technical ability: adequate training and the right nature (see also notes on 9.4). This implies that there are at least two different ways of being deficient in an art. One might lack the natural talent so that any training would be futile. Such a person could be said to lack even the potential for technical power. Alternatively, one could possess a nature suited to technical mastery but fail to receive adequate training in the principles and practices of the art. Indeed, training in an art was generally considered part of the art itself, so much so that our author, in the second passage of relevance, could claim that 'the arts are known only once they have been taught' (2.2), arguing that the very proof of their existence lies in their being transmitted from teacher to student. To be without training, then, is to be without art.

This compels a revision of the tripartite schema along the following lines. After Jouanna, I distinguish the basic categories of genuine expert, the artless, and the bad-natured. However, the artless are to be understood as those who have natural talent but lack sufficient training or exposure to an art, while the bad-natured are the emulous (φιλοτιμεομένων μὲν) among the ignorant masses (τοὺς μὴ εἰδότας) who lack any natural talent whatsoever (οὐδαμὰ δὲ δυναμένων). Our author thus creates a sort of intellectual class system with a determinate hierarchy: the expert aristocracy, possessing both talent and training, lords over the defective *dēmos*, whose members possess neither. The artless constitute an ambiguous middle class: without training they cannot join the elite, though they are by nature superior to the utterly incapable. Still, as an intellectual underclass, they join in solidarity with the bad-natured to overthrow the experts. The functional relationship, as Jori correctly perceives, is one of interdependence and mutual need (1996, 370 n. 29). But this interdependence is not so much conceptual, as Jori seems to suggest (ibid.), as it is political and practical. The artless, unable to equal their superiors in knowledge, seek to overthrow them by rousing the base. The rabble, eager to topple the 'artistocracy' but incapable of prevailing in political argument, count on the rhetorical weaponry supplied by the artless critics. Not incidentally, this would be a highly partisan—but not wholly inaccurate—characterization of Protagoras' book on wrestling and the other arts, in which, Plato tells us, he laid out for the benefit of anyone wanting to learn, 'the points one ought to raise in a debate against each craftsman himself, concerning all *technai* in general and each *technē* specifically' (*Sophist* 232d–e; see also Introduction 5).

This interdependence is key to grasping the logical structure of 1.2. Because the public offensive against the arts requires the cooperation of both the artless and the bad-natured, we may infer (recall the γάρ in μούνοισι γὰρ δὴ τοῖσιν ἀτέχνοισιν) that whoever plans to attempt such a coup either possesses a bad nature or lacks art—hence the necessity of taking κακαγγελίῃ μᾶλλον φύσιος ἢ ἀτεχνίῃ as a disjunction. The distinction is crucial not only to the governing conceit (discussed above in the general commentary on this chapter) but also to the subsidiary argument, namely, that no art could tolerate the sort of activity in which the critics and the bad-natured are engaged. The argument rests on the rationalist's premise that the intellect is no mere instrument for achieving pre-specified ends, but that it has its own unique function or end. The intellect is essentially directed toward genuine discovery, that is, the discovery of truth. No discursive activity that consists in intentionally (that is part of the force of προθυμεῖσθαι) avoiding or preventing progress toward truth could be intellectual, since it could not result in discovery, except perhaps by chance (on the contrast between art and chance, see Introduction 1). Simply put, the intent to obscure the truth is incompatible with the drive for knowledge and so cannot be adopted as the goal of any art.

With this argument, it may appear as though our author manages only to undermine the critics' specific attack on the arts. While their attack may not, in itself, constitute an art, surely it remains possible that they possess an art of discourse, speaking, or rhetoric exemplified elsewhere. In other words, the anti-intellectual disposition of their attack on the arts might be a merely incidental feature that is not found in the critics' work across the board. Thus, our author may not be entitled to the strong conclusion that they are without art. In his defense, however, I would leave open the possibility that our author is making the bolder claim (taken for granted by Jori in his analysis; 1996, 361–373) that the critics' ostensible art is not incidentally but rather essentially anti-intellectual. When he accuses them of debasing the discoveries of others without suggesting any improvements, he means that the critics' art has at its center a negative or destructive intent, that it is at best an art of refutation. A similar view of sophists as mere contradiction-mongers pervades the dialogues of Plato (e.g. *Phaedo*

91a), but, for the purposes of demonstrating the historical point about the public perception of the Greek sophists, perhaps the most telling example is Plato's *Apology*, in which Socrates is accused of denying religious dogma and corrupting the values of Athenian youth, both of which add weight to the charge that he is a sophist (18b–c). Given the apparently antagonistic orientation of some eminent sophists—recall Protagoras' famous work οἱ καταβάλλοντες, 'the arguments that overthrow,' as well as Gorgias' *On not being*—the characterization contains more than a measure of justice. Indeed, Plato questioned whether orators could lay claim to an art in the strict sense (465a; see also the following note), but in a way *de Arte* goes still further. While Plato decried the sophists for their lack of concern for the truth (e.g., *Gorgias* 454a–e and *Phaedrus* 260a–e), our author accuses them of downright hostility to it.

**1.2** φιλοτιμεομένων μὲν οὐδαμὰ δὲ δυναμένων κακίῃ ὑπουργεῖν, 'serving the mediocrity of those with ambition but utterly without power': Diels' suggestion that ὑπουργεῖν imparts a servile flavor to this description of the critics is surely correct (1914, 385). The text here is bombastic, sacrificing simplicity in syntax for the sake of a master-slave metaphor that personifies an abstraction (κακίη). Capturing the irony is essential to understanding the sentence: these critics, who aspire to usurp the status of the genuine experts, are mere lickspittle of the base. The verb ὑπουργεῖν reoccurs in this treatise (4.3, 7.2), where it connotes obedience, particularly obedience to the prescriptions of medicine, and so contributes to the sophistic themes of freedom, captivity, power and compulsion (see also, for example, 12.3). In this, *de Arte* deviates from other works of the *Corpus*, where ὑπουργεῖν and its cognates are rare; where they occur, they typically denote medical service rendered to the sick by doctors and other medical professionals (e.g., *Acut.* 66.18–20 = L. 2.370), though this meaning may be in play here, too: while doctors serve those sick and desperate for a cure, the critics serve only the vicious and power-hungry.

'Ambition' is a common rendering of φιλοτιμία (literally 'love of honor') and its cognates, but here the sense inclines more toward the archaic 'emulousness,' a coveting of someone else's position or status (the author repeatedly contrasts the desire for something with the power—or lack thereof—to obtain it; see especially 9.4). The basic charge is demagoguery, which bespeaks aristocratic sympathies and sets up a political metaphor. The *technitai* are compared to aristocratic leaders in an oligarchy: where the latter are under civil siege from democratic forces, the former are under threat from the critics, who conspire with the masses in a revolt of words. Both are leveling movements that seek to replace the excellent with the ordinary.

Again, this attitude brings our author closer to Plato, who hardly masked his disdain for democratic institutions and the demagogues who thrived in them. Moreover, by denying his opponents a real *technē* while depicting them as agents in the service of naked ambition, our author comes very near to Plato's characterization of orators as possessing not a *technē* but rather a knack for flattery (*Gorgias* 463a–b).

**1.2** τὰ τῶν πέλας ἔργα ἢ ὀρθὰ ἐόντα διαβάλλειν ἢ οὐκ ὀρθὰ μωμεῖσθαι, 'slandering their fellows' achievements when they are right or criticizing them when they are not': the formula οἱ πέλας (literally, 'those nearby') is often translated as 'neighbors,' and this sense is surely active here in *de Arte*, where the critics are to be ashamed not only because they slander, but because they are slandering those whom, as fellow citizens, they ought to regard as φίλοι. There is an implicit conceptual contrast with the preceding φιλοτιμεομένων, as the masses love fame and honor instead of their neighbors (perhaps an *ad hominem* shot at itinerant sophists), and perhaps a felt linguistic contrast with φιλοσοφία, made especially plausible by the logical contrast our author draws between those who further knowledge and those who work against it.

In the spirit of Prodicus' ὀρθοέπεια, 'correctness of words' (noted already in Jouanna 1988, 244 n. 1), our author draws a careful distinction between διαβάλλειν and μωμεῖσθαι. The distinction rests on the actual truth or falsehood of the criticism, not, as Jori suggests, the critic's awareness of such (1996, 366 n. 24), as this would imply that the critics were able to ascertain the correctness or incorrectness of technical work. Our author, who will argue in c. 7 that even lack of therapeutic success does not by itself imply the incorrectness of a doctor's prescription, would hardly attribute such competence to the artless critics (pace Jori 1996, 366 n. 27). In fact, no such competence is required: even in modern legal systems, ignorance is no defense against the charge of slander.

**1.3** τοὺς μὲν οὖν ἐς τὰς ἄλλας τέχνας τούτῳ τῷ τρόπῳ ἐμπίπτοντας, οἷσι μέλει τε καὶ ὧν μέλει, οἱ δυνάμενοι κωλυόντων, 'as for those who attack the other arts in this way, let those who are able deter such attacks when and where they care to': this passage, which introduces military imagery that will pervade the last lines of c. 1, may betray our author's professional occupation with medicine in contrast with those who have professional interests in defending the other arts. This may in turn hint (however weakly) that our author was a physician (see Introduction 5). However, there's nothing about the use of the third-person imperative form that excludes our author from the group of those with extra-medical interests. Indeed, the third-person seems to have been employed precisely to leave open that possibility, whereas such a possibility would be more difficult to read (though still not impossible) had the author used the second-person imperative. It may be objected that the following ὁ δὲ παρεὼν λόγος cements a contrast between the author and defenders of the other arts, but the Greek is ambiguous. First, the contrast does not involve the author *per se*, but rather this particular λόγος. Where the author himself may stand in relation to the defenders is, strictly speaking, not part of the picture. Second, word order is used to set up a false contrast of sorts, the sentence-penultimate οἱ δυνάμενοι in contradistinction to the sentence-initial ὁ δὲ παρεὼν λόγος. But the δὲ of the latter actually signals a contrast with τοὺς μὲν οὖν ἐς τὰς ἄλλας τέχνας … ἐμπίπτοντας. To paraphrase: 'there are people attacking the other arts, but this speech is concerned specifically with medicine.' Again, there is no indication as to whether our author himself plans to answer some of these other attacks. He may well do so. But while this passage is consistent with his having been a practicing physician, he need not have been.

**1.3** ὁ δὲ παρεὼν λόγος, 'the present discourse': the use of λόγος in c. 1 belongs predominantly to the linguistic domain (see Introduction 2), though it is difficult to secure a failsafe translation by this fact alone. Our author's penchant for poetical effect suggests he remains oriented toward oral performance, and in c. 13 he contrasts his λόγοι, which would be *heard* by the majority, with the ἔργα of medical experts, which would be *seen*. In the Introduction (section 2), I give further reasons for assimilating *de Arte* to classical logography. In any case, we should pay attention in this passage to the personification of λόγος, which our author claims has been trained in wisdom.

**1.3** τοῖσιν ἐς ἰητρικὴν οὕτως ἐπιπορευομένοισιν ἐναντιώσεται, 'will oppose those who thus march against medicine': Diels (1914, 385–386) and Jouanna stand out against most other modern editors and translators in preferring A's ἐπιπορευομένοις (which Jouanna ionicizes) to M's ἐμπορευομένοις. Neither reading can be taken literally, and so we are left to determine the relative aptness of two metaphors. Jouanna reminds us that ἐπιπορεύεσθαι, in the general sense of move or travel, appears in Polybius 4.9.2 and 1.12.4, where it signifies the marching of armies (1988, 225 n. 2). Thus, the prevailing military metaphor of the passage as a whole (about which Jouanna is too circumspect: 'there is perhaps a military metaphor,' 1988, 225 n. 2) inclines toward A. Besides ἐπιπορεῦσθαι, the verbs ἐναντιῶσθαι, θρασύνεσθαι, εὐπορεῖν, and δύνασθαι all have obvious military significance, and in fact the metaphor is put into effect already with the earlier τοὺς μὲν οὖν ἐς τὰς ἄλλας τέχνας τούτῳ τῷ τρόπῳ ἐμπίπτοντας, which τοῖσιν ἐς ἰητρικὴν οὕτως ἐπιπορευομένοισιν surely is meant to echo. Thus, there is a strong argument for keeping the senses of these two phrases consistent—so strong, in fact, that Jones, who sides with M, nonetheless translates ἐμπορεῦσθαι as 'invade.'[6]

Unfortunately for Jones, this is not the sense of ἐμπορεῦσθαι. The word has a predominantly commercial connotation: 'to travel for trade or business,' 'to deal in.' A gloss on R, apparently by Erotian, encourages us to take the passage in just this way, though it remains difficult to work this out in practice.[7] The verb may, per LSJ, take on a negative aspect, much as the English 'to traffic in,' which Jori stretches into 'intromettersi,' that is, 'to meddle in' (1996, 69). However, 'spacciare' ('to peddle') would seem more apt since Jori defends his reading by appeal to Greek cultural prejudices about the sophist as a dilettante-for-hire (1996, 340 n. 22). This risks too much in its assumptions and pays too little in its conclusions.

**1.3** εὐπορέων δὲ διὰ τὴν τέχνην ᾗ βοηθεῖ, 'well equipped through the art to whose rescue it comes': in martial contexts, βοηθεῖν is used for allies who come to the rescue of those under attack.[8] The technical turf of the physicians is under siege, and *de Arte* rushes to their aid. The physicians can defend themselves, but they cannot, properly speaking, rescue themselves. That assignment is left to our author, or at least to his speech. Many translations overlook this subtle point of diction, which weaves together both the political and military metaphors into a larger conceit. Our author projects himself as an outside ally coming to the aid of artist-aristocrats besieged by the democratic masses and sophists attempting an intellectual coup.

**1.3** θρασυνόμενος μὲν διὰ τούτους οὓς ψέγει, 'emboldened on account of these invaders, whom it blames': Diels argues that A's τοὺς ψέγειν ἐθέλοντας ('those wishing to criticize,' argued for and adopted also in Jori 1996, 70 n. 2) must be preferred to M's οὓς ψέγει, though his reasoning relies too much

[6] Tellingly, neither can Jori avoid military images when defending M: 'invaderne il campo' (1996, 339).

[7] The gloss is dismissed by Jouanna (1988, 208) and defended by Jori (1996, 340 n. 22).

[8] This is the routine meaning in Thucydides, where βοηθεῖν occurs with a predictably high frequency: ἦν οὐ δίκαιον, ἀλλ' ἢ κἀκείνων κωλύειν τοὺς ἐκ τῆς ὑμετέρας μισθοφόρους ἢ καὶ ἡμῖν πέμπειν καθ' ὅτι ἂν πεισθῆτε ὠφελίαν, μάλιστα δὲ ἀπὸ τοῦ προφανοῦς δεξαμένους βοηθεῖν [1.35]. Note, too, the military use of κωλύειν; in Thucydides, βοηθεῖν and κωλύειν function as a conceptual antithesis. See also 1.63, 6.88, and 8.40.

on ridiculing Gomperz' (admittedly misleading) translation of the Greek and not the Greek itself (1914, 386). Still, the view has some merit. The author employs the verb ψέγειν at 4.1 to characterize the critics' activity (ἐν τούτῳ ἤδη ψέγεται ἡ τέχνη), and Jori includes it in a list of terms that depict that activity as essentially negative or destructive in contrast to his own constructive project (1996, 361–362). It might be added that the military metaphor at work in this passage paints the author as a defender, not as an attacker, though M's reading would compromise the image. Finally, A's reading makes contact with the desire-power antithesis by implying that the author's opponents want to criticize the art but are too incompetent to succeed.

Against this must be weighed the following considerations. First, neither Diels nor Jori mentions the later occurrence of ψέγειν at 5.5 (εἰ τοίνυν ἐπιστήσεται ἢ ἐπαινεῖν ἢ ψέγειν ὁ νοσήσας τῶν διαιτημάτων τι οἷσιν ὑγιάνθη), perhaps because it does not clearly conform to the alleged pattern. Moreover, it is not censure, blame, or criticism *per se* to which our author objects, but rather unjust criticism and an unwillingness to suggest improvements. There is no disputing that c. 1 is dedicated to criticizing the critics, and our author may be claiming that such criticism is deserved, given the viciousness of his opponents. It is also likely that ψέγειν is meant to work with the military metaphor—our author blames the critics for starting the war, unprovoked by the art of medicine. Finally, appeal to the desire-power antithesis is weakened by our author's own admission that the art or arts are indeed criticized by his opponents (again, see 5.5), sometimes on account of genuine mistakes that have been made by experts (οὐκ ὀρθὰ μωμεῖσθαι, 1.2). That is, his opponents do not merely want to criticize. They actually do so.

As Jouanna realizes, either reading can be made to conform to the obvious intent (though A expresses the idea a bit more cleanly), which is to juxtapose the baseness of the critics with the excellence of the experts and the author himself (1988, 245 n. 3). However, M's version is superior on stylistic grounds. Accepting οὓς ψέγει, the three participial clauses form a step-wise *longueur* of increasingly many syllables (13, 14, 15), each capped by relative clauses of increasingly many syllables (3, 4, 5). To read τοὺς ψέγειν ἐθέλοντας would be not just to disrupt a delicate pattern, but also to rupture the overall parisosis. Given the inconclusiveness of the conceptual arguments in favor of either reading, such stylistic considerations take on more weight.

**1.3** δυνάμενος δὲ διὰ σοφίην ᾗ πεπαίδευται, 'powerful through wisdom, in which it has been trained': I translate consistent with the military metaphor (which, in various incarnations, persists through the treatise). In any case, 'training' captures the Greek notion of παιδεία as well as 'education' or 'cultivation,' and perhaps better, as it was sometimes applied to the training of animals. Protagoras in particular offered παιδεία that instilled εὐβουλία, or good judgment, which he was careful to distinguish from training in the *technai*, though Plato (*Gorgias* 519e) did use παιδεύειν for such training (see Woodruff 1999). Protagoras may have been the first to call himself σοφός (*Protagoras* 317b–c), and 'having been trained in wisdom' could be a reference to having studied with or learned from Protagoras, though it is at minimum a sign that our author considers himself highly educated, especially in the art of speaking (a point confirmed in c. 13). In an attempt to feign modesty, the author declines to apply the adjective σοφός directly to himself while still managing to convey that he has received the sort of training that his critics lack.

The Hippocratics do not on the whole lay claim to παιδεία. The verb παιδεύειν occurs only in *de Arte* (see also 9.4; it occurs also as a less favored textual alternative at *Morb. Sacr.* 13.17 = L. 6.370). The noun παιδεία, too, is rare in the *Corpus*. Besides *de Arte* (c. 9, where it is applied to those who learn a *technē*), it is found only in a few of the Hippocratic epistles (Maloney and Frohn 1986). Instead, the Hippocratics speak of διδάσκειν, teaching, which occurs twenty-five times in the *Corpus*. The oath in *Jusj.*, for example, includes a resolution 'to regard the one who taught me this art as equal to my parents' (4.5–6 = L. 4.628). Our author, however, does not explicitly claim to have been taught medicine as a profession; he has been merely 'well equipped,' or 'well provisioned,' by the *technē* for the current war of words, and the military metaphor is again salient.

## 2

As Jouanna observes (1988, 168), here in c. 2 our author shifts abruptly back to the topic of *technē* generally, despite having closed c. 1 with what appeared to be a transition to the topic of medicine in particular. Jori regards the apparent lapse into ontological concerns as 'a definite fracture, at least at the level of exposition' (1996, 104). He defends the digression as 'responding to a vital, fundamental exigency,' namely, showing that there exists 'a world whose configuration is compatible with the exercise of technical activity in general' (1996, 108). While this establishes the conceptual need to address the metaphysical and epistemological concerns that drive the arguments in this chapter, it does nothing to demonstrate the expository need for the excursion. But if we accept that *de Arte* is directed in part against Protagoras' attack on the arts collectively and individually (see Introduction 5), then at least some of the tension disappears. In that case, *de Arte* will presumably mirror in its 'fractured' structure the order of topics as treated by Protagoras.

The only way our author might have averted the fracture would have been to avoid mentioning medicine in his *prooimion* minor, with the rhetorically awkward result that he would have deferred the announcement of his main topic until c. 3. Instead, he ameliorates the fractured structure by transforming it into a 'fractal' structure so that the pattern of the *prooimion*—a first half dedicated to *technē* generally, a second to medicine in particular—is reiterated by the second and third chapters, the latter of which contains a second *prothesis* that echoes the first at the end of c. 1. (A third *prothesis* is found in c. 9; our author may intend the fractal pattern to govern the entire work.)

The change of topics in c. 2 is accompanied by a shift in style. The fluid sentences of the first chapter are traded for rigidly balanced clauses marching in logical lockstep. Euphonic effects are present (e.g., τὰ μὲν γὰρ ὀνόματα φύσιος νομοθετήματά ἐστιν, τὰ δὲ εἴδεα οὐ νομοθετήματα, ἀλλὰ βλαστήματα) but arguably less conspicuous and less diverse than in c. 1; antithesis and homoioteleuton are the rule. Novelty is achieved mainly through affected syntax (e.g., the interlocking chiasmus of τῶν γε μὴ ἐόντων τίνα ἄν τίς οὐσίην and the antistrophe of γινώσκεται at 2.2). Note the careful deployment of particles to convey precise logical relationships between ideas—not only the many occurrences of γάρ, but also ἐπεί, δή, and τοίνυν. The conceptual density of this *prokataskeuē* (preliminary argument in a forensic speech) is intentionally intimidating; our author knows that his arguments are barely cogent. Their logical form—rigorous reductio ad absurdum after the manner of Zeno and Gorgias—are designed to overwhelm, and the tone—imperious and patronizing—gives c. 2 an air of unquestionable authority.

**2.1** τὸ μὲν σύμπαν, 'on the whole': a common adverbial expression, this is probably a playful allusion to the charge, made by some critics, that *technē* wholly is not. See Introduction, sections 1 and 3.

**2.1** τέχνη εἶναι οὐδεμία οὐκ ἐοῦσα, 'there is no art that is not' [**2.1.a**]: the translation cannot preserve in English a grammatical indeterminacy (and perhaps also semantic and syntactic, depending on one's view) in the Greek that allows for various formal interpretations that may be divided into two groups, depending on whether the participial phrase οὐκ ἐοῦσα is construed predicatively or conditionally. Surely, the conditional construal is the less natural and, all things being equal, would be the less preferred. Still, without having settled on the sentence's meaning or on its overall significance, one cannot say that things are equal. Taking the complete ἔστι to have existential force (see Introduction 3), the sentence reads as a tautology—essentially a special case of a general form of the principle of non-contradiction:

> **2.1.a.1**: if an art does not exist, then it does not exist (that is, if there is no object, x, that is an art, then there is no x that is an art).

Restricting the complete ἔστι to its elliptical-predicative import yields the following:

> **2.1.a.2**: for anything that's an art, if it does not have any properties, then it does not have any properties (that is, for any x, if x is an art, then, for any predicate, R, if x is not R, then x is not R).

That is, there is no art that both has and does not have any properties.

If the participial phrase οὐκ ἐοῦσα is not conditional but predicative, the main verb and modifier (εἶναι οὐδεμία) may have the force of a negative existential quantifier with wide scope ranging over predicates or objects, depending on the operative function of ἔστι (i.e., either existential or predicative).[9] Thus, the sentence could mean that

> **2.1.a.3**: there is no art that does not exist, that is, every art exists.

This provocative, paradoxical and prohibitively strong claim would be the boldest possible response to the critics' presumed charge that *technē* wholly is not. Alternatively, emphasis might fall on the predicative use of ἔστι:

> **2.1.a.4**: no art fails to have any properties, that is, every art has some property.

This may have struck our author as a particularly powerful thesis. If something (medicine, for example) is an art, then it has a predicate (namely, 'is an art') and therefore 'is.' Supposing that he did not feel a sharp difference between the functions of ἔστι, he might have thought that the obvious truth of the predicative interpretation guaranteed the truth of the existential as well.

However, upon closer scrutiny, the truth of the predicative interpretation is far from obvious, at least in the way our author needs it to be. While it may

---

[9] I set aside the other possible uses of ἔστι, e.g., to connote truth, identity, reality, actuality, generic implication, duration, possibility, locative existence. Though they play a role in c. 2, they are largely irrelevant in the immediate context.

be true that, if Socrates is wise, then there is some property that Socrates has, and, thus, that Socrates himself must be or exist, to expect the same to hold of medicine is to confuse logical categories. When it is said that medicine is an art, the 'is' is to be interpreted not as indicating property-instantiation but rather inclusion. 'Medicine' does not name a particular to which one may apply some predicate or other. Rather, it names a predicate that bears a relation to other predicates: if something is medical, then it is also technical, much in the same way that we might say that a biological fact was also a scientific one. Accordingly, the correct interpretation of **2.1.a.4** is this:

> **2.1.a.5**: if it's the case that, for any x, if x has a certain property, P, then x is also an instance of *techne*, then P is instantiated, that is, there exists some y that is P.

This is a puzzling proposition that is difficult to render in natural language and, even if true (though it appears, at least prima facie, not to be), is far from self-evident. Moreover, nothing germane to the critics' presumed charge follows from it.

The least charitable reading of the passage, then, would have our author perpetrating a sophism by passing off **2.1.a.5** as **2.1.a.4**, whereas he ought to have made a clear distinction. Even if we grant him **2.1.a.4**, however, our author may still be guilty of the fallacy of irrelevance, if indeed **2.1.a.3** alone rebuts the critics' charge that *technē* wholly is not. Worse yet, he may fail to distinguish between **2.1.a.4** and **2.1.a.3** and so take himself to be giving a genuine response to the charge that *technē* wholly is not. As a rejoinder to these criticisms, it should be pointed out that our author's alleged fallacies appear to derive from a general failure to make the proper distintctions between separate and unrelated meanings of ἔστι.[10] This of course assumes that there are distinctions to be made in the first place, an assumption that has lain at the heart of logic at least since the revolution of Frege and Russell, if not before. (It is no coincidence that contemporary formal language is employed to tease out the precise differences between **2.1.a.3–5**.) A relatively recent philosophical movement has begun to challenge the authority of these assumptions and to question whether they in fact were or even ought to have been observed by ancient philosophers. By drawing upon two important claims produced by this movement, namely, Brown's notion that the Greeks conceived of ἔστι on analogy with English verbs like

[10] Vegetti recognizes, but does not analyze, what he calls the 'radicale indistinzione fra funzione copulativa e funzione esistenziale dell'essere' (1964, 348).

'teaches,' and Hintikka's insistence that the Greeks (as represented by Aristotle) thought the different 'meanings' of ἔστι to be related as different forces of a single meaning, our author's argument may be rehabilitated (Brown 1994, 224–228; Hintikka 1986). Just as 'John teaches biology' warrants, without protest, the inference to 'John teaches,' so 'medicine is an art' warrants the inference to 'medicine is,' and likewise for any art whose 'being' one might care to challenge. But having established that, for example, 'medicine is,' it becomes clear that, even if the critics are right that arts like medicine are not instantiated (e.g., that the things that doctors prescribe do not actually bring about the health of the patient), this alone does not mean that medicine or art generally 'is not,' much less 'wholly is not.' For so long as medicine is an art, it is in some way: the complete and univocal ἔστι may be legitimately applied to medicine, albeit primarily with generic-implicative, not existential, force.

However, unless this use of ἔστι has existential implications, it leaves our author open to the charge of equivocation, for the the problem raised by the critics of *technē* is the problem of its being where ἔστι has primarily existential force. On its face, the gap appears unbridgeable. To revive an exhausted philosophical *Lieblingsbeispiel*, one can know that 'bachelors are unmarried' without there actually existing any bachelors at all. The proposition 'bachelors are unmarried' is generally regarded as a conceptual truth. It is true by definition, and definitions are stipulative. Likewise, could one not know that 'medicine is an art,' even if medicine did not exist? To deny this, one would need to deny that 'medicine is an art' is an analytic truth. At least since Kripke, philosophers have become accustomed to the possibility that certain generic implicatures, specifically those that express essential relations between natural kinds, are in fact not analytic but synthetic and a posteriori.[11] They are, nonetheless, necessary. Thus, 'water is $H_2O$' is necessary but a posteriori, as is 'dolphins are mammals.' Moreover, if 'dolphins are mammals' has been discovered to be true, then surely instances of the respective natural kinds 'dolphin' and 'mammal' exist or have existed.

Would our author maintain that 'medicine is an art' is to be assimilated to a Kripkean analysis of propositions like 'dolphins are mammals' rather than to the conventionally analytic 'bachelors are unmarried'? In addition to the sense that it would make of the text, there are two reasons that weigh in favor of this hypothesis. First, if it is true that there developed in early

---

11 See Kripke 1972, especially 122–134.

Greek philosophy a distinctive function or sense of ἔστι, one which was used specifically for conjoining subjects to predicates that expressed or revealed their natural essence,[12] then it is possible that our author is working within the same tradition. Second, and relatedly, further analysis will show (see notes on 2.2–3 and 6.4) that εἴδεα, forms or natural kinds, play an important role in our author's ontology, so that on his view 'to be' in the fullest sense is to be a member of a natural kind. Medicine, it will turn out, has such a form (4.4), and he will even claim that 'there is no art that is not seen as an outgrowth of some form' (2.2). Accordingly, the proper interpretation of **2.1.a** will be expressed by the following:

> **2.1.a.6**: if something $\text{is}_n$ an art, then it $\text{is}_e$.

Here '$\text{is}_n$' represents the ἔστι of natural-essential predication, perhaps best paraphrased as 'is by nature,' while '$\text{is}_e$' signals that ἔστι is used with an existential sense (which is just to say that the natural kind named is also instantiated).[13]

So even if one ultimately resists Brown's or Hintikka's general claims about Greek views, not to mention the views themselves, one might still reconstruct, with philosophical plausibility, our author's argument in light of them. In any case, the above considerations make it more difficult to dismiss out of hand our author's position as obviously naive or fallacious. In fact, if it is correct, then it may be the critics themselves who are guilty of confusion and irrelevance, not our author. And if our author is not ultimately correct, his position is at least defensible.

**2.1** καὶ γὰρ, 'since it's just': or, alternatively, 'and in fact,' depending on the connection between the idea this phrase introduces and the foregoing. See note on **2.1.b** below.

**2.1** ἄλογον ... ἡγεῖσθαι, 'absurd to believe': something of a technical term, our author employs ἄλογον to flag the unacceptably strange or contradictory consequences of the view opposed to his. (Again, see note on **2.1.b** below).

---

[12] See Mourelatos 1970, especially pp. 56–62, where the notion of what Mourelatos calls the 'is of speculative predication' is first developed. Ultimately, my analysis does not depend on successfully identifying a unique meaning for ἔστι. Rather, it suffices that ἔστι could be used in Greek to express such relations between natural kinds, just as 'is' may do in English. My argument is simply that our author is attempting to assimilate the proposition 'x is an art' to such cases.

[13] Again, if Hinitkka's view is correct, then there is no sense to such talk of different senses of ἔστι.

Consider also the recurrence of the phrase (and the distinction made there between absurdity and impossibility) at 2.3.

**2.1** τῶν ἐόντων τι ... μὴ ἐνεόν, 'one of the things-that-are is not' [**2.1.b**]: the adjective ἄλογον introduces a *reductio ad absurdum* argument for the author's position. But the precise nature of the position opposed to our author's, not to mention its connection to the preceding claim about *technē*, requires clarification. Construing the complete ἔστι along traditional lines, as having either existential or elliptical-predicative significance, two plausible interpretations emerge.

> **2.1.b.1**: there is some property, P, such that there is some x that is P and there is no x that is P, in contradiction to which our author maintains **2.1.b.1***: for any P, it is not the case both that there is some x that is P and that no x is P; or
>
> **2.1.b.2**: there is some x such that, for some property, P, x is P, and, for any property, R, x is not R (i.e., x both has some property and has no properties whatsoever), in contradiction to which our author maintains **2.1.b.2***: for any x and P, if x is P then it's not the case that, for any property, R, x is not R.

Promisingly, these appear to be generalized forms of the conditional interpretations outlined above (see previous note) such that **2.1.a.1** and **2.1.a.2** are derivable from **2.1.b.1*** and **2.1.b.2***, respectively. This raises the possibility that the connection is straightforwardly logical, a possibility suggested (but not strictly demanded) by the Greek. Curiously, it has gone unappreciated by most commentators that γάρ could be causal and καί adverbial, emphasizing ἄλογον: 'since it's just absurd,' *vel sim*. In other words, there is at least the potential for a more rigorous logical connection here than has been imagined.

Unfortunately, such a move would appear to foreground the conditional interpretations, a result that commentators understandably have sought to avoid. Traditionally, then, καὶ has been taken as a conjunction and γὰρ as an adverb: 'and in fact,' 'and indeed.' However, there remains the burden of elucidating the relation between **2.1.a** and **2.1.b**, or, to put it another way, we are left to account for the author's motives in moving from the one to the other. As will become clear, the move is made in part to open up an opportunity for our author to voice his fundmental ontological and epistemological commitments, though certainly he might have accomplished this without an exposition of the absurdity of **2.1.b**. Moreover, the absurd proposition under consideration is no arid abstraction, but, as demanded by the rhetorical situation, the very position our author attributes to his opponents, whether explicitly or implicitly. Could either **2.1.b.1** or **2.1.b.2** be attributed plausibly to the critics? Probably not **2.1.b.1**, since they would obviously deny that those professing technical mastery practiced an art in any meaningful or successful way, and it would be difficult to accuse them of doing so even implicitly. But **2.1.b.2** comes closer, especially when considered against **2.1.a.4**, which attempted to block the critics' charge that the arts 'are not' based on the fact that some things were arts. When recast in terms friendly to **2.1.a.6**, the critics' alleged claim becomes

> **2.1.b.3**: there is an x and P such that x $is_n$ P even though x $is_e$ not, in contradiction to which our author maintains **2.1.b.3***: for any x and P, if x $is_n$ P, then x $is_e$.

This construal of **2.1.b** meets the two main desiderata. Most importantly, it attributes to the critics a view that they may have been reasonably accused of holding. Further, it explains the special logical significance of καὶ γὰρ, since **2.1.a.6** can be derived from **2.1.b.3***.

**2.1** ἐπεὶ τῶν γε μὴ ἐόντων τίνα ἄν τίς οὐσίην θεησάμενος ἀπαγγείλειεν ὡς ἔστιν, 'for what being could anyone observe of the things-that-are-not and report that they are' [**2.1.c**]: chiasmus reinforces the instinct to read a double interrogative, which has been the preference of most modern commentators (excluding Jouanna), though little sense is sacrificed if it is not.

The term οὐσίη has a particularly Platonic ring, though it cannot have the more abstract Platonic meaning here. If οὐσίη here is something that is seen, then it cannot mean simply 'being' or 'existence' *simpliciter*. Rather, οὐσίη must refer to some quality or property of the things in question (see also note on 6.4). The use of οὐσίη to mean 'property' or 'quality' suggests that the ἔστι in ὡς ἔστιν is a binary predicate requiring completion: 'it is some P,' where P names a property. After all, one could not imagine the critics committing themselves to the proposition that any of the arts 'is' without qualification, though they would likely have conceded that the various arts are something, namely, arts. Again, this likelihood hardens into certainty if we accept that the critics attacked not just the arts severally but also collectively qua art. Such a line of attack not only concedes that, for example, medicine is an art; it depends on it.

If, due to their lack of perceptible qualities, the things-that-are-not go unperceived, they likewise go unreported (ἀπαγγείλειεν). Though elsewhere in *de Arte* (10.5, 11.4, 12.6) compounds of ἀγγέλλειν are employed with emphasis on its performative aspect (reporting is an action that aims at disseminating information), here ἀπαγγείλειεν should be assimilated to the series of verbs in the immediate context denoting intentional attitudes (ἡγεῖσθαι, νομίσειε, νοῆσαι). The author's point is that the requisite intentional attitude is a necessary condition of linguistically asserting 'that it is P.' Put more succinctly, if somewhat crudely: if it is not thought, it is not (meaningfully) said. (Cf. Parmenides DK 28 B2, ll. 7–8: 'for neither could you know what-is-not, for this can't be done, nor could you [presumably as a result] say it.')

Uncompressed, the argument contained in our author's rhetorical question is the following:

1. Suppose **2.1.b.3**, namely, that there is something (call it a) that both $\text{is}_n$ something (call it F) and $\text{is}_e$ not.
2. Then a $\text{is}_n$ F.
3. Then it is perceivable (by someone) that a is F.
4. Thus, a $\text{is}_e$.

Thus, the critics' position is reduced to absurdity, since it would require that a both $\text{is}_e$ and $\text{is}_e$ not. But is the *reductio* valid? There are obvious gaps in the argument limbed above, specifically in the deduction of 3 from 2 and of 4 from 3. The former move requires a premise like the following:

2.5. if a $\text{is}_n$ F, then it is perceivable (by someone) that a is F.

The idea, while implicit in this argument, will be made explicit in our author's remarks at 2.2. More curious is the hidden premise that allows for the movement from 3 to 4:

3.5. if it is perceivable (by someone) that a is F, then a $\text{is}_e$.

Thus the route from 3 to 4 is secured, and it is encouraging, given my earlier analysis, that it is secured by adverting to the epistemological principle that a claim involving the ἔστι of natural predication must be open to verification by sense experience (premise 2.5). In other words, the sentence 'medicine is an art,' if it can be known, is known a posteriori. Still, the argument goes through only if 3.5 is true, as well, and it is to its defense that our author now turns.

**2.1** εἰ γὰρ δὴ ἔστι γε ἰδεῖν τὰ μὴ ἐόντα ὥσπερ τὰ ἔοντα, οὐκ οἶδ' ὅπως ἄν τις αὐτὰ νομίσειε μὴ ἐόντα ἅ γε εἴη καὶ ὀφθαλμοῖσιν ἰδεῖν καὶ γνώμῃ νοῆσαι ὡς ἔστιν, 'for if indeed it is possible to see the things-that-are-not, just as it is to see the things-that-are, I don't know how anyone could believe of those things that it were possible both to see with his eyes and to know with his mind that they are, that they are not' [**2.1.d**]: our author argues in support of 3.5 above, again by means of *reductio ad absurdum*.

5. But suppose that 3.5 is false so that it is perceived (by someone) that a is F and a $\text{is}_e$ not.
6. Then it is thought (by that someone) that a is F.
7. Thus, a $\text{is}_e$.

So, once again, the critics' position is reduced to absurdity, since, once again, it entails that a both $\text{is}_e$ and $\text{is}_e$ not. And, once again, there are gaps in the argument requiring supplementation. To validate the inference from 5 to 6, we must insert:

> 5.5. if it is perceived (by someone) that a is F, then it is thought (by that someone) that a is F.

Not only does this anticipate the remarks on perception, thought, and being in 2.2, but it suggests that, for our author, perception is, plausibly, an intentional attitude and, as such, may be conceived of as a kind of thinking. As it happens, this is crucial to filling in the gap between 6 and 7, since it would seem to depend on certain theses about the relation between thought and being reminiscent of Parmenides (cf. DK 28 B2; see also notes on 2.2 below).

> 6.5. If a can be thought about, then a $\text{is}_e$.

Someone who thinks that a is F demonstrates thereby that a $\text{is}_e$, if indeed thinking is a relation between mind and object and the terms of a relation must exist.

In the above reconstruction, I have rendered νοῆσαι as 'think' in order to bring out the fact that it denotes a mental state directed toward an object. This is the sense also that γινώσκεται has in 2.2, though I translate both νοῆσαι and γινώσκεται as 'know' in the sense of 'know by acquaintance,' where the emphasis falls on 'acquaintance.' The phrase καὶ ὀφθαλμοῖσιν ἰδεῖν καὶ γνώμῃ νοῆσαι introduces an antithesis between perception and knowledge that will play a major role in c. 2 (see 2.2), though the specific cognitive issues it raises will not surface until 11.2. Both νοῆσαι and γινώσκεται stand in close relation to γνώμη, which I translate throughout as 'mind,' since the English word preserves the idiomatic contrast with the perceptual faculties in particular and the physical body more generally (cf. 7.3). Moreover, it is suitably vague. Our author says nothing explicit about the relation of γνώμη to σύνεσις or λογισμός (see notes on 1.2 and 11.3, respectively), though one is inclined to suppose that σύνεσις is the faculty of γνώμη that carries out the activity of λογισμός, since σύνεσις is said at 1.2 to be responsible for making discoveries, and λογισμός is the process by which the doctor discovers the causes of disease that are hidden from perception (11.3), a task that our author has assigned in general terms to γνώμη (11.2). Moreover, γνώμη appears in both cc. 2 and 11 to do more than just reason; it presides over all mental representation. Where vision allows for perceptual acquaintance with objects or states of affairs (the eyes are said to see both a thing having a property—e.g., a 'a red cyst'—and that there is a thing with the property—e.g., 'that there is a red cyst'), γνώμη allows for mental acquaintance with objects or states of affairs.

**2.2** ἀλλ' ὅπως μὴ οὐκ ᾖ τοῦτο τοιοῦτον, 'isn't it rather more like the following?': the Greek is an unusual but documented idiom expressing cautious affirmation, as noted by Jouanna (1988, 246 n. 9), who cites a parallel in Plato at *Cratylus* 430d. I translate as a question to capture the author's conciliatory (and perhaps patronizing) tone, which he likely adopts *en lieu* of a formal argument for the philosophical pronouncements that follow.

**2.2** τὰ μὲν ἐόντα, 'whereas the things-that-are': given that the ultimate concerns of preceding arguments revolved around the problems resulting from the claim that one could see or know that which is$_e$ not, the phrase τὰ ἐόντα, as a form of ἔστι, ought to be understood as having primarily existential force. The neuter plural commits our author to some variety of ontological pluralism. Had he wished to remain neutral on the question, he might have employed the construction τὸ μὲν ἐὸν, literally, 'what is,' which could have maintained consistency with either monism or pluralism. However, as will become clear shortly, 'the things-that-are' refers not necessarily to basic physical elements (our author takes no clear position on what those may be) but includes also anything that has an εἶδος, e.g., any one of the various arts.

The particle μέν is often translated as 'whereas' or 'while' in paratactic contexts. Our author is chiefly concerned with the second clause (starting with τὰ δὲ μὴ ἐόντα), since it is the premise on which the foregoing argument turned. The first clause, introduced by τὰ μὲν ἐόντα, while not in itself trivial, provides metrical balance for and conceptual contrast with the more important second.

**2.2** αἰεὶ, 'always,' 'in every case': while for Parmenides 'what is' exists in a timeless present (DK 28 B8), the post-Parmenidean philosophers attribute to their fundamental being or beings an eternal existence, which they indicate with the verb ἔστι and the adverb ἀεί (Ion. αἰεί). So, according to Anaxagoras, mind 'is always' (ἀεί ἐστι, DK 59 B14), while Melissus insists that whatever is, is always (ἔστιν ἀεί, DK 30 B3).[14] For Empedocles the roots 'in this way always are, unchanged in a circle' (ταύτῃ δ' αἰὲν ἔασιν ἀκίνητοι κατὰ κύκλον, DK 31 B17; see also 25.35). The line from Empedocles is especially intriguing, since the word order allows αἰὲν to modify ἔασιν independently of ἀκίνητοι, obtaining thereby an entailment: they are unchanged in a circle, and thus they are always. I propose that our author employs a similarly poetic arrangement to split αἰεί between τὰ μὲν ἐόντα (where it will have temporal significance: 'the things-that-are always') and ὁρᾶταί τε καὶ γινώσκεται (where it will have a triple significance: '(1) without exception, (2) every time they are seen and known, they are seen and known to have the same properties (3) invariably'). Indeed, the poetic exploitation of ἀεί to philosophical ends goes back at least to Heraclitus, who offers the closest linquistic parallel to *de Arte*: 'though this *logos* is always, always do humans turn out to be uncomprehending of it' (τοῦ δὲ λ'γου τοῦδ' ἐόντος ἀεὶ ἀξύνετοι γίνονται ἄνθρωποι, DK 22 B1; see McKirahan 116 n. 3; for a potential Hippocratic parallel in style, see the Heracleitean *Alim.* 147.17 = L. 9.120). It is possible, too, that the placement of the disyllabic αἰεὶ is motivated in part by our author's desire to mirror the disyllabic οὔτε of the parallel colon.

Melissus, Anaxagoras, and Empedocles probably were motivated to make their being or beings eternal in an effort to conform to the Parmenidean constraint that 'what is' should never cease to be, since that would require some adversion to what is not (DK 28 B8). Since, as the fragment of Heraclitus makes plain, the pre-Socratic penchant for eternality predates even Parmenides, it is difficult to say whether our author shares their particular concerns, though the sometimes Eleatic language and logic of c. 2 (more on this below) probably indicates he is aware of the problems posed by Parmenides.

**2.2** ὁρᾶταί τε καὶ γινώσκεται, 'are seen and known': this is not the present tense of ongoing or repeated action but rather of timeless action, or, more precisely, of temporally unspecified action (probably with some modal import; 'are visible and knowable' might be a defensible rendering). The

---

[14] The line from Anaxagoras is a contentious emendation by Diels (see further Curd 68 n. 68). Melissus writes more than once that what is was always and will be always (DK 30 B1 and B2).

things-that-are always will, without exception, be seen and known at some time. The specific antithesis surfaces elsewhere in pre-Socratic thought, most conspicuously in Antiphon and Melissus (see Introduction 3), and much ink has been spilled discussing the latter,[15] though my own inclination is to read *de Arte* in part as a repudiation of Parmenides.

> For never can this be victorious, that the things-that-are-not are (εἶναι μὴ ἐόντα),
> but you, block your thought from this path of inquiry,
> and do not let habit, derived from much experience, force you down this much-experienced path[16]
> to guide your sightless eye (ἄσκοπον ὄμμα) and clanging ear
> and tongue, but judge by reason (κρῖναι δὲ λόγωι) the much-contested refutation uttered by me. (DK 28 B7)

Where our author begins his argument by accusing his opponents of claiming (absurdly) that the things-that-are are not, Parmenides begins his by accusing his opponents of claiming (absurdly) that the things-that-are-not are. But Parmenides diagnoses his opponents' fallacy differently: they are deceived by their senses, which, being 'blind' or 'sightless,' do not see what is. It is the judgment of reason alone that can oppose the senses and discern what is. Our author, by contrast, does not dismiss the senses as dysfunctional, but regards their sight as a legitimate path to knowledge of the things-that-are. For him, there is no rift between the seen and the known. If his opponents' position pits them against perception, then so much the worse for them.

Whether or not our author is alluding consciously to Parmenides' poem, there is no doubt that he advocates a brand of empiricism at odds with Eleatic doctrine. The things-that-are are given to us by perception, and, if something is not perceivable, then it is not. This programmatic statement, seemingly naïve in its lack of nuance, will be refined in c. 11 to accommodate the practical reality of medical situations. For there our author will have to cope with the fact that some diseases have causes that are not directly perceivable. Part of the solution will rely on our author's limitation of the-things-that-are to those that exist always. This makes it unlikely that our author is concerned with particular existents as such (e.g., this fire, that

[15] Jori, for example, makes much of the alleged connection to Melissus (1996, 115–125), as does Vegetti (1964, 360–366). Gomperz, too, thought it significant (6).

[16] The Greek is ἔθος πολύπειρον ὁδοῦ, and I take the adjective to modify both nouns, which I think is consistent with the poetic genre and yields a richer sense. Conveniently, it also mirrors my construal of αἰεί in 2.2.

medical intervention), which, as had been recognized well before Plato, routinely come into being and then leave again. It is much more likely that he has in mind the universal kinds—what he will call 'forms' (εἴδεα)—of which particulars are instances: fire, medicine, etc. All of these are always seen to have the same properties without changing. Fire is always hot; medicine always heals the sick (except when it does not—see 3.2). Thus, the best paraphrase of our author's idea would run something like the following: 'the instances of those things that exist always (that is, the natural kinds) are, without exception, perceived and known (by all who perceive and know them and in every case) to have the same properties invariably.'

**2.2** τὰ δὲ μὴ ἐόντα, 'the things-that-are-not': these do not exist and, therefore, are not anything, i.e., have no predicates or properties, including, as we shall see, the properties of being seen and known.

**2.2** οὔτε ὁρᾶται οὔτε γινώσκεται, 'are neither seen nor known': the significance of this sentence, and of this key clause, has inspired much commentary. Its similarity to a line from a fragment of Melissus (ὥστε συμβαίνει μήτε ὁρᾶν μήτε τὰ ὄντα γινώσκειν, DK 30 B8 (3)) has seemed to some an impossible coincidence. In the Introduction (section 3), I give reasons for placing less weight on the connection than have some, though I concede that our author nonetheless may be signaling his familiarity with and desire to participate in the ongoing philosophical debate about being to which Melissus is an heir. As I have already discussed (Introduction 3), this debate had many participants, and echoes of several of them have been detected here, including also Gorgias, Protagoras, and Antiphon. The debate itself can be traced back to Parmenides, and some have thought that here the author of *de Arte* is laying bare his commitment to Eleatic doctrine (Taylor 225), though without explaining exactly how or why this would be.

I claimed earlier that our author's views were incompatible with some Eleatic doctrines, though one should not infer therefrom the complete absence of sympathy. Indeed, this part of *de Arte* resembles, both in its subject matter, language and oracular tone, lines from the poem of Parmenides as much as anything else.

> For neither could you know what-is-not, for this cannot be done,
> nor could you say it. (DK 28 B2, ll. 7–8)
>
> οὔτε γὰρ ἂν γνοίης τό γε μὴ ἐὸν (οὐ γὰρ ἀνυστόν)
> οὔτε φράσαις.

What-is-not is utterly unknowable or unthinkable. If we deem this the fundamental insight of Eleatic philosophy,[17] then we shall label our author an Eleatic as well, since he clearly accepts this proposition in some form.

However, the usual suspects of Eleatic mischief—Parmenides, Zeno, and Melissus—strenuously denied the verity of sense perception, while our author claims not only that the things-that-are-not are not known, but also that they're unperceived. Contraposed, the audacity of the thesis is startling: if a (or a's being F) is perceived (by someone), then a is$_e$ (or even is F, or perhaps both). One might interpret this, not unreasonably, as approaching an extreme form of subjectivism that denied the possibility of falsehood for perceptual judgments. This seems to have been what led Gomperz to compare this passage with Protagoras' *homo mensura* (22), a comparison that encouraged the initial conjecture of Protagorean authorship (Introduction 5). But one need not read our author as recommending such a radical epistemology. All he means, I submit, is that the natural kinds that do not exist (e.g., spontaneity, as he asserts at 6.4) are never instantiated and so are never seen or known to have the putative properties attributed to them. This is consistent with a common-sense view of knowledge that allows for a world populated by various kinds of natural objects. The things we see all around us are really there, and they have the qualities we perceive them to have. This does not, of course, answer all the questions one might raise about such an epistemology, and a satisfactory exposition of our author's epistemology would have to account for them. While *de Arte* is philosophically informed, its primary concern is practical, and so we should not be surprised if our author sketches a physician-friendly epistemology without filling in the philosophical details.

**2.2** γινώσκεται τοίνυν, 'accordingly, the arts are known': note the antistrophe, which signals the close relationship between this sentence and the preceding, a relationship reinforced by the particle τοίνυν. Not only is the thought continuing, but there is a strong logical connection—not one of entailment, but rather a tacit *modus tollens* syllogism moving from 1) the general principle that the things-that-are-not are neither seen nor know and 2) the claim that the arts are both seen and known to the (unstated) conclusion that 3) the arts are. This is the second distinct argument in c. 2 that all the arts are.

[17] Victor Caston has argued—rather convincingly in my view—that something like this is the case (2002).

Full appreciation of this (as it seems to me) fairly obvious point has been hindered by the apparent lack of a grammatical subject for γινώσκεται. Some commentators have suggested emendations that would change ἤδη to some variation of εἴδεα (e.g., Littré, 6.4.7) while others have found it easier to insert something similar (e.g., Gomperz, 38, and Diels 1914, 388). Eschewing a change to the text, still others have supplied τὰ ἐόντα ('the things-that-are') as the implicit subject,[18] a tempting solution until one realizes that the subject of the immediately preceding clause is not τὰ ἐόντα but τὰ μὴ ἐόντα (the things-that-are-not). Jouanna, however, plays down the urgency of finding the missing subject (1988, 247 n. 1). We have in γινώσκεται a passive impersonal construction (cf. 11.2) that allows us to understand the genitive absolute τῶν τεχνέων as the logical subject. I would add only that our author's motive for the periphrastic construction is probably rhetorical. The nominative αἱ τέχναι would have rendered γινώσκεται ungrammatical and so the precise antistrophe of the passage impossible.

**2.2** δεδιδαγμένων ἤδη τῶν τεχνέων, 'only once [the arts] have been taught': the MSS diverge here, with A giving δεδιδαγμένων and M δεδειγμένων, which has been the choice of editors (save Daremberg, 1855, 39, and Diels, DK 87 B1) until Jouanna, who prints δεδιδαγμένων, citing in defense of his reading the principle of *lectio difficilior* (1988, 247 n. 2) and arguing also that δεδιδαγμένων could more easily have become δεδειγμένων through the inattention of a copyist than *vice versa*. I agree with Jouanna's decision, though I wonder whether δεδιδαγμένων should not be recommended in part because it is the more natural reading. We know that the arts characteristically were considered to be transmissible from master to pupil (see Introduction 1), and surely it follows from something's being taught that it is also known (cf. *Meno* 87c). Thus, δεδιδαγμένων speaks directly to the logic of the argument, supplying just what our author needs to make his case that the arts are. Lastly, I would note that δεδιδαγμένων delivers a more precise parisosis. Either way, little meaning is compromised, as our author uses the two verbs seemingly interchangeably at 9.1.

**2.2** οὐδεμία ἐστὶν ἥ γε ... οὐχ ὁρᾶται, 'there is no art that is not seen': supplying the understood subject, τέχνη, where the author does not, presumably motivated by his obsession with metrical balance. There are echoes here of the

---

[18] This is Vegetti's preference (1964, 373), followed by Jori (1996, 70), whose interpretation of the passage is indebted to it. See especially his third 'ontological and epistemological thesis' on p. 130.

chapter's opening line (τέχνη εἶναι οὐδεμία οὐκ ἐοῦσα), signaling a renewed argument for the claim that there is no art that is not. The sentence-final, passive verb recaptures the ὁρᾶται of the preceding sentence (thereby filling out the logical syllogism) and offsets the sentence-initial γινώσκεται in a stylistic flourish.

**2.2.** ἔκ τινος εἴδεος, 'as an outgrowth of some form': the preposition ἐκ is a puzzling choice of words, and no editor or translator has satisfactorily explained its significance here. Most give some variation on the literal but utterly opaque 'from.' In a footnote to his version (1923, 103 n. 2), Jones suggests the ingenious alternative 'springing from' to resonate with the author's peculiar use of βλαστάνειν + ἀπό ('grow out of') in the following lines; the forms (εἴδεα) are subsequently referred to as βλαστήματα (see notes on 2.3 below). My translation attempts to preserve Jones's intuition and our author's imagery while avoiding such seemingly nonsensical locution as 'there is no art that is not seen growing out of some form.' The art itself is not the outgrowth of the form; rather, it is the seeing of the art that is made possible by the fact that it has a form. Accordingly, the preposition ἐκ indicates the origin or source of the result described by the main verb (ὁρᾶται), and so the causal overtones of the English 'outgrowth' are fitting.

Certainly, the suitability of the translation depends in no small part on the meaning ascribed to the Greek noun εἶδος. Scholars have puzzled over both its abrupt intrusion into our author's argument as well as its gradual creep into the lexicon of early Greek thought generally.[19] I will not here trace the historical evolution of the term in detail nor quibble with the specific claims made by scholars. Their studies show what is confirmed even by a casual review of εἶδος in context: the term accrued a diverse extension as

[19] Informative studies include Taylor 1911, Gillespie 1912, and Diller 1971, 1975 and Langholf 1990, 194–208. Jori develops his conclusions out of an admirably complete review of the secondary literature, though his account largely avoids engagement with primary source material, including, lamentably, the illuminating fragments from Empedocles' *On nature*. To summarize, Jori stakes out two interpretive antitheses, that of Taylor, who draws parallels to the use of εἶδος and related concepts in Pythagorean thought, and so is inclined to understand εἶδος as 'real essence' (1911, 226, implemented in translation by Jones 1923, 102). Against Taylor is set Gomperz' view that the εἶδος of a thing is the content of its phenomenal character ('der Inbegriff wahrnehmbarer Attribute') which, together with its δύναμις, or underlying quality ('verborgene Eigenschaft'), consitutes its essence (1910, 100). Jori synthesizes these opposing intepretations into a view of εἶδος as '*la proprietà specifica* di una realtà e, parallelamente, *la forma peculiare* della sua presenza, del suo collocarsi nella visibilità' (1996, 149, emphasis in original). This is generally consistent with my own view of the meaning of εἶδος in *de Arte*, if less precise, though I cannot agree with Jori's equation of εἶδος and δύναμις (1996, 149), which I take to be closely related yet distinct.

the nuances of its original meaning of 'shape' or 'form' (in a non-technical sense) were exploited by Greek physicists, philosophers, physicians and mathematicians. It is obviously related to the verb ἰδεῖν (and so to ὁρᾶται), and εἶδος often referred to the visible aspect of a thing. Insofar as shape or form was considered characteristic of a thing, an εἶδος could be that kind, type or class to which various individual things belonged in virtue of exhibiting a certain shape or character (Gillespie 1912, 183–184). In medical usage especially, εἶδος operates sometimes as a synonym for φύσις conceived of as a physical constitution, at others as a characteristic quality or set of qualities (Diller 1975, 86; Gillespie 1912, 181–183).

It is this last sense of εἶδος that is of interest to the study of *de Arte*, a sense that signals a movement toward a more abstract notion closely connected to the idea of causal qualities or powers. (At **4.4**, our author argues that, insofar as they have agreed to be treated by the art of medicine, patients 'observed its form' and 'came to know its power.') There is direct evidence of this movement both in philosophy (cf. Melissus' reference to 'forms and power' [εἴδη τε καὶ ἰσχὺν] at DK 30 B8) and in other, seminal works of the *Corpus*.

> I promised to show that these things, which I claim to be human constituents, are always [reading αἰεὶ ταῦτα ἐόντα], both by convention and by nature. These are, I claim, blood, phlegm, and yellow and black bile. First, I claim that the names (ὄνομα) of these things are distinguished according to convention (κατὰ νόμον) and that no one has the same name as another; second, that their forms (ἰδέα) are separate in accordance with nature (κατὰ φύσιν), and that phlegm does not resemble blood, nor blood bile, nor bile phlegm. For how could these things be similar to one another when their colors are not seen to be the same and they do not seem to be similar to the touch? Nor are they similarly warm, cold, dry or wet. So of necessity, when they differ in respect of their form (ἰδέα) and power (δύναμις), they are not a unity, if indeed fire and water are not one.
>
> (*Nat. Hom.* 174.11–176.9 = L. 6.40–42; cf. also *Alim.* 142.20–22 = L. 9.104)

The powers spoken of here are causal powers—as in *VM*, especially c. 22, where power is equated with strength (149.3–10 = L. 1.626)—capable of effecting change, including especially changes in the perceptual organs of an observer. The four humors differ in form insofar as they differ in their characteristic causal-phenomenal powers, but while qualitative similarity or difference can be verified through empirical observation—one can observe the powers in question—one cannot determine a thing's form by naïve observation alone. The form of phlegm, for example, is a unique complex of powers such that each member of the complex is exhibited by all and only by particular instances of phlegm. One can detect a certain degree of dryness, bitterness, etc., and in this sense it would be possible to speak of 'seeing' the form of phlegm. But knowing what the form of phlegm is—indeed, knowing that phlegm has a distinctive form at all—requires an inference based on systematic observation and comparison of a range of phenomena. Having regularly observed a certain dryness and bitterness and color regularly conjoined, we have grounds for speaking of the form of phlegm. For the author of *Nat. Hom.* as for the author of *de Arte*, that phlegm has a form is proof that it 'is always' and, we might add, simply 'is.'

There is a separate front of philosophical discourse on the subject of forms that is equally important to making sense of *de Arte*. As noted above, our author writes in the ultimate sentence of the chapter that εἴδεα are βλαστήματα, natural outgrowths or offshoots. The imagery and metaphor has its roots in Empedocles' poem *On nature*.[20]

> Out of these (ἐκ τῶν, sc. 'roots') sprouted (ἐβλάστησε) all things that were, are and will be hereafter (ὅσα τ' ἦν τ' ἔστι καὶ ἔσται ὀπίσσω), trees, and men and women .... (DK 31 B21)
>
> Out of these (ἐκ τῶν, sc. 'colors') [the painters] prepare forms (εἴδεα) resembling all things, fashioning trees and men and women. (DK 31 B23)
>
> Out of these (ἐκ τῶν, sc. 'roots') came to be blood and other forms (εἴδεα) of flesh. (DK 31 B98)
>
> And once (the roots) were mixed together, ten-thousand tribes (ἔθνεα) of mortals poured out, arranged in all kinds of forms, a sight to see (παντοίαις ἰδέῃσιν ... θαῦμα ἰδέσθαι). (DK 31 B35)

By Empedocles' account, the forms are the natural kinds that emerge out of the mixture and separation of the natural elements (which he calls ῥίζοι, 'roots'), and as such they underwrite taxonomical distinctions between and within species (there are many 'forms of flesh,' for example). That these forms are, as in the Hippocratic case examined above, closely connected to the perceptual faculties is strongly suggested by the analogy with painting, as well as by phrases such as ἰδέῃσιν ... θαῦμα ἰδέσθαι. (Cf. *de Arte* 2.1, τίνα ... οὐσίην θεησάμενος, and 2.2, ἔκ τινος εἴδεος οὐχ ὁρᾶται.) It is less clear whether the form could encompass phenomenal properties such as color or temperature, as they do in *Nat. Hom.* For Empedocles, form in the the sense of 'shape' or 'structure' is dominant. The emphatic repetition of natural kind terms may signal that Empedocles sees forms not just as the shapes of individuals but as structures characteristic of kinds, belonging not just to

---

[20] A second clear case of Empedoclean influence on the Hippocratic discussion of forms is found at *Alim.* 140.16–17 = L. 9.100. See Introduction 4.

individuals but to groups of individuals. Indeed, by noting that it is in virtue of their forms that splotches of paint resemble living exemplars of the natural kinds, Empedocles appears to be on the cusp of recognizing that a single form is capable of being realized in multiple individuals or instances.[21]

I will return shortly to the question of what other considerations motivate our author to utilize peculiarly Empedoclean terminology in his argument. For now, it is enough to have drawn attention to these medical and philosophical points of contact, both of which converge on a notion of εἶδος as a natural kind determined by the observable character of the things-that-are always.

**2.3** οἶμαι δ' ἔγωγε, 'in my opinion': a hint of condescension suggests that the contradictory view is hardly worthy of serious consideration, a sentiment our author makes explicit in what follows. Further, the restrictive particle indicates that the views he is about to articulate are his own. Strictly speaking, this does not necessarily mean that they are original to our author. However, after Lloyd's demonstration that first-person language is the hallmark of innovation in the Greek enlightenment from the early philosophers on (1987, 59–70), we have a prima facie reason for taking οἶμαι δ' ἔγωγε as a claim to originality.

**2.3** καὶ τὰ ὀνόματα αὐτὰς διὰ τὰ εἴδεα λαβεῖν, 'they acquire their names, too, because of their forms' [**2.3.a**]: not only is the visibility of the arts attributable to their having forms, but so are their names. The remainder of the chapter is dedicated to sketching a theory of the correctness of names, though there is little consensus on either the precise logic of his argument in its defense or his reasons for laying out the theory as though it constituted some sort of conclusion to his argument that all the arts are.

The pivotal phrase is διὰ τὰ εἴδεα, which indicates that the forms of the arts somehow cause their names (cf. the use of διά τι at 6.4).[22] If forms cause names in some sense, then it would be reasonable to infer that hav-

---

21 Mourelatos 2006 argues that, if the standard cyclical interpretation of Empedoclean cosmology is correct, Empedocles must have had the type-token distinction clearly in view (64–65).

22 The word 'cause' here should be given a wide range, given both the vagueness of the idea in early Greek thought as well as its flexibility in contrast to the modern notion, which is often colored by mechanistic or materialistic assumptions. The biological analogy suggested by the image of plant development further underscores the need for caution, since the (apparently) teleological aspects of growth blur the lines between causes (in the modern sense) and other kinds of explanatory element. For a comprehensive study of causation, explanation, and related issues in ancient Greek thought, see Hankinson 1998.

ing a form is a necessary condition of having a name; without a form as cause, there is no name as effect. Our author may be giving a defense of the immediately preceding claim that every art has a form. Inferring cause from effect, he infers the existence of the forms (and thus of the arts themselves) from the fact that they have names.[23] However, our author does not claim that all names are caused by forms, but rather only that the names of the arts are so caused. Later, at 6.4, he alleges that spontaneity (τὸ αὐτόματον) has no being other than a name. If spontaneity can have a name without having a form, then our author cannot hold, without contradiction, the view that forms cause names. In any case, our author treats the forms as given. It is their relation to names, not their existence, that is at issue.[24]

The author's argument against spontaneity raises the alltogether more plausible possibility that he is responding here to the charge that the arts have no being other than a name, or exist 'in name only.'[25] While he never uses the exact phrase or even an equivalent, this apparent lapse could be written off as yet another casualty of the highly compressed logic of the chapter. After all, if our author is assuming that his reader is familiar with the original charges brought by the critics, the need to enumerate the specific criticisms becomes less urgent. Alternatively, he may be anticipating a rejoinder from the critics to his argument that, insofar as each art is an art, it is *simpliciter* (see notes on 2.1 above). To concede that the arts are in this sense is to say only that words such as 'medicine' are meaningful. It does not follow that 'medicine' successfully refers to any objects or events in the world, and it is this question of objective existence that the critics are raising. Yet, again, we encounter the problem of redundancy. For the author has already claimed that the arts have forms, and this by itself implies that medicine is more than a (merely meaningful) name. Had our author wanted to buttress his case for the forms, he should have made an argument resembling the one in *Nat. Hom.* for the formal uniqueness and phenomenal existence of the four humors (see notes on 2.2). It is difficult to see how his position on the correctness of names here at 2.3 adds anything new or interesting to the argument as it stands.

---

[23] This is a proposal made independently by Jouanna (1988, 177), Hankinson (1998, 77), and Jori, the latter of whom claims that the names of the arts serve a testimonial function that 'rappresenta una garanzia ontologica «debole»' (1996, 380).

[24] Gomperz makes a similar, if less rigorous, case (1910, 102).

[25] Taylor, for example, seems to take this view (1912, 225), though elsewhere he reformulates it in terms closer to Jori's (1996, 227–228).

On the whole, there are few internal clues as to the author's motive here. However, it is my contention (defended at greater length in the Appendix) that scholars have long overlooked compelling external clues. Briefly, structural similarities between Sextus Empiricus' *Against the Professors* and *de Arte* suggest that later Sceptical attacks on the arts preserve at least something of the criticisms to which our author is responding. One such criticism, which Sextus lodges against all the arts collectively, is rooted in the ostensible failure to make sense of the way in which arts are taught (1.35–38). If they are taught, then they must be taught either through direct acquaintance with what is evident or through linguistic description. But what is evident is evident to all and so cannot be taught. If the arts are taught through linguistic description, the language used must signify either by nature or by convention. But it does not signify by nature, Sextus concludes, because Greeks and barbarians do not understand each other's speech; that is, a naturalist theory of the correctness of names would imply the existence of a common language, or at least of a common understanding. If it signifies by convention, then the meaning of a term must be established by ostension. Thus, if a student knows the meaning of the words spoken by his teacher (as he must if he is to be taught), he will know already the objects to which the words are applied. Since one cannot be taught what one already knows, teaching will be impossible.

If a convincing case could be made for a naturalist theory of the correctness of names that accomodated linguistic diversity, that is, the apparent 'conventionality' of language, Sextus' argument would lose its force. While scholarly opinion diverges widely on the logic of our author's argument about names at 2.3, a broad consensus has emerged that our author's use of the paradoxical phrase 'conventions imposed by nature' [φύσιος νομοθετήματά] is intended to redraw the battle lines of the νόμος-φύσις debate over the correctness of names so as to concede the diversity of language while maintaining that linguistic correctness is not determined simply by human *fiat*.[26] Our author thereby clears away the objection to the possibility of genuine teaching, an objection that would threaten his claim at 2.2 that 'the arts are known only once they have been taught' and thus jeopardize his argument for the arts' being.

[26] Gomperz and Diels apparently saw the locution as a confusion rather than an innovation, impelling them to emend the text, a move followed by Heinimann (see note below). The trend since has been to leave the text as it stands and interpret the apparent paradox as an attempt to transcend the conventional limits of the νόμος-φύσις debate (Joly 1956, 200; Vegetti 1964, 367; Sedley 2003, 72).

**2.3** ἄλογον γὰρ … ἡγεῖσθαι, 'for it's absurd … to think': we encounter this phrase for the second time in c. 2, again employed to introduce a *reductio* argument for a general proposition that provides justification for the author's position as expressed in what immediately precedes (**2.3.a**).

**2.3** ἀπὸ τῶν ὀνομάτων … τὰ εἴδεα βλαστάνειν, 'the forms grow out of names' [**2.3.b**]: the author's position must be **2.3.b***: forms do not grow out of names. The challenge is to understand βλαστάνειν in such a way that **2.3.b*** underwrites (perhaps supplemented by additional premises) **2.3.a.** For this, let us return to the fragments of the poem of Empedocles, the apparent source of our author's terminology. Recall that, in the fragments presented earlier, forms (εἴδεα) were depicted as growing out of (βλαστάνειν) the four elements, or roots (ῥίζοι). The imagery unmistakably evokes plant growth. Empedocles probably takes the roots of a plant to be the material source out of which the shoots and leaves develop (think of any perennial species, an especially apt analogy given Empedocles' doctrine of recurrent cycles); likewise, the four elements are the material out of which the natural kinds are composed. Surely our author does not take seriously the hypothesis that forms or names may be the material cause of the other. I submit instead that he is borrowing language from Empedocles to express a less specific notion of causal or developmental dependence, of which material causation is only one variety (e.g., if a is the material cause of b, then b is developmentally dependent on a). Accordingly, we might interpret **2.3.b*** as follows:

**2.3.b.1***: forms do not depend on names for their development.

Still, if this is correct, then **2.3.b.1*** must play a role in some plausible reconstruction of our author's argument for **2.3.a.** Clearly, **2.3.a** does not follow from **2.3.b.1*** alone. I propose that our author is making an inference to the best explanation, namely, to the best explanation of the fact, broached at 2.3, that the name of an art (e.g., 'medicine') corresponds to a form. The immediately intuitive explanations of this correspondence in the case of any given art would include the following:

1. the name of the art depends for its development on its form; or
2. the form of the art depends for its development on its name; or
3. the correspondence is a mere coincidence.

Supposing that 3 is rejected out of hand on grounds of its improbability, our author is left with 1 and 2, the latter of which is excluded by **2.3.b.1***. The only viable explanation, then, is 1. This explanation adds nothing to our author's argument that there is no art that is not except insofar as it affords him the rhetorical opportunity to interject his theory of the correctness of names in response to an objection from the method of teaching.[27]

**2.3** καὶ ἀδύνατον, 'not to mention impossible': there is nothing about the argument to suggest that our author finds it genuinely impossible even to think that the forms grow out of names. Rather, he seems to regard the thesis itself as physically impossible given the nature of forms and of language. (Cf. 8.2, where those who expect art to accomplish what it is by nature unable to accomplish are called mad.)

**2.3** τὰ μὲν γὰρ ὀνόματα φύσιος νομοθετήματά ἐστιν, 'names for nature are conventions imposed by and upon nature' [**2.3.c**]: the position (and inclusion) of φύσιος in this sentence is much debated. Gomperz' transposed φύσιος after βλαστήματα, a decision seemingly rooted in the conviction that 'outgrowths' were natural, and that these were intended to stand in contrast to conventions, which were routinely opposed to nature by fifth-century philosophers and sophists (see Introduction 2). Pigeonholing our author in the context of this debate motivated Heinimann to dub the emendation 'quite understandable, but superfluous' in his canonical study, *Nomos und Physis* (1945, 157 n. 30), and ultimately to follow Diels' outright seclusion of the word. Diels had defended his emendation with two observations about the manuscript tradition (1914, 389–390). First, while M gives the Ionic form φύσιος, A gives the Attic form of the genitive, raising the possibility that φύσεως is a *koinē* intrusion. Second, he notes that A's gloss on the passage comes on the bottom of one page and that φύσεως is the first word at the top of the next. He takes the original gloss to have been τῇ εἰσιν τὰ ὀνόματα καὶ τῇ τὰ εἴδεα φύσεως. As noted above, scholars have reached an informal consensus that the *lectio difficilior* be left to stand, and I would offer the following stylistic observations in support. We should reject Gomperz' transposition outright on the grounds that νομοθετήματα and βλαστήματα are surely being exploited for their homoioteleuton. More important, though, are the striking figures that result from inclusion of φύσιος: chiasmus with ὀνόματα and νομοθετήματα, perfect isocolon between the τὰ μὲν and τὰ δὲ cola (18 syllables per), not to mention the deliciously sophistic oxymoron 'conventions of nature.' All of these (which are favorite figures of our author) are utterly

[27] This should be distinguished from Heinimann's claim that parts of the argument (namely, those I label **2.3.c–d**) are logically superfluous, justified only by the author's interest in articulating a theory of language (1945, 157).

destroyed by transposing or excluding φύσιος. Against Diels' specific objection to the Attic form, I will say only that A and M often give similarly divergent readings (e.g., 1.2, where A reads συνέσιος and M ξυνέσεως).

If the poetic predisposition of our author is granted, then a horizon of polysemantic possibilities opens up. The phrase φύσιος νομοθετήματα is intended first and foremost to be construed as a subjective genitive formula (**2.3.c.1**): names are conventions imposed by nature.[28] Yet there is precedent in the contemporary νόμος-φύσις debate (cf. Antiphon F44(a)IV.2–7 τὰ μὲν ὑπὸ τῶν νόμων κείμενα δεσμοὶ τῆς φύσεώς ἐστι) for an objective genitive construal (**2.3.c.2**): 'names are conventions imposed upon nature.'[29] My translation puts both construals in play, a decision I defend on thematic grounds (see following notes). For now, it suffices to distinguish between the normative and descriptive aspects of the word νομοθέτημα that underwrite this approach. An enactment or regulation may be referred to in the course of describing the actions, as a matter of fact, of a community: 'I have heard reports that the Athenians voted to enact a regulation against impiety.' Such references do not recognize the regulation as obligatory; they do not even ask the question, as it were. Alternatively, a regulation may be invoked with normative force, namely in contexts concerned with conformity or noncomformity to its specfic content: 'you broke the Athenian regulation against impiety. We thereby sentence you to death.'[30] On my view, the subjective genitive construal highlights the normative aspect: 'nature places constraints on the correctness or incorrectness of linguistic conventions.' The objective genitive, then, would correspond to the descriptive aspect: 'human beings institute regulations for the application of words to nature.' Finally, it's worth noting that φύσιος is located so that it may be taken also as genitive complement to ὀνόματα (see my remarks on αἰεί at 2.2 above): 'names of nature.'[31] Our author is concerned not with the names for

---

[28] Vegetti (1964, 367) and Sedley (2003, 72) see an illuminating parallel in Plato's *Cratylus*, where Socrates hypothesizes a νομοθέτης who originally legislated the correct names for all things (388e).

[29] This is the preference of Morrison 1976 (527), who, not surprisingly, uses the passage in support of his interpretation of the fragments of Antiphon.

[30] This corresponds to Hart's distinction between 'internal' and 'external' statements about laws and legal validity (1961, 89–91), though one might also appeal to the traditional grammatical *cum* philosophical distinction between imperatives and indicatives, taking sentences like 'nature places constraints, etc.' as veiled commands, e.g., 'obey nature in your adoption of linguistic conventions.' The point would be that words like the Greek νομοθέτημα might play a (different) role in each kind of sentence.

[31] Jori (1996, 74 n. 3), too, following Mondolfo (1958, 135 n. 1), recommends that this possibility be kept in view.

artificial things, but for natural things (or, more specifically, for εἴδεα, 'natural kinds'). Thus, when each element of the semantic ensemble is given a voice, the phrase ὀνόματα φύσιος νομοθετήματα yields a striking thematic harmony: the correctness of names applied to natural kinds is established by nature's authority, to which humans ought to look when establishing the conventions that govern the application of names to natural kinds.

**2.3** τὰ δὲ εἴδεα οὐ νομοθετήματα, ἀλλὰ βλαστήματα, 'whereas forms are not conventions but outgrowths' [**2.3.d**]: the difference between βλαστήματα and νομοθετήματα is key to understanding the logical connection between **2.3.c–d** and **2.3.b**. There is little question that the former is allied with φύσις, as are the εἴδεα. So Heinimann insisted that βλαστήμα is nothing but a poetic synonym for φύσις, and likewise for νομοθετήμα and νόμος (1945, 157). Joly went still further, proposing that the εἴδεα are the natural essences or realities to which at least some names correspond (1956, 201ff.), and most commentators have followed suit.[32] The consensus of scholars on this point is surely correct, even though their conclusions have been formulated without taking advantage of the illuminating parallels with Empedocles' poem. Still, while many have traced with some success the basic skeleton of our author's position, fleshing out the logical connective tissue remains a challenge. To quote the recent evaluation of a leading scholar of ancient philosophy, 'the logic of this is obscure,' (Sedley 2003, 72; cf. Hankinson 1998, 77: 'some sense may be sucked from that mire'). I agree that the argument is obscure, though it is not impenetrable so long as we keep in view another set of textual parallels found in the fragments of the sophist Antiphon.[33]

---

[32] That names do or ought to reflect the forms found in nature is granted (in on form or another) by Vegetti (1964, 367), Morrison (1976, 527), Fabrini and Lami (1979, 130–133), Jori (1996, 132 n. 33), and Sedley (2003, 72), among others, though the idea that nature is the ultimate source of names goes back to Littré (6.4–5 n. 1). Jori gives an exhaustive summary of the history of scholarship on the question (1996, 71 n. 3).

[33] To my knowledge, surprisingly few scholars have developed the thematic connections between Antiphon's writing and c. 2 of *de Arte*. Diels and Kranz print the chapter in its entirety as an appendix to fragment F1 but offer little comment. Untersteiner slyly prints the text from c. 2 as something Antiphon 'may well say' (1948b, 237–238). Cherniss, meanwhile, collects numerous intriguing parallels between *de Arte* and Antiphon's fragments while concluding, inexplicably, that 'all of this and more too would not constitute evidence that Antiphon wrote the De Arte, which he certainly did not' (202 n. 10). J.S. Morrison utilizes *de Arte* in an attempt to emend and interpret a fragment of Antiphon's (F1) with only tenuous relation to the theory of names outlined here (1976, 526–528). Morrison remarks in passing on the similarity between c. 2 and one of the fragments I will discuss (F44(a)IV.1–7), but he makes little of it, and he seems to think that *de Arte* is the more transparent text and so ought to be used to explicate Antiphon, whereas quite the reverse is true

Antiphon, like Empedocles, saw nature as fundamentally a process of growth and development.

> For those things belonging to convention are impositions, while those that belong to nature are necessary. Further, the agreements of convention are not natural growths, while the growths of nature are not agreements.
> (F44(a)I.23–33)
>
> τὰ μὲν γὰρ τῶν νόμων ἐπίθετα, τὰ δὲ τῆς φύσεως ἀναγκαῖα · καὶ τὰ μὲν τῶν νόμων ὁμολογηθέντα οὐ φύντα ἐστίν, τὰ δὲ τῆς φύσεως φύντα οὐχ ὁμολογηθέντα.

Conventions are supplementary, things 'added on' to what is natural by the authority of human agreement. Natural things are growing and developing. Antiphon dubs them 'necessary,' presumably because their patterns of change are indifferent to the contingencies of human decision and agreement. This prompts him elsewhere to characterize nature as inherently autonomous: 'advantages conferred by convention are shackles on nature; those by nature, free' (τὰ σὲ ξυμφέροντα, τὰ μὲν ὑπὸ τῶν νόμων κείμενα δεσμοὶ τῆς φύσεώς ἐστι, τὰ δ' ὑπὸ τῆς φύσεως ἐλεύθερα, F44(a)IV.2–7).

Antiphon illustrated these general principles with a thought experiment recorded by Aristotle in the second book of his *Physics*.

> Antiphon says that a sign of this [i.e., that matter is to be identified with the nature of a thing] is that, if someone buried a bed and the rotten wood acquired a power so that as a natural result it sent out a shoot [ἀνεῖναι βλαστόν], it would not become a bed but rather wood. This shows that the accidental quality is its arrangement according to convention and art [τὴν κατὰ νόμον διάθεσιν καὶ τὴν τέχνην], while its substance is that which remains constant through these affections. (193a12–18)

Outgrowths are expressions of nature, then, insofar as they manifest an innate impulse to change. The pattern of change is autonomous in that it cannot be artificially altered; even after a carpenter has carved a tree into a bed, it retains its potential for growth into a tree. The bed, then, is, necessarily and by nature, a tree (or, as Antiphon puts it, wood, emphasizing its material composition, since, to use the language of *de Arte*, it 'is always' wood, and so its evident form is wood). It is a bed only by convention—nothing about the tree *qua* wood compelled it to take the form of a bed. Instead, it was compelled to take this form by external intervention, that of

---

(530). Heinimann 1945 refers only briefly to Antiphon's fragment in his discussion of medical 'Sprachphilosophie' (162), while Pendrick denies, implausibly, any connection whatsoever (251). Gagarin 2002 notes, somewhat dismissively, the stylistic similarities between Antiphon and *de Arte* (90). See also Introduction (sections 3, 5).

the craftsman who fashioned it. Its 'bedness' is not at all necessary; without the craftsman's interference, the tree would never have become what we call 'bed.' Antiphon might even have argued that, strictly speaking, it never really became a bed at all. It was always really wood, though for a time it was referred to conventionally as a bed, its 'bedness' having been posited on top of and in addition to, that is, imposed upon, its nature.[34]

If we read *de Arte* against the background of Antiphon's views on the νόμος-φύσις antithesis, then we might reconstruct the argument for **2.3.b.1*** as follows.

1. Forms are natural outgrowths, developmentally independent of conventions (**2.3.d.1**).
2. Names are conventions imposed upon nature (**2.3.c.2**).
3. Therefore, forms do not depend on names for their development (**2.3.b.1***).

Note, however, that this argument remains logically distinct from any theory about the correctness of names, the main tenet of which is expressed not by **2.3.c.2**, but by the normatively charged **2.3.c.1**. Conveniently, the language of freedom and slavery employed by Antiphon in his fragments has a normative dimension applicable to the debate over the correctness of names. Names that do not correspond to natural kinds shackle nature by imposing upon it a false taxonomy, thereby obscuring and distorting its true structure. Short of dispensing with the conventions of language altogether, the most effective way to minimize the linguistic violence done to nature would be to establish names that mirror as closely as possible the structures of nature, namely, the forms. Thus, while the phonetic composition of particular names may be determined by convention, the structure of natural kinds will place constraints on the way these names are used.

## 3

The chapter marks a transition from general concerns about *technē* to medicine in particular by way of a second *prothesis*. But in giving a definition of medicine that will serve as the foundation for his *apodeixis*, or logical demonstration, our author moves beyond a mere declaration of intent and into the territory of formal argument. Hence, c. 3 is functionally ambiguous;

---

34 My understanding of Antiphon's conception of nature is indebted to Paul Woodruff (whose views on the subject are summarized in his 2004) and R.J. Hankinson (1998, 126–127).

it contains the closing statement of the *prooimion* as well as the opening remarks of the *lusis*, or refutation, which begins officially with c. 4.

Attention is momentarily diverted away from the critics, and a subtle anacolouthon (περὶ δὲ ἰητρικῆς—ἐς ταύτην γὰρ ὁ λόγος—, ταύτης οὖν τὴν ἀπόδειξιν ποιήσομαι) moderates the tonal and stylistic intensity. Poetic effects are few (the euphony of παντὸς ποιεῖν, περὶ τούτου μοι ὁ λοιπὸς λόγος being the obvious exception), and our author for the first time in the speech yields priority to conceptual clarity over creativity of expression.

**3.1** περὶ μὲν οὖν τούτων, 'concerning these matters, then': the intended referent of 'these matters' (i.e., the foregoing, including c. 2 and perhaps also c. 1) is unclear. It might be the question of the being of *technē* generally, or perhaps with specific application to medicine in particular. Most likely, though, 'these matters' refers to the dense epistemological, ontological, and linguistic (that is, philosophical) arguments limned in c. 2. The question is closely connected to the question concerning the referent of ἐν ἄλλοισιν ἂν λόγοισιν. See notes below.

**3.1** εἴ γέ τις μὴ ἱκανῶς ἐκ τῶν εἰρημένων συνίησιν, 'should anyone not have reached a sufficient understanding from what has been said': an allusion to the obscurity of the arguments in c. 2, this does not imply that 'these matters' are exclusively philosophical, since the obscurity of the philosophical arguments will affect the cogency also of our author's conclusions about *technē*.

**3.1** ἐν ἄλλοισιν ἂν λόγοισιν, 'in other discourses': one might be inclined to understand this as a transitional device that foreshadows the subsequent battery of arguments in defense of medicine. While the philosophical arguments of c. 2 are sufficient to prove the point, they are too abstruse for most audiences, compelling our author to reformulate his arguments 'in other words.' The sharp contrast between other discourses and 'this discourse' (ὁ λόγος) rules out this interpretation, however. The other discourses are some other work or works on a much more general theme than *de Arte*, which is concerned solely with medicine. Jouanna maintains that our author is attesting to 'discourses that defend the arts against its detractors by means of a more developed general argument' (1988, 248), while Gomperz thinks that the discourses are 'a written work with metaphysical or epistemological content' (1910, 106). In proposing that the reference is to a single text, Gomperz supposes too much. There could easily be several that address these topics individually, or that address different aspects of these topics (λόγοισιν is plural, after all). Still, he notes that Herodotus employs this sort of locution (e.g., at 1.106: ἐν ἑτέροισι λόγοισι δηλώσω) where the historian is undoubtedly referring to another, self-contained work of his own on the Assyrians. Similar phrases employing future passive verb forms occur in the Hippocratic *Corpus*, most notably in *Artic.* (4.174.17–18, 4.190.7–8), where the author seems to be alluding to other works of his own, though this is impossible to verify.

Based on the internal evidence alone, I see no way to settle these questions about the other discourses. That they dealt in some measure with the philosophical problems raised in c. 2 is surely right, but as to their number (whether one or several) and precise topical orientation we must remain silent. The authorial intrusions at 2.1 (δοκεῖ δή μοι) and 2.3 (οἶμαι δ' ἔγωγε) weigh ever so slightly in favor of the hypothesis that he is the author of the 'other discourses' on 'these matters,' but this is hardly conclusive.

**3.1** τὴν ἀπόδειξιν ποιήσομαι, 'I will now give a demonstration': the quasi-technical use of ἀπόδειξις bespeaks a basic awareness of logical form typical of the sophistic movement and the accompanying attention paid to principles of argumentation. If we may extrapolate from the context and compare with the occurrence of ἐπίδειξις at 1.1 and 13.1, we will hypothesize that a demonstration is, for our author, a linguistic artifact, a λόγος, presumably exhibiting a formal logical structure. At least, it is about (περὶ) something—but not just anything. The proper focus of a demonstration is a proposition, in this case the proposition that medicine is. The implication is that a demonstration is meant to provide reasons for accepting a certain conclusion, and this is distinct from, but not irrelevant to, refuting arguments in support of the contradictory position.

**3.2** διοριεῦμαι ὅ νομίζω ἰητρικὴν εἶναι, 'I will define what I think medicine is': Jori hears echoes of ὁρίζειν in its original connection to boundary stones set down to mark off one field from the next (1996, 152). Accordingly, we should understand our author as delimiting the field of medicine in multiple respects that include differentiating between the various *technai* as well as establishing limits on medicine's power (see following notes). This may be true in some sense, as is the observation that the definition given is determined in part by the content of his argument (Jori 1996, 155), but none of this precludes our author's statement from serving as a definition *stricto sensu*, which Jori explicitly denies (1996, 154). Our author gives his account of 'what medicine is,' and this is continuous with the classical notion of what it means to give a definition. In *Phaedrus*, for example, Plato has Socrates commence his speech against love with a definition, chiding those who do not follow this procedure for beginning their discussions without agreeing on terms (237bff.). A definition on this account is supposed to establish the true nature of something, and this is not far from Aristotle's view of definitions as conveying 'what a thing is' (e.g., *APo.* 90b4ff.). All these fall in line with the Socratic quest for definitions that would lay bare what piety (in the *Euthyphro*), courage (in the *Laches*), justice (in the *Republic*), and the like 'are.' Indeed, the practice of giving precise definitions of terms came into vogue in fifth-century sophistic circles, epitomized by the preoccupation of the sophist Prodicus with making fine distinctions in meaning between words that were regarded as practically synonymous. (Plato parodies Prodicus at *Protagoras* 337a–c.)

Our author's promise to divulge 'what medicine is' is reminiscent of the discussion of being and form in c. 2. In effect, he promises to enumerate the characteristic properties of medicine, that is, to describe its form. Its form will comprise a set of three perceptually verifiable powers that constitute a triad of jointly necessary and separately sufficient conditions that distinguish genuinely medical activities from the non-medical.

3.2 τὸ δὴ πάμπαν ἀπαλλάσσειν τῶν νοσεόντων τοὺς καμάτους καὶ τῶν νοσημάτων τὰς σφοδρότητας ἀμβλύνειν καὶ τὸ μὴ ἐγχειρεῖν τοῖσι κεκρατημένοισιν ὑπὸ τῶν νοσημάτων, 'totally removing the sufferings of the sick or alleviating the violent effects of their diseases, as well as not handling the sick who have been overwhelmed by their diseases': following Jones (1923, 193), one may feel tempted to translate τὸ δὴ πάμπαν as an adverbial phrase (cf. τὸ μὲν σύμπαν at 2.1) introducing a general definition. The source of this temptation is the apparent incongruity that results from taking πάμπαν to modify ἀπαλλάσσειν: the author appears to claim that the physician's job is to completely cure diseases and ameliorate their violent effects. But which is it? Both, I think. Our author here gives an account of the three distinct kinds of activity that are to be included under the aegis of medicine, and, as noted above, we should think of these as disjunctive conditions, not as a single, compound condition. That is, a certain activity is medical just in case it is *either* the complete removal of disease *or* the amelioration of violent effects *or* the refusal to treat a hopeless case (the occurrences of καί should not be taken as signaling logical conjunction). Grammatical considerations only reinforce this construal. The neuter definite article belongs to both substantive infinitives, and πάμπαν falls within its scope. It must modify ἀπαλλάσσειν.

This leads to the question about the definition that has most occupied commentators. The third disjunct is a negation, and since antiquity this fact has prompted some to deny our author's account of medicine the status of a proper definition.[35] However, we may take some direction from what seems to be a concessive ordering of the the three conditions. Ideally, the physician will completely cure the sick person. When that is not possible, he will seek to manage the disease. When even that is impossible, he will refrain from treatment altogether.[36] In conceding the natural barriers to a complete cure, our author's definition of medicine resembles Isocrates' account of rhetorical training in *Against the Sophists*, where he writes that his pedagogy is capable of perfecting the speech of those with talent and to improve the speech of the untalented.

> For ability, whether in speaking or any other activity, depends upon a good nature and hands-on experience (εμπειρία). Education (παίδευσις) makes such people more skilled (τεχνικός) and equips them for research. For it teaches them to apprehend immediately the things they otherwise only stumble upon (εὐτυγχάνειν). But it cannot develop those of an inferior nature into fine debaters or wordsmiths, though it can improve them and make them more sensible about many things. (13.14–15)

Still, some may object that Isocrates does not propose a condition analogous to our author's third; he does not concede that there may be people whose speaking abilities he cannot at least improve. But surely it is understood that such a class exists, for not even the self-aggrandizing Isocrates would boast of improving the rhetorical skills of those with acute mental infirmities, to mention one extreme example.

The analogy with rhetoric suggests further that the three conditions enumerated by our author correspond to three distinct and exhaustive classes of patient: those whose disease is curable, those whose disease is merely manageable, and those whose disease is neither curable nor manageable. It is the practical situation of the doctor with respect to this last class that gives substance to the allegedly negative component of the definition. Such patients will come before him, begging for relief. Relatives will weep and plead. The doctor will use his art to make a diagnosis and give a (presum-

---

[35] Pseudo Galen, *Introductio sive medicus*, 14.687.3–8: ὃν γάρ τινες ὅρον ἰητρικὸν ᾠήθησαν, οὐκ ἔστιν ὅρος · τό τε μὴ παράπαν ἀπαλλάσσειν τῶν νόσων τοὺς κάμνοντας καὶ τὸ τὰς σφοδρότητας ἀμβλύνειν καὶ τὸ τοῖς κεκρατημένοις μὴ ἐγχειρεῖν · οὐ γὰρ ἐξ ὧν μὴ δύναται αἱ τέχναι, ἀλλ' ἐξ ὧν δύναται οἱ ὅροι αὐτῶν εἰσιν. (Some have had in mind a definition of medicine that is not a definition: 'totally removing the sufferings of the sick or alleviating the violent effects of their diseases, as well as not taking in hand the sick who have been overwhelmed by their diseases.' For it is not from medicine's incapacities, but from its capacities, that definitions are composed.)

[36] On the idea of relative health in Greek medicine generally, see Müri (1936, 10–14); van Brock (1961, 147–150, 157–165); and Kudlien (1973).

ably unpopular) prognosis, acknowledging that treatment is futile.[37] That such practices constitute a substantive component of the medical art may be illustrated by imagining the consequences of mistaken prognosis. The patient would, under such circumstances, be subjected to rounds of treatment (almost certainly uncomfortable if not painful) that would increase his overall suffering and raise his expectations of eventual relief. Thus, he will die having suffered more, both physically and psychologically, than he would have had the doctor 'not taken him in hand.'[38] On the most charitable interpretation, then, the 'negative' condition in our author's definition of medicine refers neither to a simple failure to treat nor to therapeutic *aporia*, but rather to an informed and deliberate decision, made in the best interest of all concerned, not to intervene.[39] Hence, it is clear that all three conditions given in our author's definition, far from being arbitrary or merely expedient, follow necessarily from the three classes of patient and the implicit *telos* of the medical art, recognized throughout the *Corpus Hippocraticum* but expressed most memorably in *Epid. 1*: 'regarding diseases, to practice two things: benefit or do no harm' (ἀσκεῖν περὶ τὰ νοσήματα δύο, ὠφελεῖν ἢ μὴ βλάπτειν, 2.634.8–636.1; cf. 5.5).

The author of *de Arte* is not alone in his convictions. The Hippocratic writers are well aware that some patients are beyond help, and the *Corpus* is remarkably uniform in its explanations of incurability (Von Staden 1990, 85–97). Commonly, Hippocratics describe such situations in the same agonistic language that we find here in *de Arte*.[40]

> To make every patient healthy is impossible. To accomplish this would be better even than prognosticating what is about to happen. But as it turns out people do die, some from the strength of the disease before calling in the

[37] I agree whole-heartedly with Jouanna's characterization of non-intervention as epistemic mastery of the disease where physical mastery is impossible (1988, 249), though one must still show that epistemic mastery is essential to medicine and not a mere parlor trick. Certainly, knowing the details of a patient's condition will be key to evaluating the usefulness of medical intervention. (See also von Staden 1990, 104.) But this shows only that knowledge is necessary as a means to the purely practical ends of the physician; it is not conceptually necessary, that is, it is not part of the definition of *technē*, as it would be for Plato. See further Mann 2008b.

[38] I am indebted to von Staden 1990 for bringing to my attention the Hippocratic provenance of this rationale for non-intervention (104–105). See also Müri (1936, 4–9) and Kudlien (1967, 118–124).

[39] However, the charitable interpretation is potentially compromised by the argument at 8.5, where our author defends the doctor's decision to discontinue treatment following the patient's failure to improve. But see also 11.5.

[40] See further von Staden (1990, 97–102).

> doctor, others immediately after having called for help, living either for a day or a little longer, but dying before the physician contests the disease with his art. (*Prog*. 2.110.8–112.3)

At first, it may seem as though the recognition of medicine's limitations is inconsistent with the optimism that is characteristic of the *Corpus*, where medicine 'in fact has the extraordinary capacity to return all who are sick to health, to secure the condition of those who are already healthy, to bring about fitness in athletes and to deliver what each person desires' (*Acut*. 39.21–40.1 = L. 2.244). However, to suppose that no disease is incurable in principle, that is, by nature, is compatible with the fact that some particular cases of disease may, due to circumstances, be incurable in practice (Von Staden 1990, 91–93). There is little reason to think that our author's reference to incurability is out of place as an element in a definition generally or in the definition of medicine in particular.

3.2 πάντα ταῦτα δύναται ἰητρική, 'all these things are in medicine's power': the text is somewhat uncertain. Diels goes to great lengths to extract his reading (ταῦτα πάντ' αδύναται) from Pseudo-Soranus (1914, 390–395), but I am perplexed by editors who are intent on inserting a negation (cf. Gomperz, οὐ δύναται), since, as Jouanna points out (1988, 209–210), the reading without the negative is perfectly acceptable. The reading Diels suggests would (to avoid complete outlandishness) require that ταῦτα πάντ' refer to the diseases, not to the attributes of medicine elaborated in the definition, though this is the more natural way of taking it. On Jouanna's reading, the author simply means to reinforce that medicine has the capacities he's claiming for it. This accords well with his subsequent attempts to attest to the power (δύναμις) of the art later in the treatise (e.g., 4.4), as well as with the general idea that the form of a thing is constituted by its characteristic powers.

3.3 ποιεῖ τε ταῦτα καὶ οἵη τέ ἐστιν διὰ παντὸς ποιεῖν, 'it does these things and always is able to do so': with διὰ παντὸς the author hints at the proper function of a definition, namely, to identify those characteristics that the *definiendum* cannot fail to have. This brings the notion of definition into line with a the Greek conception of nature, since, as was evident in Antiphon's fragments (see comments on 2.3), the nature of a thing is constituted by those qualities which persist through change, that is, that are always in the subject (cf. τὰ μὲν ἐόντα αἰεὶ at 2.2). Gillespie is very nearly correct when he concludes that the definition provides 'the essence or nature or εἶδος of the art' (1912, 198), though I cannot agree that 'the εἶδος is the system of rules by which the art of medicine actually does heal' (1912, 198). In accordance with what I have argued above (see notes on 3.2), the extension of the term 'medicine' is a set of actions, procedures, or operations, not bits of knowledge or rules. The use of the verb ποιεῖν here confirms this. Moreover, these procedures are the kinds of things that one can see happening—at least, the evidence of perception will be required to gauge whether or not they are occurring (cf. 2.2: τὰ μὲν ἐόντα αἰεὶ ὁρᾶταί; οὐδεμία ἐστὶν ἥ γε ἔκ τινος εἴδεος οὐχ ὁρᾶται). But they are not just perceivable; they are in fact perceived. Our author exploits the verb ποιεῖν for the sense of actuality it imparts: 'medicine really does these things.' He thereby advances beyond a mere definition and, against those who deny the existence of the art, makes an existential claim that directly counters the existential charge that medicine is not.

3.3 ᾗ ἂν ἕκαστος αὐτῶν πρήσσειν τι οἰόμενος τυγχάνῃ, 'on the very points where any one of them happens to think they are accomplishing something substantial': there is perhaps an intentional ambiguity in ᾗ.[41] Our author means not only that he will refute medicine's detractors where they think they've accomplished something (that is, he will address their specific arguments), but also in the same way, that is, by turning their arguments against them. Thus, his strategy is to concede his opponent's premises while disputing their conclusions. True, patients sometimes recover without a physician. But this is itself proof of the art's existence (c. 5), as is the physician's unwillingness to undertake hopeless cases (c. 8).

The critics merely think they have accomplished something, though they have not. This idea is meant to contrast with the accomplishments of the art mentioned in the preceding (see notes above), but the language here is meant also to recall 1.1, where the competence of the critics is called into question on account of their failure to achieve the ostensible aims of their discourses. The sentence-final τυγχάνῃ transitions into the author's defense against a series of arguments from chance, τύχη. In addition, it subtly turns the tables on the critics: any success they may appear to enjoy is attributable to chance, not art.

[41] Many thanks to Lesley-Dean Jones for bringing this to my attention.

## 4

With c. 4 begins the *lusis*, or direct refutation of the opponent's charges. Our author himself marks this beginning with the word ἀρχή, but, as I argue below, the choice of words bespeaks an attention to logical function that requires something stronger than 'beginning' when translating (contrast with *Loc. Hom.* 38.4 = L. 6.278). I opt for 'premise,' which correctly indicates the place of the succeeding sentence within the formal structure of the treatise. A premise is supposed to be true, at least within the context of the argument in which it is a premise, which is not to say that it is self-evident. *De Arte's* ἀρχή, then, is more than a premise in the modern sense, I think, insofar as it seems to be the sort of proposition to which all would agree without demanding further justification. Thus, it anticipates to some degree the Aristotelian notion, with the important exception that our author's ἀρχή need not be a scientific axiom but may simply be the premise of an argument (cf. *APo.* 71b19–33). For, unlike Aristotle's demonstrations, *de Arte* is not an explanation, but only an argument—what Aristotle would have called a dialectical deduction (though 'deduction' is perhaps too formal a label for *de Arte*).

In summary, then, we can develop a fuller picture of the *apodeixis* as it appears in *de Arte*. It is a λόγος based on a universally accepted premise, or ἀρχή, where ἀρχή is to be understood, ideally, as both a discursive and a logical starting point. It is constructed with the intent to prove a certain conclusion, the terms of which are clearly specified in a definition given at the outset. Though we do not know whether universal acceptability, much less self-evidence, is the author's criterion for adopting definitions or premises, he, like Diogenes of Apollonia, foreshadows the Aristotelian and Stoic idea (Sextus Empiricus, P 2.135–143) that an *apodeixis* moves from what is evident or immediately known to a conclusion that is less evident (see also notes on 13.1). While we cannot know that he would have given this account of demonstration generally, we can still credit him here with a practical example of an *apodeixis* that emphasizes its logical features over rhetorical style. In this, at least, he exceeds our expectations of a 'mere' sophist.

Having acknowledged the point of agreement between the critics and himself, our author turns immediately to their disagreement, specifically to the charge that medicine's apparent successes are to be attributed not to *technē* but to *tuchē*, 'chance.' The claim seems to have been supported by a family of related but distinct arguments that provoke from our author several independent *pisteis*, or argument-proofs, which are delivered over the next three chapters of *de Arte*. There are, in fact, two distinct proofs in c. 4. The first is given in response to the theoretical objection that medical treatment is not always accompanied by recovery (4.1–2), while the second is oriented to a situation familiar to any practicing physician: a patient, though having undergone treatment for his illness and recovered, subsequently refuses to credit the doctor with his recovery (4.3–4; see also my notes on 5.5).

Our author's responses aspire to deductive rigor (witness the renewed frequency of the particle γάρ), but his diction reveals also a calculating talent for exploiting the nuances of language. The central question is one of responsibility (αἰτιήσασθαι, 4.3), a concept of obvious moral and juridical provenance. Who is responsible for the patient's recovery? Our author argues his case as though at trial, and the chapter is littered with legal jargon and double-entendres. But for maximum rhetorical effect, our author inspires his legalese with a religious zeal.[42] He alleges that the patients turned themselves over to medicine (ἐν ᾧ τῇ τέχνῃ ἐπέτρεψαν σφᾶς αὐτούς, 4.3), as though they were putting themselves in the hands of a god—the phrase ἐπιτρέπειν τῷ θέῳ is a commonplace in Homer (*Od.* 22.289, 19.502).[43] Thus, *de Arte* poses the causal controversy as a theological crisis: which god should be thanked for the patients' recovery? Should it be Τύχη? Or should Τέχνη receive our praise? These patients consulted Τέχνη when they were in trouble,[44] but now they give the glory to Τύχη. The religious overtones may explain also the curious use of the verb ὑπουργεῖν,[45] as well as other words that, while not intrinsically religious, have obvious religious application (e.g., πιστεύειν, θεᾶσθαι).

**4.1** μοι ἀρχὴ τοῦ λόγου, 'my discourse starts from the following premise': the phrase ἀρχὴ τοῦ λόγου has a distinctly philosophical ring, though it is not a particularly common formula among Pre-Socratic thinkers and is found

[42] Ducatillon notes this in passing, without explanation or deeper analysis (1977a, 46). The religious element is consistent also with Lulofs' analysis of chance in c. 4, which connects *de Arte* to tragic themes concerning human beings and fate (1923, 161–162).

[43] In Attic legal discourse, ἐπιτρέπειν is used frequently to signal that a dispute is being turned over to a third party for arbitration or judgment (Thucydides 4.54, 4.83; Demosthenes 27.1, 59.45). Accordingly, our author is reminding the patient that he agreed to treat the doctor's judgment as the final word on the matter of his health.

[44] Cf. χρᾶσθαι θεῷ, Aeschines, 3.124; Aristotle, *Pol.* 1323b21–25; Herodotus 4.78.4.

[45] Cf. Pausanias, *Graeciae descriptio* 6.6.9 τοῖς μὲν δὴ τὰ ὑπὸ τοῦ θεοῦ προστεταγμένα ὑπουργοῦσι; elsewhere in the *Corpus*, it is the doctor who is depicted in the service of medicine, e.g., in the first book of the *Epidemics* (2.636.2).

mostly in the fragments of more literary-minded figures. Ion of Chios (DK 36 B1) identifies his ἀρχή τοῦ λόγου with the thesis that 'all things are three and nothing is more or less than these three things.' The use of ἀρχή may have some logical import here, indicating a proposition that serves as a basis for all further deductions about the nature of things, though we can only speculate, since exceedingly little of the λόγος that followed is extant. In the case of Gorgias (*Helen*, DK 82 B11 §5), the phrase does not seem to indicate anything more than the beginning of his speech. In any event, neither Ion nor Gorgias seems to require that his ἀρχή is universally accepted. Of all the Pre-Socratics, *de Arte* recalls most vividly the physiologically preoccupied philosopher Diogenes of Apollonia, who employs the notion of an ἀρχὴ τοῦ λόγου in a similar way: 'it seems to me that a person beginning any argument (λόγου παντὸς ἀρχόμενον) must provide an indisputable premise (τὴν ἀρχὴν ἀναμφισβήτητον), as well as an explanation (ἑρμηνεία) that is simple and serious' (DK 64 B1). The ἀρχή of our author's argument is a proposition, namely, the observation that some of those who are treated regain their health (see following notes), and this has obvious logical import for any subsequent argument about the efficacy of medicine. For if it is not admitted that there is at least some minimal correlation between medical treatment and recovery, it is unclear how our author could argue that medicine is responsible for the recovery of patients. Thus, the remainder of *de Arte*, which attempts to elucidate and defend the features of this correlation, is dependent upon this premise.

4.1 ἐξυγιαίνονται, 'fully recover': in remarks on this passage, Jouanna draws attention to the vexed question regarding instances of ἐξυγιαίνεσθαι in the *Corpus* (1988, 249–250). It has been argued that they are corrupt and should be emended to ἐξυγιάζεσθαι (van Brock 1961, 1507–507, 269–271), though this view has met with persuasive opposition (Schmidt 1980). I see no reason to diverge from the MSS, both of which give some form of ἐξυγιαίνεσθαι, though I have resisted the passive constructions often employed in translating ἐξυγιαίνονται. They are subtly misleading insofar as they suggest a legitimate case of agent causation (e.g., Jones' 'healed,' 1923, 195). But our author is not simply assuming what he wants to prove. Instead, his choice of words is more careful: the patients have 'recovered,' or 'come to be healthy,' and the author's task is to show that medical treatment was the primary agent in effecting this change. The sentence cannot mean: 'some of those treated by medicine are healed by it.' (That this would be the more natural sense if ἐξυγιάζεσθαι were the correct reading speaks against it, I should think.) As the following passages make plain, our author is arguing against detractors who would in fact deny that medicine ever heals anyone. What they cannot deny, however, is the fact that there are cases in which a patient is treated *and* recovers. The author's task is to show that this was *because* of the treatment.

The completive prefix ἐξ- recalls its use at 1.2 and alludes to the first disjunctive condition in our author's definition of medicine, 'totally removing the sufferings of the sick' (3.2). There are indeed cases in which medicine appears to have achieved its highest aim. But not all (οὐ πάντες) patients fully regain their health. Perhaps some find their conditions merely improved—think here of the second disjunctive condition in the definition of medicine. This may leave some room for criticism (ἐν τούτῳ ἤδη ψέγεται ἡ τέχνη), but most threatening are those criticisms that focus on patients whose conditions have not improved or have worsened (τοὺς ἁλισκομένους need not refer to fatalities, but may also include those 'taken prisoner' by their diseases), since these represent genuine failures of the art, as opposed to cases of informed, intentional non-intervention as defined by the third disjunctive condition.

4.1 οἱ τὰ χείρω λέγοντες, 'those who speak more meanly of it': the comparative may indicate a contrast between critics who find fault with the art because it sometimes fails to cure completely and those who hold that medical therapy is never responsible for a patient's recovery. The former is compatible with the limited efficacy, and therefore being, of medicine, while the latter attributes the apparent successes of medical intervention to *tuchē*, mere coincidence (see following notes below). This is certainly a less charitable position, and perhaps also a weaker one, supposing that χείρω here has the semantic range of formulas such as αἰσχροεπεῖν and λόγων οὐ καλῶν τέχνη in c. 1. If so, then it is further possible that our author is alluding to Protagoras, or at least to the sophistic business of making the weaker or worse argument stronger,[46] which in turn may be a sign that our author does not take the criticism terribly seriously.

4.1 τοὺς ἀποφεύγοντας αὐτὰ τύχῃ ἀποφεύγειν καὶ οὐ διὰ τὴν τέχνην, 'those who escape [their diseases] do so by chance and not because of art': the author introduces chance, a subject that occupies him for the next three chapters.

[46] Per Aristotle's testimony in the second book of his *Rhetoric*: 'and this is what it means to make the weaker argument (τὸν ἥττω δὲ λόγον) stronger; thus, people justly objected to Protagoras' promise' (1402a23 = DK 80 A21 = B6b). Cf. Plato, *Apology* 18b.

In c. 4 (unlike c. 5), chance is identified as a mutually exclusive alternative to the art; either recovery is caused by medical intervention, or it is brought about by the agency of chance. But is chance to be construed as itself a genuine cause, or rather as denoting a certain way of being caused? The reconstruction of the critics' argument offers some guidance.[47]

1. Not all cases of medical intervention correlate with patient recovery.
2. Thus, medicine is not the cause of recovery in any particular case.
3. Therefore, the correlation in some cases between medical intervention and patient recovery is by chance.

If they are to constitute a valid argument, the above claims must be supplemented by additional premises.

1.5. If, in any particular case, medicine is the cause of a person's recovery, then all cases of medical intervention will correlate with recovery.

This warrants the move from 1 to 2 by *modus tollens*. Further, the inference from 2 to 3 is guaranteed by the implicit definition of chance.

2.5. Chance is mere coincidence, that is, the correlation of two events that are causally unrelated.[48]

The most economical reconstruction of the critics' argument, then, relies on a notion of *tuchē* as coincidence. It relies also on a respectable and long-standing intuition that the validity of causal explanations must appeal in some way to laws or law-like principles or regularities.[49] In the current context, however, the critics badly misapply this intuition, an error that perhaps justifies our author's seemingly casual dismissal of the objection. For it will be obvious to most that questions about the causal efficacy of a certain form of treatment will be referred to the law-like relations (or lack thereof) that obtain between various outcomes and that particular form

---

[47] Jori, too, correctly identifies these as the three prongs of the critics' attack, though he does not probe the presuppositions that warrant their logical interrelations (1996, 160). As a result, he misunderstands our author's defense.

[48] That chance is defined partly in negative relation to causation explains the mutual exclusivity of the two categories. That the definition is taken over from the critics justifies our author's taking it for granted, pace Jori (1996, 163). Indeed, it would have been dishonest had he not met his critics on their own terms.

[49] The paradigm of which is the influential deductive-nomological model of scientific explanation as outlined in Hempel and Oppenheim 1948. It is consistent with the author's view that, in order to be constitutive of a thing's εἶδος, a power must be regularly or necessarily connected with it (cf. 12.3).

of treatment, not medical treatment *simpliciter*. The question of whether I should credit the prescribed antibiotic with curing my bacterial pneumonia depends on whether antibiotics correlate with recovery from pneumonia across the population. Surely proof of the effectiveness of the antibiotic does not require that every medical therapy correlate in every case to full recovery.

**4.2** ἐγὼ δὲ οὐκ ἀποστερέω μὲν οὐδ' αυτὸς τὴν τύχην ἔργου οὐδενός, 'I myself do not deprive chance of its accomplishment': our author implies a contrast between his own even-handed and sensible view, which leaves room for both *tuchē* and *technē*, and the critics' radical view, which denies altogether the efficacy and reality of *technē*. Moreover, ἔργον may connote function or purpose. To put the point more colloquiually, chance 'plays a role,' or 'has a job to do.'

**4.2** τοῖσι μὲν κακῶς θεραπευομένοισι νοσήμασι τὰ πολλὰ τὴν ἀτυχίην ἕπεσθαι, τοῖσι δὲ εὖ τὴν εὐτυχίην, 'for the most part misfortune follows upon the poor treatment of a disease, while good fortune follows upon good treatment': my translation of ἀτυχίην and εὐτυχίην using the English 'fortune' reflects an attempt to capture the play on words. When the author speaks of good fortune for those who are treated well, he does not mean that their recoveries are the result of chance (i.e., coincidences), but rather that their outcomes are good. The resulting 'ambivalence' about the role of luck in medicine strongly echoes a passage from *Loc. Hom.*

> Further, what need has medicine of luck? If there are drugs clearly appropriate for illnesses, I think that drugs do not depend on luck to turn the illnesses into health .... Anyone who will exclude luck from medicine or any other activity, alleging that it is not those who have good knowledge of a thing who have good luck, seems to hold a view completely opposite to mine. For in my view only those who know how to do something well or badly have good or bad luck (ἀτυχεῖν). For good luck is doing something well, and those with knowledge do this; and bad luck is doing something badly, through lack of knowledge. (85.25–35 = L. 6.342)

Wordplay naturally raises worries about equivocation, and some have thought that by sliding between two different senses of *tuchē*, our author's reply is rendered irrelevant to the critics' original objection.[50] This, however,

[50] Jori, for example, alleges that the easy transition from one sense to another leaves the argument, in his words, 'privo di un fondamento adeguato' (1996, 162). To my knowledge, the play on words itself was first recognized by Joos (1957, 246).

is to misunderstand the force of the author's claim, which should be compared to remarks on chance and the being of medicine in *VM*.

> Some practitioners are poor, while others are much better. This would not be the case if medicine absolutely were not, nor if its observations and discoveries had never been made. Rather, all would be similarly inexperienced and ignorant, and all the affairs of the sick would be administered by chance (τύχη). (118.10–119.1 = L. 1.570)

Lack of variation in the success rates of physicians is consistent with the claim that health is meted out by chance, not art, and both of these scenarios would come to pass if there were no art. But success rates do vary, and this indicates that medicine has real consequences for the health of its patients. There really are procedures that causally affect a patient's health for the better, and some physicians have managed to identify them and incorporate them into therapeutic practice.

Our author's articulation of a similar point is neither arbitrary nor irrelevant, but is aimed with strategic precision at premise 1.5 from the critics' argument from chance (see note on 4.1 above): 'if, in any particular case, medicine is the cause of a person's recovery, then all cases of medical intervention will correlate with recovery.' As noted earlier, the efficacy of a particular type of treatment is demonstrated not by the overall success of medical treatment generally, but by its regular correlation with positive outcomes. (Hence the formula τὰ πολλά, 'for the most part,' though the demand for regularity is already contained in our author's notions of forms as 'the things that are always;' see 2.2). In this respect, *de Arte* is more careful even than *VM*, since the relative overall success rates of physicians will not serve as a perfectly reliable proxy for the efficacy of the specific treatments they employ. In principle, a range of doctors could have the same overall rate of success while employing vastly different therapies, so long as each doctor had comparable records of successful therapeutic application.

**4.3** ἔπειτα δὲ καὶ πῶς οἷόν τ' ἐστὶ τοῖσιν ἐξυγιανθεῖσιν ἄλλο τι αἰτιήσασθαι ἢ τὴν τέχνην, 'how, then, could those who fully recover hold something other than the art responsible for this': the focus shifts from skepticism about the efficacy of medicine generally to particular cases in which a fully recovered patient questions the efficacy of the specific treatment applied by the doctor. Jori is thus correct that the argument is 'partial' and 'episodic,' and 'incapable, therefore, of constituting an appropriate basis for reaching a conclusion of *general* import' (1996, 163), though he is wrong to expect this in the first place. Our author's concerns expand beyond academic questions of medicine's being to include all attempts to question the power of medicine.

Accordingly, *contra* Jori (1996, 160), the argument he begins here is directed not at the general theoretical objection from chance outlined above but is intended for deployment in more practical contexts, specifically, those in which a patient denies that the prescribed therapy is responsible for his recovery.

4.3 εἴπερ χρεώμενοι αὐτῇ καὶ ὑπουργέοντες ὑγιάνθησαν, 'if indeed they recovered while using and submitting to it': it may seem as though our author begs the question by assuming that the patients recovered by using and submitting to medicine when this is precisely what's at issue. However, as the translation indicates, the participles χρεώμενοι and ὑπουργέοντες do not indicate means but rather simultaneity of action with respect to the action of the main verb. Our author is reiterating the fact that these patients recovered when they were treated, not merely asserting that they recovered because they were treated. That is nothing new but rather a restatement of the ἀρχὴ τοῦ λόγου (see note on 4.1 above).

4.3 τὸ μὲν γὰρ τῆς τύχης εἶδος ψιλὸν ... θεήσασθαι, 'to observe the form of pure chance': another instance of hypallage (cf. 1.2), the adjective ψιλὸν (bare, naked, unadorned or unaccompanied) agrees with τὸ εἶδος though it is understood to modify τῆς τύχης. The correlation between recovery and therapy was not a mere coincidence; medicine had something (if not everything) to do with it, and the author contends that the patient is committed to acknowledging this on some level. The verb θεᾶσθαι is familiar from 2.1, where it means 'observe perceptually,' and its occurrence here seems consistent, especially as the object of perception is an εἶδος, a form or natural kind as determined by its observable character (see notes on 2.2). It is a further question whether our author indeed allows for a form or natural kind of chance in the sense of coincidence. His strategy here is purely dialectical, and it is possible that his reference to a form of chance is made purely for the sake of argument and nothing more. It is conceivable that, as a relational property holding between causal events, chance achieves a limited status as a natural kind. On the other hand, one might regard the criteria for judging two events a coincidence as containing an irreducibly subjective element, since, by definition, any correlation cited in making such a judgment would not be a causal relation. That is to say, a coincidence of events occurs when the two events might strike an observer as causally related, even though they are not. But, given the variety of potential observers and the range of criteria such observers might apply, it is difficult to imagine that this would constitute a natural class.

4.3 οὐκ ἐβουλήθησαν, 'they did not wish': at first it may seem odd to talk of wishing to observe or not to observe something, since, under normal conditions, a person does not stand in a volitional relation to his sense perceptions. One does not have control over whether the tower appears to him white or round, etc. However, whether one looks at the tower at all is under his control, and this plays into our author's point: one may choose to avoid acknowledging certain realities, but they remain realities nonetheless.

In any case, the argument is focused on the realities implicitly acknowledged by the fully recovered but recalcitrant patient.

1. The patient made a voluntary decision to undergo the prescribed therapy.
2. If the patient made a voluntary decision, then he had a reason or set of reasons for making the decision.
3. Thus, he had a reason or set of reasons.
4. This set of reasons either included the expectation that the therapy would benefit him, or it did not.
5. If it did not, then the patient is guilty of recklessness, stupidity, intemperance, *vel sim.*
6. If it did, then he has no grounds for now overturning his previous conviction that the prescribed therapy is beneficial, i.e., causally effective in curing his condition.

Or as Gomperz puts it, given the patient's decision to go forward with treatment, 'one may not, at least not without compelling analysis of the case, introduce direct empirical evidence that the recovery would have occurred even without medical treatment' (1910, 111). Such is the trap our author has laid for the hypothetical patient-critic. Gomperz dubbed it 'advokatenhaft,' and surely there is something lawyerly about it. Understandably, our author is less concerned with demonstrating the efficacy of any particular treatment than with deflecting, by any rhetorical means, attacks on the efficacy of prescribed therapy that a doctor might encounter in the course of his practice. His strategy betrays a flair for courtroom drama: the patient-critic is accused of giving inconsistent testimony, and the jury is left to speculate as to his motivation for changing tunes. The diction only reinforces the juridical imagery. The detractors 'hold chance responsible' (αἰτιᾶσθαι) for their recoveries. Our author does not, though he is careful not to 'rob' (ἀποστερεῖν) chance of its 'property' (ἔργον), in contrast to the critic who deserted chance when ill but hails its power now that he has recovered.

4.4 ἐς τὴν τύχην ἀναφορῆς ἀπηλλαγμένοι εἰσί, τῆς μέντοι ἐς τὴν τέχνην οὐκ ἀπηλλαγμένοι, 'they are freed from their reliance on chance, though their debt to the art is not discharged': the phrase has long baffled translators. For the phrase ἐς τὴν τύχην ἀναφορῆς ἀπηλλαγμένοι, Gomperz gives the puzzling 'free from domination by chance' (1910, 41). Jones and Vegetti work from the literal sense of ἀναφορά, 'a turning back to,' from which its legal meaning of 'recourse' probably derives: the former translates 'freed from dependence upon luck' (1923, 195), while the latter 'freed from having to turn to chance' (1965, 441). Jouanna seems to sense here an assignment of credit, though his translation is non-commital: 'removed from relating health to chance' (1988, 228). Probably the difficulty arises from another play on words. The first occurrence of ἀναφορά requires the sense of 'recourse' while the (understood) second occurrence is better suited by Jouanna's translation. The patient owes credit to the art. I would add that in legal contexts, ἀπαλλάσσειν means 'to discharge' (see Demosthenes 36.25, 37.21), and, according to the LSJ, ἀναφορά is used in third-century legal papyri and epigraphy with the meaning 'payment' or 'installment.' Extending the metaphor introduced earlier, when he promised not to deprive chance of its due, our author treats the question of causal efficacy as though he were prosecuting a breach-of-contract case before a court of law. The patients agreed to treat medicine as a legitimate party to the contract, only to renege once services had been rendered. With this, our author moves from the theoretical, through the practical, and into the downright quotidian; his argument could be used by a doctor refused payment for his services. The subtle *ad hominem* assault on medicine's detractors is merciless and possibly hilarious—their objections proceed not from a genuine concern for the truth but are part of a pathetic ploy to avoid paying their medical bills.

4.4 καὶ τὸ εἶδος ἐσκέψαντο καὶ τὴν δύναμιν περανθέντος τοῦ ἔργου ἔγνωσαν, 'they observed its form and, once the deed was accomplished, they came to know its power': the verbal pair καὶ ἐσκέψαντο καὶ ἔγνωσαν echoes ὁρᾶταί τε καὶ γινώσκεται at 2.2. By demonstrating that medicine is both seen and known, the author puts the fact of its being beyond dispute, at least according to his own philosophical principles. By submitting to treatment, the patient acknowledges, at least implicitly, the treatment's empirical claim to repeated success. That is to say, the treatment possesses the power to cause recoveries in patients suffering from a certain condition as one of its defining characteristics, and so by acknowledging the reports of its causal power the patient 'sees' also its form in that he consents to *a posteriori* claims about its effectiveness. When he recovers after having been treated, he becomes directly and personally acquainted with its causal power. He 'knows' it. Moreover, he must recognize that his own case only confirms the efficacy of medicine. At least, it gives him no grounds for skepticism.

## 5

Our author continues his argument against the claim that medicine's apparent successes are due to chance. Again, the chapter contains at least two distinct *pisteis*: patients who recover without consulting a doctor have merely healed themselves by chancing upon what a doctor would have prescribed for them (5.1–5.5); and even the mistakes of doctors testify to the art's existence (5.5–5.6). This second *pistis* is a digression from the main topic, and it demonstrates how heavily the problem of failure weighs on our author's mind.

The rhetoric relies, as in c. 4, on the religious potential of key terms such as χρεωμένους ('having consulted,' i.e., a doctor, but, in religious contexts, an oracle), ἀπιστέω ('I do not doubt'), μεγάλη ('great' or 'powerful'), σῳζόμενοι ('saved' or 'redeemed'), etc. Medicine is exalted as a benevolent and magnanimous god, willing to save even those wretches who disrespect it. The detractors, meanwhile, are depicted as ungrateful agnostics who spit in the face of their protective divinity while hypocritically reaping the benefits of his care. Agnosticism about medicine (he conspicuously places the participle νομίζοντες under the scope of the negation here, not the infinitive εἶναι) is assimilated to agnosticism about the gods. The impiety that leads to open skepticism about the gods' existence (cf. Protagoras, DK 80 B4) is of a piece with the hubris that encourages the denial of medicine's existence. There is a touch of the tragic in our author's response to the critics. Like Oedipus, who thought he could escape the reach of the gods, the skeptical patient who recovers without a doctor flaunts his autonomy from medicine. Both are wrong, and in fact they are living proof of the divinity's and doctor's power, respectively. Thus, *de Arte* takes on the character of a choral lament as our author chides the obstinate and ignorant protagonist for failing to show proper reverence for the *technē* that cured him.

Stylistically, c. 5 is more subdued than most other sections. Euphony and syntactic figures are rarer, perhaps sacrificed to the demands of precise logical expression. The notable exception comes in the form of a sophistic flourish at chapter's end (5.6), where alliteration abounds and the clauses are carefully crafted to mirror each other, exhibiting both chiasmus and isocolon.

**5.1** ὁ τἀναντία λέγων, 'he who makes the opposite argument': the verb λέγειν must mean 'to make an argument,' not merely 'to say' or 'to claim,' which is the sense accorded the nominal form λόγος which occurs also in the same sentence. As in c. 4, the author concedes the critics' premise, though not the validity of the arguments constructed on its basis. It is perhaps significant that Protagoras is reported to have claimed that on every matter there are two arguments opposed to each other (δύο λόγους ... ἀντικειμένους ἀλλήλοις, DK 80 B6a) and to have written two books of 'antilogies' (DK 80 B4), a practice which seems to have exerted some influence. Consider, for example, Antiphon's tetralogies.

**5.1** πολλοὶ ἤδη καὶ οὐ χρησάμενοι ἰητρῷ νοσέοντες ὑγιάνθησαν, 'many who were sick have recovered even without consulting a doctor': our author continues his defense against another version of the argument that recovery is due to chance in the form of spontaneity (τὸ αὐτόματον), though the word itself will not be mentioned until 6.3. In c. 4, the critic attempted to question the correlation between medical treatment and recovery by highlighting those cases in which patients failed to recover. Now, his opponent tries to build a case around the fact that many recover without consulting a doctor, suggesting that medical treatment will not pass even the minimal test of counterfactual dependence—treatment is not even a necessary condition of recovery. Our author will counter by arguing that, even when diseases clear up 'on their own,' i.e., spontaneously, the cure does not occur without antecedent, external causes, and these causes are thoroughly understood (and thus can be manipulated) by doctors.

**5.1** ἐγὼ τῷ λόγῳ οὐκ ἀπιστέω, 'I do not doubt the claim': this sentence, in which our author agrees with an empirical claim put forward by the critic, echoes the first sentence of c. 4, in which our author puts forward an empirical claim that he expects to be accepted by all. As at 4.2, our author attempts to position himself as the champion of reasonableness and common sense, in contrast to the extravagant skepticism of the critic.

**5.2** ἰητρικῇ περιτυχεῖν, 'to chance upon medicine': from the translator's standpoint, one of the top priorities must be to convey the etymological relation to *tuchē* borne by the verbs περιτυχεῖν and ἐπιτυχεῖν. To accomplish this in English, I have employed the phrase 'chance upon' for περιτυχεῖν;

ἐπιτυχεῖν connotes perhaps more strongly the notion of success or accomplishment, and so I use 'hit upon by chance.' As at 4.2, the use of compounds containing *tuchē* signals a shift in the sense of the word. (See also following notes.)

**5.2** οὐ μὴν ὥστε εἰδέναι ὅ το ὀρθὸν ἐν αὐτῇ ἔνι ἢ ὅ τι μὴ ὀρθόν, 'this does not, of course, actually result in their knowing what is correct in it and what is not': as in some other Hippocratic treatises, chance does play a role in medicine, though a narrowly circumscribed one (see Introduction 1). Chance in this sense anticipates Aristotle's notion of an act that brings about a wished-for end without having been done for the sake of that end (*Phys.* 196b33–197a8). A patient comes across medicine by chance when he happens to apply the correct remedy, even though he does not know what medical treatment is proper to the condition from which he is suffering. Our author is careful to note that a patient who happens to bring about his own recovery does not thereby gain knowledge of what is correct or incorrect—and this is deemed essential to practicing an art. The firm line between layperson and professional has been in place since 1.2 ('slandering the discoveries of those who have knowledge in front of those who do not'), and this may reflect some attempt by the critics to blur the lines.

The author's point depends upon the tripartite definition of medicine from c. 3. It is crucial that the first condition of the definition—complete cure of the patient—makes no epistemic demands on the medical practitioner. The patient may serve the cause of medicine even in ignorance, just so long as he carries out the physical procedures that actually bring about a cure.

**5.2** ἀλλ' ὥστε ἐπιτυχεῖν, 'but rather in their hitting upon by chance': as Jones remarks in a footnote, 'the sense is clear but the reading uncertain' (1923, 196 n. 1). The MSS make a strong case for reading ἀλλ' ὥστε: A gives ἄλως τε; M ἄλλως τε; A[3] and Vat correct to ἀλλ' ὥστε. This sits comfortably neither with the ἐπιτύχοιεν of A and M[2] nor the ἐπιτύχειεν of M and Vat, though Jouanna opts nonetheless for the former, printing ἀλλ' ὥστε ἐπιτύχοιεν. (For Jouanna's justification, refer to 1988, 251 n. 2. See also the discussion by Jori, 1996, 75 n. 4). Following a suggestion by Jones (which he himself did not take, probably out of respect for the *lectio dificilior* principle), I print the infinitive form, yielding a simple actual-result clause that parallels the οὐ μὴν ὥστε εἰδέναι of the preceding and delivers the precise sense expected. Actuality is key, since our author claims that the patient is 'in the presence' of medicine even when he does not know it.

5.3 καὶ τοῦτό γε τεκμήριον μέγα τῇ οὐσίῃ τῆς τέχνης ὅτι ἐοῦσά τέ ἐστι καὶ μεγάλη, 'and this is powerful evidence of medicine's being—evidence that it both is and is powerful': our author gives what is said to be a τεκμήριον, a piece of evidence or a proof. A τεκμήριον serves as a solid foundation from which one may τεκμαίρεσθαι, draw conclusions or make inferences about what is not obvious to us. Though medicine itself is an abstraction, its effects are evident, and so its power is manifest (cf. 4.4). A strikingly similar expression occurs in the later Hippocratic treatise *Praec.*: 'with all these things it would appear powerful evidence for the being of the art (μέγα ἂν τεκμήριον φανείη [σὺν] τῇ οὐσιῃ τῆς τέχνης) if some excellent practitioner did not refrain from the following greeting, bidding the sick not to think disturbed thoughts in their haste to reach the opportune moment of their recovery' (33.17–18 = L. 9.264). This would seem to be more evidence that *de Arte* was familiar to some later medical writers.

We should not forget that τεκμήριον is a legal term as well as a medical one; Antiphon's court speeches are rife with it. As in c. 4, the author sounds as though he were trying to convince a jury that medicine has being. What force does this piece of evidence have? Logically, not much. If we accept that an unbeliever was saved by medicine, then it goes without saying that medicine is capable of saving, that is, that it has being. This is a valid but trivial deduction that runs the risk of begging the question. (See following note.)

5.3 φαίνονται καὶ οἱ μὴ νομίζοντες αὐτὴν εἶναι σῳζόμενοι δι' αὐτήν, 'even those who do not believe that it is are evidently saved by it': the agnostic patients are not 'apparently' saved but 'obviously' so. Such is the force of φαίνονται, which again invokes the connection between visibility and being. The unbelievers themselves are the unequivocal evidence of the incorrectness of their own view. The juxtaposition is exploited principally for its irony; there is no appreciable difference, from a strictly logical point of view, whether the layperson who chances upon medicine recognizes the existence of medicine or not. Hence, agnosticism (as opposed to ignorance) does not figure in the argument as it plays out in the rest of the chapter.

Though it is incidental to the main argument, there is a serious, if overly mannered, point: medicine is no mere name that may be applied to events or withheld at the whim of convention. In the language of c. 2, medicine is an outgrowth; its characteristic causal processes or effects, and thus its being, are independent of human belief in that being.

5.4 πολλὴ γὰρ ἀνάγκη καὶ τοὺς μὴ χρεωμένους ἰητροῖσι, νοσήσαντας δὲ καὶ ὑγιασθέντας, εἰδέναι ὅτι ἢ δρῶντές τι ἢ μὴ δρῶντες ὑγιάνθησαν, 'even those who did not consult a doctor but recovered after falling sick must surely know that they recovered by doing or not doing something': the γὰρ flags this as a premise in an argument for an earlier claim, namely, that those who recover without consulting a doctor nonetheless are saved by medicine. The premise itself depends on the pair of aorist participles, νοσήσαντας δὲ καὶ ὑγιασθέντας, which introduce a specific temporal sequence: at time $t_0$ the person fell ill then at $t_n$ recovered. Even the sick person can infer from this (with a high degree of certainty: πολλὴ ἀνάγκη εἰδέναι)[51] that something happened at $t_{m:0<m<n}$ to effect the change in condition. This is reasonable enough, so long as one subscribes to some general causal principle governing changes in condition, but there remain three questions about this 'something' that 'happened.' First, how does one validly infer from the fact that something happened that the sick persons were the agents of their own recovery, as the author clearly does (ἤ δρῶντές τι ἤ μὴ δρῶντες ὑγιάνθησαν)? Second, and related, if something happened, that is, if 1) some event occurred that 2) came about through the agency of the sick person and 3) effected the change in condition from sick to healthy, whence the potentially negative characterization of the event as 'not doing something?' Either the author imagines that a change in condition is possible without an intervening event, in which case the above interpretation of the argument's premise is incorrect, or we must understand the phrase 'not doing something' in a way that is compatible with the occurrence of an intervening event brought about through the sick person's agency. Finally, there is a question about the sick person's knowledge of the intervening event. Does he know only that something effected the change in condition, or does he know specifically what it was that so effected the change?

With respect to the first question, the author may assume that the sick person is operating in an environment over which he has substantial control. Thus, any change or lack of change in environment or diet could be attributed to his agency. Even if the body were somehow on course to heal itself 'spontaneously,' the internal causal processes at work would require insulation from external interference. (Surely there are things a person can

---

[51] I cannot agree with Jori that the phrases πολλὴ ἀνάγκη εἰδέναι and πολλὴ ἀνάγκη ἐγνωκέναι at 5.4 and 5.5, respectively, indicate that our author attributes infallible perception to the sick person (1996, 175 nn. 26 and 27). The necessity invoked is logical: given that 1) changes in condition are brought about through some cause; 2) the sick person experienced a change in condition; then it follows necessarily that 3) there was a cause of the sick person's change in condition. If the author means further that the sick person knows *what specifically* caused the change in condition, as I believe he does, then the syllogistic structure will be still more complex.

do to inhibit his body's recuperation from a cold, for example.) The sick person's choice of environment or diet, then, would emerge as a legitimate necessary condition of the allegedly spontaneous recovery. Further, if he knows specifically what effected his change in condition, then he may know for a fact that it was something he did. Thus, our answer to the first question may depend on our answer to the third, which, along with the second, I will address in the following notes.

5.4 ἢ γὰρ ἀσιτίῃ ἢ πολυφαγίῃ, ἢ ποτῷ πλέονι ἢ δίψῃ, ἢ λουτροῖσιν ἢ ἀλουσίῃ, ἢ πόνοισιν ἢ ἡσυχίῃ, ἢ ὕπνοισιν ἢ ἀγρυπνίῃ, ἢ τῇ ἁπάντων τούτων ταραχῇ χρεώμενοι ὑγιάνθησαν, 'for it was by fasting or by overeating, by drinking much fluid or by abstaining from it, by bathing or by not bathing, by vigorous exercise or by rest, by sleep or by wakefulness, or by using some combination of these that they recovered': Gomperz calls the passage 'stürmisch hastenden' (violently rushed) and 'häufenden' (cluttered) but this is flatly contradicted by the painstaking construction of its language, namely, the parisosis and homoioteleuton that our author uses to provide a rhythmic and euphonic structure for this list. The dative pairs follow a highly stylized syllabic pattern: 10, 9, 9, 9, 10. The three 9-syllable pairs are specially crafted so that the first member of the pair comprises three syllables and ends in -οισιν, while the second member comprises four syllables and ends in -ίῃ. The sentence exhibits bursts of alliteration (πολυφαγίῃ, ἢ ποτῷ πλέονι) and is governed overall by assonance on the vowel *ēta*. Where he might otherwise lull his audience with a laundry-list of potentially beneficial activities, our author aims to keep it entertained with the poetic effects of the language.

Both Jouanna (1988, 251) and Gomperz (1910, 113) remark on the unusual (but not unique) use of ταραχή, which here has not the pejorative sense of 'disturbance,' but only 'mixture' or 'combination.' Still, Ducatillon sees a potential problem here.

> To use the components of regimen without compelling oneself to balance those that wither with those that strengthen, those that deteriorate with those that restore, is pure silliness. It is to ignore the doctrine both of Cos and Cnidos, whose experts prescribe the establishment of a rigorous *summetria* between its constituents. It is to risk aggravating the disease. (1977a, 73)

Dedicated to the proposition that our author is a practicing Greek physician, Ducatillon invents a motive for his diction: he is writing in the words that an untrained layperson would if he were wondering what caused his recovery (1977a, 74). But no special explanation is required, since the passage seems rather to endorse the view of medical therapy as a matter of targeting a precise mean between extremes. The examples cited by our author are excesses and deficiencies (e.g., overeating and fasting) in activities (e.g., taking in nutrition) that, under normal (that is 'healthy') conditions, may be said to have a mean or measure insofar as there is a proper balance to be struck between fasting and overeating in order to maintain health. This, it turns out, is just what the author means by 'doing or not doing something' (see the second question of the preceding note). With respect to a particular component, one may adjust his regimen in the direction of the excessive extreme ('doing something') or in the direction of the deficient extreme ('not doing something'). That restoring health may be a matter of hitting the mean on multiple dietetic axes (i.e., of 'using a ταραχή of all these things') underscores the complexity of medicine, but it does not call into question the 'metric' principle of dietetics. Regardless of whether our author was a practicing physician, then, clearly he is familiar with this axiom of medical therapeutics.

The various extremes enumerated can be found in other treatises in the Hippocratic *Corpus*. With the exception of πολυφαγίη, an unusual word that occurs only in *de Arte*, the other terms are ubiquitous in the *Corpus* as factors affecting health and sickness. Gomperz compares the list to the famous 'relativity of goods' speech by Protagoras at *Protagoras* 334a–c (1910, 112). He further contends that both the Protagorean remark and this list of therapeutic factors demonstrate the relative nature both of the qualities of things and of the means available to us for influencing them. However, while it is true that different treatments are appropriate to different conditions, I detect here nothing more than a sophistic *topos* (cf. 12.6) that has little if any impact on the logic of the argument (in contrast to *VM* 3.4, for example, which stresses the relative healthiness of certain regimens to different physiological types).

5.5 καὶ τῷ ὠφελῆσθαι πολλὴ ἀνάγκη αὐτούς ἐστιν ἐγνωκέναι ὅ τι ἦν τὸ ὠφελῆσαν, καὶ εἴ τί γ' ἐβλάβησαν, τῷ βλαβῆναι, ὅ τι ἦν τὸ βλάψαν, 'in virtue of having been benefited, they surely must have known what it was that benefited them; and likewise, if they were harmed somehow, then, in virtue of being harmed, what it was that harmed them' [**5.5.a**]: turning to the third remaining question ('does the recovered sick person know only that something effected the change in conditions or does he know specifically what it was that so effected the change?'), we find that the answer rests in part on a difficult stretch of text. The quandary is this: shall we read ὅτι ἦν τι τὸ ὠφελῆσαν/ὅτι ἦν τι τὸ βλάψαν, following Gomperz? Or ὅ τι ἦν τὸ ὠφελῆσαν/ὅ τι ἦν τὸ βλάψαν, with Jones and Jouanna? The first option produces the modest claim (henceforth, the 'Weak Interpretation') that whoever was benefited or harmed must acknowledge that something was doing the benefiting or harming. On the second, our author is much bolder: whoever was benefited or harmed must know precisely what it was that caused it (the 'Strong Interpretation'). The difference between the two interpretations is just the difference between a *de re* and *de dicto* construal of the patient's purported knowledge. Does he know of some particular thing that it caused his recovery? Or does he know merely the proposition that something caused it?

Textually, we are torn. One of the main manuscripts, A, has the second τι but not the first. Other manuscripts have neither. There is any number of plausible stories that could be confected to explain how an original text with τι in both places or neither place could have been the ancestor of the surviving MSS. Gomperz and Heiberg emend to read two occurrences of τι, though I must add that the indefinite pronouns are somewhat beside the point. While their inclusion demands that we read ὅτι, not ὅ τι, we may read ὅτι even without the τι and still limit our author to only the more modest of the two assertions, though the syntax is a trifle more awkward. Between ὅτι and ὅ τι we cannot decide on textual grounds alone.

That being the case, let us examine the interpretive grounds for adopting ὅ τι. Jones curtly dismisses Gomperz' version:

> It would surely make the sentence a flat repetition of the preceding one. I take the sequence of thought to be this. Cures apparently spontaneous are not really so. The cure has its cause, e.g., a bath or a sleep, and the fact that the cure followed the bath or sleep proves that the latter was the cause. To distinguish the beneficial in this way is not guesswork, but implies the existence of an art. (1910, 197)

Thus, Jones attributes to our author a sophomoric analysis of causation, the principle of *post hoc propter hoc* criticized by the author of *VM*.

> I know that, if the patients happen to have done something atypical around this day [of their decline in health], either bathing or walking around or eating something strange (supposing it had been better to do all these than not), nonetheless many doctors, just like laypersons, put the blame on one of these things and remain ignorant of the cause, canceling what treatment might have proven most beneficial. Instead, they should know what an untimely bath does or what fatigue does. For the distress associated with either one of these is never associated with the other, nor with those that originate from repletion or from such and such a food. So whoever does not learn how these things stand in relation to a human being will be able neither to know their results nor to use them correctly. (148.7–19 = L. 1.624–626)

In Jones' defense, *VM*'s criticism might constitute evidence that this was a prevalent approach to diagnosis in Greek medicine. Particularly striking is *VM*'s reference to the extremity or abnormality of the alleged causes,[52] which is consistent with my hypothesis that our author's list of dietetic examples is governed by a metric principle of therapeutics (see note on 5.4 above). I would add to Jones' analysis that immediate temporal antecedence is not enough to establish that some event caused the recovery; if at time $t_0$ the person fell ill and at $t_n$ recovered, we cannot infer an event to be the cause of the recovery simply on the grounds that it occurred at $t_{m: 0<m<n}$. To be correctly identified as the cause of recovery, the event must also represent a deviation from the norms of a moderate regimen in health.

What is the Weak alternative to this interpretation? Our author turns to highly abstract language at 5.5 to make a metaphysical point. His reliance on articular infinitives and participles is not gratuitous. He identifies τὸ ὠφελῆσθαι, a 'being benefited,' which implies the existence of τὸ ὠφελῆσαν, a 'thing benefiting.' He uses the passive infinitive to indicate a predicate term (call it F). When some person recovers from illness, he or she has been benefited, and so Fc, where c is the constant designating the person who has undergone the benefiting. Our author's claim would be that the passive construction implies that F is a two-place relation, and hence that Fc (perhaps better F _c) is an incomplete expression as it stands. Another term is required to complete it. The recovered person does not know what in particular benefited him, so he cannot fill out the expression with a constant, for example, Fac. But insofar as 'being benefited' is a correct use of language, he knows that 'benefits' is a two-place predicate, and he must acknowledge the need for a second term (a subject term, if you will). That is, even though he does not know that Fac, he does know that $\exists x(Fxc)$. There is something that stands in the benefiting relation to him.

Thus far, both the Strong and Weak Interpretations are internally coherent. To choose between the two, then, will require that both be tested against the remaining text of c. 5.

**5.5** τὰ γὰρ τῷ ὠφελῆσθαι καὶ τὰ τῷ βαβλάφθαι ὡρισμένα, οὐ πᾶς ἱκανὸς γνῶναι, 'for isn't everyone capable of knowing the things determined through his benefit or harm' [5.5.b]; as at 3.2, ὡρισμένα recalls its original connection to boundary-marking. In this case the boundary is one between two classes, one of which includes those components of regimen that have harmed

[52] Without using the word, the author is criticizing the prevalent tendency, exhibited also by writers in the Hippocratic *Corpus*, to formulate diagnoses based on a πρόφασις, an antecedent cause that triggers an existing disposition to illness in the body (see also my commentary on 6.3).

the sick person, the other of which includes those that have benefited his health. In either case, class membership is determined by an empirically ascertainable causal power, and though the technical term εἶδος is not used, it seems reasonable to read into the distinction between these two classes a distinction between forms, or natural kinds as determined by characteristic causal powers. It may be of further significance that these two kinds are not assigned unique names, thereby illustrating the claim at 2.3 that forms are not dependent upon names and reinforcing the implicit message of 5.3: medicine is a natural entity, not a conventional designation.

To some, the Strong Interpretation has seemed to collapse under the weight of **5.5.b**, which, on the historically favored reading, takes the indicative, not the interrogative, mood and so states categorically that not everyone can know exactly what caused his benefit or harm. The recovered person must know that something benefited or harmed him, but special technical knowledge—knowledge of causes and what is correct or incorrect—is exactly what the self-recovered lack, according to our author. This was stated unequivocally at 5.2, but similar sentiments appear later in the treatise. At 7.3, our author characterizes patients as knowing neither what they are suffering nor because of what they are suffering, and at 11.4 he will charge that if patients knew what caused disease, they would never have gotten so sick.

The Weak Interpretation respects the epistemic gulf that separates the layperson and the doctor, a respect that is reflected in its consistency with **5.5.b**. However, this consistency should not distract us from the fact that, as it stands, the precise logical relation between **5.5.a** and **5.5.b** is inscrutable. The curious γάρ cannot carry out its usual function of introducing a reason or justification for the preceding, since the fact that not everyone is qualified to recognize the causes of disease or recovery in no way entails that patients know that something benefited or harmed them. The meaning of γάρ in **5.5.b** requires thorough and convincing explication, if we are to preserve the Weak Interpretation, but I do not see what that could be. Though γάρ sometimes serves an explanatory function, I cannot make sense of **5.5.b** as such a case. In the absence of a convincing account, then, the most responsible option will be to posit a lacuna immediately after **5.5.a**. Whatever the claim that **5.5.b** was meant to justify, it has not survived in the MSS.

Those who opt for the Strong Interpretation face two challenges. First, they must somehow resolve the apparent contradiction of this interpretation in **5.5.b**. Second, they must show that our author is equipped to allow the sick person precise knowledge of what benefited or harmed him while keeping sufficient distance between the layperson and the doctor. On the first point, Ermerins and Reinhold suppressed the negative particle οὐ in **5.5.b**, a sort of surgical removal of the offending contradiction. However, a less invasive alternative was proposed by Denniston (1929). He remarked that the sentence makes perfect sense if understood as a rhetorical question, noting that our author is fairly liberal with this device (cf. especially 2.1, but also 4.3, 5.6, 7.4–5, 8.4).[53] The logic falls into place with the slightest adjustment of punctuation: patients know what benefited or harmed them—after all, does not everybody?

Denniston's is an attractive solution, provided that we can explain why our author cedes such specialized knowledge of causes to laypersons. In a word, he does not. Or, rather, he recognizes a difference between knowing what caused one's disease and knowing what explains it. He is in good company. For the author of *VM*, who seemed above to take exception to approaches like that described in *de Arte*, relies on this very distinction. When he excoriates *post hoc* practitioners for supposing they have found what is responsible (αἴτιος) for the patient's change in condition, his criticism is not that the causes they identify are utterly irrelevant (though sometimes they are), but rather that they are not explanatory and therefore are uninformative. He is perfectly comfortable with the recognition *that* a surfeit of cheese made me ill. In fact, on his view, this kind of recognition was the first step in developing the art of medicine (121.2–15 = L. 1.574–576). But a complete causal statement, properly speaking, is more than this. It is explanatory. It tells us *why* (that is, in virtue of what) the cheese had this effect on me, and in doing so it must involve τὰ αἴτια, 'those things that, when they are present, a specific condition arises, but, when their combination changes, the condition ceases' (*VM* 144.2–5 = L. 1616–1618). There is a difference between knowing that cheese harmed me and knowing *in virtue of what* the cheese harmed me, and it is this latter sort of knowledge that constitutes an explanation of my illness. This may be reflected also in our author's deployment of terminology: the doctor's task is to discover τὰ διά τι (6.4) and τὰ αἴτια (11.4), while the laypersons know only τὸ βλάψαν.[54]

---

[53] Not coincidentally, Denniston's suggestion was made in the midst of a dispute over the function of the particle γάρ.

[54] Consider in this context the line drawn by Mackie between 1) 'merely' causal statements, which are based on the perception of particular chains of events, and 2) causally explanatory statements, which specify those features in virtue of which the effect in question was produced. Such features will, on Mackie's account, feature in the universal propositions that determine causal relations (1974, 248–269).

The distinction between causal *that*-statements and explanatory *why*-statements implicit in *de Arte* and *VM* was made explicit by Aristotle.

> But yet we think that *knowledge* and *understanding* belong to art rather than to experience, and we suppose artists to be wiser than men of experience (which implies that wisdom depends in all cases rather on knowledge); and this because the former know the cause, but the latter do not. For men of experience know that the thing is so, but do not know why, while the others know the 'why' and the cause.
>
> (*Metaph.* 981a24–30, trans. Ross in Barnes 1984)

For Aristotle, too, knowing *that* is a matter of perceiving individual cases, whereas knowing *why* is a matter of forming universal judgments involving classes of things.

> And art arises, when from many notions gained by experience one universal judgment about similar objects is produced. For to have a judgment that when Callias was ill of this disease this did him good, and similarly in the case of Socrates and in many individual cases, is a matter of experience; but to judge that it has done good to all persons of a certain constitution, marked off in one class, when they were ill of this disease, e.g. to phlegmatic or bilious people when burning with fever—this is a matter of art. (981a5–12)

At first, **5.5.b** may appear to put forward an eccentric, not to mention implausible, claim about the transparency of causal relations to everyday observation. After closer study, however, it reveals itself as the fifth-century seed of an idea that came to fruition with Aristotle. Unlike Aristotle, or for that matter Plato, our author will not admit that there is anything special about the knowledge by experience that arises from the observation of individual cases. Aristotle insisted that the man of experience often has the power to succeed where the man of *technē* does not (981a13–24), and Plato allowed that rhetoricians had some real knack, though he denied that this was an art (*Gorgias* 462b–c). Our author champions an even more restrictive view, according to which experience is a cheap commodity. There are only two intellectual castes: laypersons who know *that*, and experts who know *why* (cf. 1.2).[55] If the reasonableness of this distinction is granted, then the Strong Interpretation appears no less viable than the Weak.

[55] So Jouanna, who rejects Denniston's suggestion, is compelled to read Aristotle back into *de Arte* in differentiating between the skilled doctor, the ignorant layperson, and 'entre les deux se situe le malade qui, en s'étant guéri lui-même, a rencontré le savoir propre à l'art' (1988, 252).

**5.5** εἰ τοίνυν ἐπιστήσεται ἢ ἐπαινεῖν ἢ ψέγειν ὁ νοσήσας τῶν διαιτημάτων τι οἷσιν ὑγιάνθη, πάντα ταῦτα τῆς ἰητρικῆς ἐστι, 'so if the sick person knows how to praise or blame any of the components of regimen by which he recovered, then all these belong to medicine' [**5.5.c**]: the invocation of praise and blame reflects how closely the terms of causal analysis were tied to their juridical origins (cf. 4.3),[56] though one should note that slippage between concepts of moral or legal responsibility and scientific causation occurs even today. In any case, causation is the subject here in **5.5.c**, which encapsulates the main argument of the chapter.

1. If a layperson recovers without a doctor, then, though he did not know in advance what would improve his condition, he knows in retrospect that something improved his condition (**5.5.a**).
2. If he knows that something caused his recovery, then he knows there is something with the power to effect patient recovery.
3. Therefore, by the first condition of the tripartite definition given at 3.2, if a layperson recovers without a doctor, he knows medicine exists.

As it stands, the argument is consistent with the Weak Interpretation, but it is out of step with the text on two separate but related points. First, it makes no mention of regimen or dietetic components. Second, while the conclusion in 3 demonstrates that medicine exists in one sense, it falls short of proving the author's thesis, given at 5.2, that those who recover without a doctor hit upon 'by chance the very treatments that would have been applied had they consulted a doctor.' Given the definition of medicine at 3.2, the author understands that his task in fully rebutting the critics is two-fold: first, he must show that the set of events or objects picked out by the definition is non-empty; second, he must show that this set is roughly identical with the set of events or objects (or a subset thereof) to which the term 'medicine' is actually applied in practice. To effectively counter the charge that medicine is not, it is not enough for him to establish that fasting cures a certain kind of fever; fasting must also be just what the doctor (would have) ordered.[57]

Let us recast the argument, then, in terms friendly to the Strong Interpretation, with particular emphasis on its deviations from the Weak version above.

---

[56] See further Vegetti 1999.

[57] Jori's distinction between 'medicine as such' and 'medicine professionally characterized' represents an attempt to articulate the two-fold task (1996, 168), though it suggests, incorrectly, that our author is wielding the word 'medicine' in two different senses.

1'. *Every person whose condition improves knows precisely what caused the improvement* (5.5.b).
2'. If a layperson recovers without a doctor, then, though he did not know in advance what would cure him, he knows in retrospect *precisely what caused his recovery* (*call it* c) *and, further, it will be the case that* c *was a component of his regimen* (5.5.a).
3'. If he knows that c caused his recovery, then he knows that c has the power to effect patient recovery.
4'. Therefore, by the first condition of the tripartite definition given at 3.2, if a layperson recovers without a doctor, he knows medicine exists *in virtue of the dietetic components of which he made use.*

This version of the argument stays closer to the text and is on the whole more cogent. Moreover, it puts our author in a considerably better position to argue that the recovered person made use of what the doctor would have ordered, had he been consulted, though he will not state this conclusion explicitly until 6.1.

I am inclined, then, to endorse the Strong Interpretation as the stronger interpretation of c. 5, though, whichever alternative one adopts, it is interesting that both turn on the knowledge attributable to the recovered person. One could be forgiven for thinking that the author's best counter to his critics would not depend at all on the content of the recovered person's propositional attitudes. Rather, one might expect a simpler argument such as the following.

1". Some people recover without consulting a physician (5.1).
2". In each case, some component of regimen will have been the cause of the recovery.
3". Thus, there will have been something with the causal power to effect patient recovery.
4". Therefore, by the first condition of the tripartite definition given at 3.2, medicine exists in virtue of the dietetic components of which use was made.

If the earlier arguments were sound, then, *a fortiori*, this one will be sound, as well, and we are probably meant to feel its weight even without hearing it. Why does our author go to the extra trouble? As he did in c. 4, he moves beyond the obvious response to an abstract theoretical objection to build a dialectical trap for an antagonist situated within the scenario described by the theoretical objection. When faced with the objection that, because not all who are treated recover, those who recover do so by chance, he first disposes of the general complaint and then proceeds to make a special dialectical argument that will apply to a person who, having himself recovered following treatment, credits his recovery to chance. Here in c. 5, instead of answering the critic directly with the simple argument above, he assembles an elaborate dialectical argument from which the simple argument may be extracted but which will have special resonance for the person who has recovered without a doctor. *De Arte* appears designed not just to offer a general theoretical defense of medicine, but also to provide ammunition for the doctor forced to fight against the protests of mendacious patients and lying laypersons, whose public recriminations contradict what they themselves know, or at least believe, to be true.

Finally, note that my reconstruction of the above arguments makes reference only to dietetic components that contribute to recovery (and thus deserve praise) but does not mention components that inhibit recovery or worsen the sick person's condition (and so deserve blame). Indeed, it seems odd to blame some part of the regimen by which one recovered, and this has prompted some to emend the text. Ermerins inserts ἢ ἐβλάβη after ὑγιάνθη, while Heiberg adds ἢ οὐχ ὑγιάσθη. The latter should be ruled out on the grounds that the instrumental dative οἷσιν suggests that the dietetic components had some real effect, even if an undesirable one, not that they were causally inefficacious with respect to recovery. Moreover, as Jouanna observes, the chapter's emphasis on cases of recovery speaks against the emendation (1988, 252). Ermerins' interpolation is vulnerable to the same objection and, in addition, is thematically problematic. If 'blaming' correlates to 'harming,' then our author is claiming that harmful dietetic measures are a part of medicine, which runs afoul of both common sense and the tripartite definition of medicine. Indeed, in the next few lines the author will argue that harm done to a patient demonstrates the existence of medicine precisely because they do *not* belong to medicine correctly practiced.

Instead, I propose that we understand the phrase τῶν διαιτημάτων τι οἷσιν ὑγιάνθη to refer to what I have called the 'dietetic axes' integral to the metric principle of therapeutics (see notes on 5.4 above). Thus, food consumption is a dietetic axis, as is bathing, sleeping, etc. By praising fasting for contributing to the improvement of his condition, one concedes the causal relevance of food consumption levels to his health. Likewise, to blame oversleeping for inhibiting one's (eventual) improvement is to concede the causal relevance of the sleep axis, implying that there is an appropriate measure of sleep, even if one has failed to hit it. It is in this sense that blaming a dietetic component will secure its status as a part of medicine.

**5.5 καὶ ἔστιν οὐδὲν ἧσσον τὰ ἁμαρτηθέντα τῶν ὠφελησάντων μαρτύρια τῇ τέχνῃ ἐς τὸ εἶναι**, 'the mistakes of medicine, too, no less than the benefits, are testimonies to its being': again we encounter legal terminology, as μαρτύριον would have been a word familiar from the law courts, where it referred primarily to evidence gleaned from witness testimony or the testimony itself. In his defense of medicine, our author is turning the prosecution's own witness (i.e., medical failure) against it.

In so doing, he appears to sacrifice the reputation of the doctor, who, he freely admits, makes mistakes, though it is possible that the argument remains purely hypothetical: if doctors make mistakes, then there is an art of medicine (see notes on 5.6 below). This is the treatise's most explicit expression of the distinction between the doctor and the art he practices. That the doctor sometimes gets it wrong surely impugns his medical expertise; that there is something to get wrong surely implies medicine's existence. This is true even in the most extreme form of physician error, iatrogenic harm. The argument differs importantly from what precedes; no longer is our author contemplating the situation of sick people who have recovered without consulting a doctor. Nor does the argument turn simply on issues of causal responsibility. What connects this new argument to the foregoing is the notion of blame, which in **5.5.c** is used to indicate causal responsibility. Here, the notion resurfaces in our author's reference to mistakes, τὰ ἁμαρτηθέντα, for which the patient will hold the doctor accountable. But blaming a doctor for harming a patient raises questions not just of causal responsibility but also of conformity to some normative standard, and it is to the question of such standards that our author now turns.

**5.5 τὰ μὲν γὰρ ὠφελήσαντα τῷ ὀρθῶς προσενεχθῆναι ὠφέλησε, τὰ δὲ βλάψαντα τῷ μηκέτι ὀρθῶς προσενεχθῆναι ἔβλαψε**, 'for what is beneficial brings benefit through correct application, while what is harmful causes harm through incorrect application' (**5.5.d**): the benefit-harm antithesis recalls characterizations of the two-fold *telos* of medicine such as that found in the *Epidemics* (see notes on 3.2): to benefit and not to harm. However one understands the notion of benefit, no doctor, including the doctor who operates under our author's tripartite definition, would defend iatrogenic harm under any circumstances. Reference to the *telos* is crucial for establishing the guidelines for correct and incorrect procedure. Whatever causal means achieve the *telos* are correct; whatever hinders or contravenes that same *telos* is incorrect. The incorrect, then, is logically parasitic upon the correct, and in fact the incorrect procedure that harms the patient implies the existence of a minimally correct procedure, namely, non-performance of the harmful procedure. In cases where it would be possible to provide palliative care or even a complete cure, there will be maximally correct procedures that constitute a proper subset of the minimally correct, but that is peripheral to our author's immediate concern. Most important is the fact that allegations of iatrogenic harm implies the existence of and difference between the correct and incorrect.

**5.6** καίτοι ὅπου τό τε ὀρθὸν καὶ τὸ μὴ ὀρθὸν ὅρον ἔχει ἑκάτερον, πῶς τοῦτο οὐκ ἂν τέχνη εἴη, 'and where the correct and incorrect each has its own determination, how could this not be art' (**5.6.a**): when our author writes that art is implied by the existence of a border between the correct and incorrect (ὅρον ἔχει ἑκάτερον), this is not just a way of saying that the arts include some notion of correct and incorrect procedure. Rather, he means, first, that such procedures exist and, second, that the classes of correct and incorrect procedures should not overlap. Thus, one might paraphrase **5.6.a** as follows: for any specific *telos*, t, if in a particular case there are both determinably correct and incorrect procedures for achieving t, then the case falls within the scope of a *technē*.

As noted in the Introduction (section 1), a *technē* was supposed to possess clear guidelines as to what was correct procedure and what was incorrect procedure. One might go further and say, as does our author, that, insofar as the existence of correct and incorrect procedures implies both a coherent *telos* and the physical possibility of achieving that *telos* by causal means, they provide a sufficient condition for the existence of an art. This of course leaves aside the question of whether any doctors actually know which procedures are correct and incorrect, a question that must be answered if the critics are to be refuted in full. Still, it secures a necessary step in that refutation, and it does so using a premise that one would expect to find at the heart of the critics' argument: doctors sometimes harm patients.

The argument in its entirety runs as follows.

1. For any procedure, p, performed by a doctor in a particular case, if p harms the patient, then p is determinably incorrect and there is some determinable set of minimally correct procedures, namely, all those that do not include performing p (**5.5.d**).
2. With respect to the *telos* of avoiding harm, if in a particular case there are both determinably correct and incorrect procedures for achieving it, then the case falls within the scope of medicine (from **5.6.a**).
3. Therefore, for any procedure, p, performed by a doctor in a particular case, if p harms the patient, then the case falls within the scope of medicine.

If medicine finds application in real cases, then clearly it exists. Thus, anyone who accuses a doctor of harming a patient implies thereby the existence of medicine and cannot, at least not without contradiction, assert that it does not.

**5.6** τοῦτο γάρ ἔγωγέ φημι ἀτεχνίην εἶναι ὅπου μήτε ὀρθὸν ἔνι μηδὲν μήτε οὐκ ὀρθόν, ὅπου δὲ τούτων ἔνεστιν ἑκάτερον, οὐκέτι ἂν τοῦτο ἔργον ἀτεχνίης εἴη, 'there is artlessness, I claim, where there is neither correctness nor incorrectness; but where each of these is present, the work of artlessness would be absent' (**5.6.b**): the sentence structure echoes that of 2.2 and serves to emphasize the logical interdependence of the contradictory antitheses under discussion, namely, τέχνη-ἀτεχνίη and τὸ ὀρθόν-τὸ μὴ ὀρθόν. I follow Jones' contrast between 'present' and 'absent' to reflect the paraphrastic alpha-privative formulations of the Greek (1923, 199). The noun ἔργον deserves special attention, too, since the oxymoron it engenders together with ἀτεχνίης is striking. For the Greeks, the arts were precisely those crafts aimed at producing some product. 'Lack of art' would denote, among other things (see my notes on 2.2), the inability to properly produce such a product. In English, I hope that 'work of artlessness,' as a pun on the phrase 'work of art,' captures the paradox without misleading.

Shorn of its poetic adornments, **5.6.b** can be analyzed into two distinct claims:

1. for any specific *telos*, t, if in a particular case there are neither determinably correct nor incorrect procedures for achieving t, then the case does not fall within the scope of a *technē*; and
2. for any specific *telos*, t, if in a particular case there are both determinably correct and incorrect procedures for achieving t, then the case falls within the scope of a *technē*.

This adds little of substance to the overall argument, though it does explain the occurrence of γὰρ in **5.6.b**, since 2 above is identical to **5.6.a** and so obviously is deducible from the conjunction of 1 and 2.

## 6

In c. 6 our author shows more restraint, in rhetorical terms, than he will in the following sections, and he devotes less effort to impugning the character of the critics (though he does imply at 6.2 that they are more ignorant even than laypersons). Again he gives two distinct *pisteis*. First, he defends against the anticipated objection that, even if dietetic measures can cure disease, the medical community's dependence on drug therapy entails that in practice doctors are ignorant of medicine, or at least of a significant part of it. Second, he counters the charge that recoveries are utterly spontaneous—they do not have any cause or explanation whatsoever.

Stylistically, the chapter is dominated by syntactical symmetry (e.g., ὑπὸ φαρμάκων τῶν τε καθαιρόντων καὶ τῶν ἱστάντων in 4.1; ἐν τοῖσι πλείστοισι τῶν τε φυομένων καὶ τῶν ποιευμένων in 4.3) and antithesis (οὐσίην ἔχον οὐδεμίαν ἀλλ' ἢ ὄνομα in 6.4), repetition (e.g., γινόμενον ... γινόμενον and φαίνεταί τε καὶ φανεῖται in 6.4), and the occasional alliterative outburst (e.g., ὅπου οὖν οὐδὲν οὔτ' ἐν τοῖσιν ἀγαθοῖσι τῶν ἰητρῶν οὔτ' ἐν τῇ ἰητρικῇ αὐτῇ ἀχρεῖόν ἐστιν in 6.3).

**6.1** ἔτι τοίνυν εἰ μὲν ὑπὸ φαρμάκων τῶν τε καθαιρόντων καὶ τῶν ἱστάντων ἡ ἴησις τῇ τε ἰητρικῇ καὶ τοῖσιν ἰητροῖσιν μοῦνον ἐγίνετο, ἀσθενὴς ἦν ἂν ὁ ἐμὸς λόγος, 'still, if doctors and their art brought about cures only by means of purgative and binding drugs, my argument would be weak': the natural inclination is to see in ἀσθενὴς ἦν ἂν ὁ ἐμὸς λόγος a peculiarly sophistic concern for the strength of arguments, recalling the charge of 'making the weaker argument stronger,' which is leveled at Socrates in the *Apology* (18b) and which Aristotle associates with Protagoras at *Rh.* 1402a17 ff. That this particular phrase was in use among fifth-century orators and writers is attested to by the speech of Nicias at Thucydides 6.9: ἀσθενὴς ἂν μου ὁ λόγος εἴη. The adjective ἀσθενής, which could mean 'weak' in the sense of 'sick,' may be intended as a joke: if doctors cure only with drugs, then my argument is a hopeless case! Perhaps our author is comparing himself to a doctor: like the doctor who makes weak people stronger, he makes weak arguments stronger.

Commentators generally disagree on which λόγος our author has in mind. Ducatillon, following in the footsteps of Kudlien (1967, 134), maintains that in this chapter the author anticipates a new criticism, namely, that doctors limit themselves to prescribing only purgative and constipating substances as therapy (1977a, 52). However, a good doctor will advise a more complex therapy that involves changes to patient regimen; reliance on the most obvious and elementary drugs indicates a merely cursory grasp of the art, and here Ducatillon invokes Plato (1977a, 53).

> SOCRATES: All right, tell me this. Suppose someone came to your friend Eryximachus or his father Acumenus and said: "I know treatments to raise or lower (whichever I prefer) the temperature of people's bodies; if I decide to, I can make them vomit or make their bowels move, and all sorts of things. On the basis of this knowledge, I claim to be a physician;

> and I claim to be able to make others physicians as well by imparting it to them." What do you think they would say when they heard that?
> PHAEDRUS: What could they say? They would ask him if he also knew to whom he should apply such treatments, when, and to what extent.
> SOCRATES: What if he replied, "I have no idea. My claim is that whoever learns from me will manage to do what you ask on his own"?
> PHAEDRUS: I think they'd say the man's mad if he thinks he's a doctor just because he read a book or happened to come across a few potions; he knows nothing of the art.
> (*Phaedrus* 268a–c, trans. Nehamas and Woodruff in Cooper 1997)

Like inferior doctors in *de Arte*, the pharmacologist in the Platonic dialogue has discovered a few drugs that have certain effects. Certainly, Ducatillon is right that Plato wants a *technē* to be a fairly complex body of knowledge. However, Plato's criticism in the *Phaedrus* does not seem to be that the pharmacologist's knowledge is not complex enough in the sense that his therapeutic repertoire lacks variety. To the contrary, the pharmacologist is initially portrayed as a show-off, someone who claims to be able to make a body do whatever he wants by a variety of novel means. It is not that the pharmacologist uses too few remedies, but that he does not know how to apply those remedies to achieve the proper goal of his art.

Gomperz' interpretation follows much the same current, though at a slightly different pitch. He paraphrases: 'the probative force of his speech would be inferior, so believes our anonymous author, if the medical art relied only on those older methods of healing, comparably inferior in number, that eliminate the symptoms more than they remove the underlying causes' (1910, 116–117). Like Ducatillon, Gomperz takes λόγος to refer to the treatise as a whole, which is dedicated to proving the reality of medicine. Chapter 6 defends medicine against a new and specific charge: medicine relies on a mere handful of outdated therapies that treat the symptoms of diseases rather than their deeper causes. Gomperz' distinction between the treatment of symptoms and diseases is curious, since nothing in *de Arte* points us in this direction. It turns out, however, that he is more interested in pursuing the distinction between old, outmoded drugs and new, refined dietetic approaches. Plato, it seems, respected this distinction but preferred to conserve the old ways. Socrates criticizes the dietetic approach in his discussion with Glaucon in *Republic* III.

> Not if you recall that they say that the kind of modern medicine that plays nursemaid to the disease wasn't used by the Asclepiads before Herodicus. He was a physical trainer who became ill, so he mixed physical training with medicine and wore out first himself and then many others as well.
>
> How did he do that?

> By making his dying a lengthy process. Always tending to his mortal illness, he was nonetheless, it seems, unable to cure it, so he lived out his life under medical treatment, with no leisure for anything else whatever. If he departed even a little from his accustomed regimen, he became completely worn out, but because his skill made dying difficult, he lived into old age.
>
> That's a fine prize for his *technē*.
>
> One that's appropriate for someone who didn't know that it wasn't because he was ignorant or inexperienced that Asclepius failed to teach this type of medicine to his sons, but because he knew that everyone in a well regulated city has his own work to do and that no one has the leisure to be ill and under treatment all his life. It's absurd that we recognize this to be true of craftsmen while failing to recognize that it's equally true of those who are wealthy and supposedly happy.
>
> How is that?
>
> When a carpenter is ill, he expects to receive an emetic or purge from his doctor or to get rid of his disease through surgery or cautery. If anyone prescribed a lengthy regimen to him, telling him that he should rest with his head bandaged and so on, he'd soon reply that he had no leisure to be ill and that life is no use to him if he has to neglect his work and always be concerned with his illness. After that he'd bid good-bye to his doctor, resume his usual way of life, and either recover his health or, if his body couldn't withstand the illness, he'd die and escape his troubles.
>
> (406a–e, trans. Grube and Reeve in Cooper 1997)

Whether or not Plato is right that there was an older style of medicine that eschewed dietetic prescriptions—*Acut.* appears to second Plato (37.2–4 = L. 2.224)—there does seem to be some basis for the distinction between a method that embraced regimen in therapy and one that rejected it in favor of purgatives and surgery. Gomperz may be correct, then, that our author is taking sides in a contemporary debate, though his reasons for allying himself with dietetic medicine are not made explicit beyond the remark that doctors who employ such techniques are more celebrated. He is careful not to accuse the pharmacologists of being utterly worthless as doctors. Likewise, Plato does not allege that complicated dietetic prescriptions are ineffective; he concedes that Herodicus lived to a ripe old age. Rather, he thinks they are simply not worth the time and energy. The carpenter is better off dead than gingerly tending to a fragile body for the rest of his life, even if that life were a long one. Neither in Plato nor in *de Arte*, then, do we find a technical explanation as to why one method is to be preferred to the other. The *Republic* lacks such an explanation because it is beside the point, and we might suspect the same of *de Arte*. It will not do, in any case, to invent one, as does Gomperz.

Gomperz' fascination with Herodicus is understandable given his agenda: to persuade us that Protagoras or a Protagorean wrote *de Arte*. (Protagoras praises Herodicus at *Protagoras* 316e). Jouanna, too, cites the *Republic* passage, though mainly by way of contrast with the regimen-friendly *de Arte*. He gives more attention to the Hippocratic *Corpus*. *De Arte* follows other Hippocratic works in holding medicine to be 'a complex art that marries a diverse dietetics to pharmacology' (1988, 253). Jouanna cites *VM* as one treatise that 'denounces the simplifying theories of its adversaries and insists on the complexity of dietetics' (1988, 253). However, *VM* pursues those who 'reduce the principle of explanation for human disease and death, hypothesizing that it is the same one or two things in all cases' (118.4–6 = L. 1.570). This may well be a critique of simplification, but not of therapeutic simplification. And it is not simplification as such that is rejected. Simplification is rejected because it is generally wrong, and the author goes on in the ninth chapter of that treatise to detail the errors of the reductionists. He does not favor complexity for the sake of complexity. No doubt he would find complication just as problematic as simplification.

The Hippocratic treatise that comes closest to espousing the view Jouanna attributes to the author of *de Arte* is *Acut*. In the opening chapters, the author takes a work called the *Cnidian Sentences* to task.

> Whenever [the authors] discuss symptoms in order to determine how each disease ought to be treated, in these cases my judgment differs exceedingly from their account. Not only for this reason do I withhold my praise, but also because the remedies they applied were few in number. For they advised almost exclusively (except in cases of acute disease) the giving of purgative drugs and the drinking of milk and whey at the proper time.
> (36.11–15 = L. 2.224)

> Surprisingly, the ancients [presumably the Cnidian doctors, but maybe not] wrote nothing of value concerning regimen. And indeed they left out quite a bit. (37.2–4 = L. 2.224)

Perhaps, then, *Acut.* confirms Plato's story in the *Republic*. On the other hand, we should bear in mind that the Hippocratic author's distinction is less than firm. The Cnidians do employ more than the few remedies mentioned, just not on a regular basis (and it should be appreciated that milk and whey are not distinguished from drugs). What the ancients wrote about regimen was not particularly helpful. That does not mean that they wrote nothing at all.

The main obstacle to foisting the dietetic-pharmaceutical distinction on *de Arte* is that our author nowhere clearly distinguishes between two groups of practitioners or methods of practice. In fact, 6.1 asserts a counterfactual: *if* medicine and doctors cured only by drugs, my argument *would be* weak. This entails that doctors do not cure by drugs alone. After all, as he will state at 6.2, neither doctor nor layperson would dare claim that regimen was not a form of medical treatment. Only the phrase 'most highly praised doctors' suggests some sort of contrast with an inferior group, but it need not. Our author simply and sensibly takes the more celebrated doctors as representative of the profession. As for the less celebrated, who really cares what their methods are? Perhaps their methods are the same as those of the most celebrated physicians but poorly applied. What matters is only that the reputable practitioners all employ changes in regimen as treatment.

Still, why does this matter? In my earlier comments on 5.5, I divided our author's project in that chapter into two components. He must show 1) that the set of events or objects picked out by the definition is non-empty; and 2) that this set is roughly identical with the set of events or objects (or a subset thereof) to which the term 'medicine' is actually applied in practice. In c. 5, he was concerned primarily with 1. Now he anticipates an objection based on the criterion in 2: what if medicine cured only with drugs? Then we would be faced with a case in which a recovered patient attributed his recovery to some genuinely effective procedures, namely those included in his regimen, though these procedures were not the sort of thing prescribed by physicians. That is, 1 would hold though 2 would fail. However, since doctors make use of regimen, a potentially fatal objection to 2 is thwarted, clearing the way for our author's claim at 5.2 that self-recovered patients recovered not just by using medicine but by using what a doctor would have prescribed. Thus, these first few sentences of c. 6 are intended just to sure up 2, not to extol medicine's complexity or comprehensiveness, as most scholars have supposed.

Jori is to my knowledge the only commentator who has correctly discerned the thrust of our author's argument here (1996, 178), though we must still explain why our author would worry about such an objection in the first place. Who would think that medicine did not include dietetic measures? Or, to put it another way, why do drugs pose a special problem for our author? It may be that the above passages from Plato and the *Corpus* indicate that medicine had a long-standing association with pharmacology in the public mind. Jori further suggests that drugs, as synthetic products, must be produced and administered intentionally and strategically; one cannot happen upon them simply by chance (1996, 177). However, Hippocratic pharmacology shows us that many drugs were not synthetic in the required sense, but rather were completely natural and utterly mundane.[58] Moreover, there is no textual evidence that our author conceives of drugs as primarily synthetic (see further my notes on 6.3 below). Usually ignored, however, is the fact that the hypothetical objection refers not to drugs generally, but specifically to purgative and binding drugs, though these two categories are by no means exhaustive of ancient Greek pharmacology.[59] Presumably, they are singled out because they would not be included in a typical regimen and so would not be chanced upon by a sick person.

**6.2** οὐδὲ ἰδιώτης ἀνεπιστήμων ἀκούσας, 'nor unknowledgeable layperson (provided the latter had even heard of them)': the layperson's lack of knowledge is a recurrent theme in *de Arte* (cf. 5.2 and especially 11.4). A non-professional might be ignorant of what is correct and incorrect in medicine, but even he will know what sorts of things doctors prescribe. The participle ἀκούσας is probably conditional ('if he had heard (of the treatments)'); the only limit to the layperson's ability to identify elements of the doctor's therapeutic repertoire is his exposure to medical practice. It is possible, however, that ἀκούσας could mean 'upon hearing (of the treatments)', though this would yield a much stronger, and less plausible, claim.

**6.3** οὖν οὐδὲν οὔτ' ἐν τοῖσιν ἀγαθοῖσι τῶν ἰητρῶν οὔτ' ἐν τῇ ἰητρικῇ αὐτῇ ἀχρεῖόν ἐστιν, 'nothing is useless for good doctors or for medicine itself': the distinction between good doctors and the art itself depends again on the two-fold task outlined above (see notes on 6.1 and 5.5). Whatever procedure the sick person uses to heal himself will be something a good doctor, i.e., one who has broad knowledge of correct and incorrect procedure in medicine, would have recommended. Even if this is not the case, the procedure will belong to medicine proper, insofar as it is a correct procedure. In fact, everything one could do to one's body is a potential medical procedure insofar as it will have some effect on the body and thus could play some role in a causal process that brought about one of the ends of the art.

Notice the re-emergence of poetic affectation in our author's language, specifically in the alliterative assonance of οὖν οὐδὲν οὔτ' and the metrical balance of the two οὔτε clauses (12 syllables per).

---

[58] In fact, Greek medical writers were at pains to clearly distinguish foods from drugs. See Scarborough 1983 for an account of the theoretical background of Hippocratic pharmacology that validates the general description in *de Arte*.

[59] However, Plato gives them special attention in the passages from the *Republic* and the *Phaedrus*, and, as Craik observes (1998, 234), the author of *Loc. Hom.* regards them as the two main types of drug (see Introduction 4).

**6.3** ἐν τοῖσι πλείστοισι τῶν τε φυομένων καὶ τῶν ποιευμένων ἔνεστιν τὰ εἴδεα τῶν θεραπειῶν καὶ τῶν φαρμάκων, 'forms of treatments and drugs are present in most things, both natural and synthetic': this is the second occurrence of εἶδος in c. 6 and the last occurrence in the treatise overall. Gillespie is not wrong when he translates the term at 6.2 as 'kind' and here at 6.3 as 'nature' (1912, 197), though I use the English 'form' to preserve continuity within the treatise and to emphasize that we are dealing not with different meanings of εἶδος as our author conceives it, but rather with different aspects of a central, unified concept. 'Natural kind' would be in many respects the best translation, so long as we understand that this includes anything that has causal power *qua* the type of thing that it is. Accordingly, 6.2 depends on the 'kind' in 'natural kind,' whereas 6.3 depends on the kind's being 'natural.' The natures of therapies and drugs are present in all (ἐν τοῖσι πλείστοισι must be literary understatement) the things that grow and are made. This means just that some subset of a thing's causal powers—whether it be a natural or synthetic thing—will be relevant to healing the human body when applied in a certain way, some as drugs and some otherwise. Moreover, and more important for the argument as it will unfold (see following note), the actions of these treatments and drugs will be explicable and, thus, predictable.

It is tempting to follow Jori in reading a conceptual connection into the syntactic parallels between τῶν φυομένων and τῶν θεραπειῶν, on the one hand, and τῶν ποιευμένων and τῶν φαρμάκων on the other (1996, 178 n. 35). The implication would be that therapies are natural, while drugs are synthetic, contrived, or artificial. That Hippocratic medicine routinely used natural substances as drugs should suffice to refute this reading, though I would also add that, strictly speaking, the forms of *both* therapies and drugs are said to be present in *both* natural and synthetic things. The case for a stronger conceptual correlation between drugs and synthetics would require a stronger grammatical correlation. At the very least, one would expect a τε-καί contruction in the text: τὰ εἴδεα τῶν τε θεραπειῶν καὶ τῶν φαρμάκων.

**6.3** οὐκ ἔστιν ἔτι οὐδενὶ τῶν ἄνευ ἰητροῦ ὑγιαζομένων τὸ αὐτόματον αἰτιήσασθαι, 'not a single person who has recovered without a doctor can still give the credit to spontaneity': we encounter again the verb αἰτιᾶσθαι meaning 'to hold responsible' or 'to identify as cause' (the first occurrence is at 4.3), though here it has the unusually positive sense of 'give credit to.' As discussed, the verb and its cognates, αἰτία and αἴτιος, eventually became the primary terms of Greek causal analysis, though they started out with legal and moral connotations of blame. But blame does not map neatly onto all instances of causation, and for obvious reasons: often we want to identify something as a cause though we do not want to blame it for anything. *De Arte* is a case in point. Our author wants to hold medicine responsible for patients' recovery, but he does not seek to defame medicine. We are much closer, then, to a purely causal investigation than a moral or legal one. On the other hand, our author is clearly exploiting the forensic connotations of αἰτιᾶσθαι (but more so in c. 4, of which the use in c. 5 is an echo) for rhetorical effect. Thus, the term finds novel 'scientific' application while retaining its courtroom cachet.

Indeed, causation continues to be the pressing concern, as indicated by the sudden introduction of τὸ αὐτόματον, or spontaneity, which commands our attention insofar as it serves as a concrete point of contact with other works in the Hippocratic *Corpus*.[60]

> When patients discharge blood spontaneously (ἀπὸ ταὐτόματου) this indicates a rupture of the vessel in the kidney. (*Aph.* 4.530.10–11)

> If the spinal marrow is diseased either from a fall, or from some other πρόφασις, or spontaneously (ἀπὸ αὐτόματου), the person loses control over his legs, so that when touched he does not feel it, and loses control over his stomach and bladder, so that for the first few days he passes no stool or urine, except under compulsion. (*Prorrh.* 2 9.42.9–13)

Spontaneity might be understood in different ways, however, as *Alim.* demonstrates: "humors degrading both the whole and part, both from without and from within, spontaneous (αὐτόματον) and not spontaneous: spontaneous to us, but not spontaneous as far as the cause (αἰτία) is concerned" (141.20–23 = L. 9.102). We are faced not with two different senses of the term spontaneity so much as with two different aspects that arise when αὐτόματον (which in Greek applies to anything that occurs of itself or on its own) is employed in two distinct contexts. The first aspect is epistemic: spontaneous events have causes, but their causes are difficult to discern because, being internal to the human body or whatever dynamic system is under consideration, they are unobservable in practice, even if not in principle. The second aspect is metaphysical: spontaneous events are categorically uncaused.[61]

---

60 There is one piece of evidence in support of τὸ αὐτόματον as a legal category. In Lysias' *Against Andocides*, the speaker demands: καὶ τούτων πότερα τοὺς θεοὺς χρὴ ἢ τὸ αὐτόματον αἰτιᾶσθαι (6.25).

61 I shall leave aside for now Aristotle's more nuanced notion of τὸ αὐτόματον as described in the second book of his *Physics*. See Johnson (2010) and Mann (2010) for a comparison of the

Many Hippocratic writers clearly use τὸ αὐτόματον of internally generated—but nonetheless causally determined—phenomena.

> But whenever bile breaks out spontaneously (αὐτόματον) up and down, without any purgative or emetic drug, it is more difficult to stop. For the spontaneous flow is compelled by a force within the body, while a drug-induced flow is not compelled by an innate (συγγενής) force.
>
> (*Loc. Hom.* 72.12–15 = L. 6.326.1–4)

But other instances of spontaneity are not so transparently epistemic. Events that occur spontaneously are often contrasted with those that occur with a πρόφασις: 'a little better than these are such [pupils] as are clearly smaller or broader, or are angled, whether such conditions arise from a πρόφασις or are spontaneous (αὐτόμαται)' (*Prorrh. 2* 9.48.4–6). Much turns on what is meant by πρόφασις. The exact meaning and origin of the word is a vexed question among scholars. The prevailing view gives it primarily epistemic significance ('evident cause'), though it is possible also that its epistemic value lay partly in its temporal antecedence to the effect, in which case the qualifier 'without a πρόφασις,' which occurs at various places in the *Corpus*, will have metaphysical implications.[62]

For his part, our author rejects metaphysical and epistemic spontaneity in virtue of the arguments in c. 5 that every recovery comes about through doing or not doing something, and further that the recovered person can and ought to recognize exactly what it was that did so. Despite initial appearances, the argument of 6.3 does not merely continue the same line of thought but rather addresses a third aspect of τὸ αὐτόματον: explanatory

---

Aristotelian and Hippocratic views on spontaneity. A recent and insightful discussion of the Hippocratic notion, which complements some of my remarks here, can be found in Holmes (2010, 142–147).

[62] On the connection between πρόφασις and evidence (e.g., to the senses), see the linguistic studies in Deichgräber (1933), Pearson (1952), Rawlings (1975) and Irigoin (1983), as well as the discussions in Weidauer (1954) and Rechenauer (1991). Cochrane (1929) and Kirkwood (1952) stress the temporal antecedence of a πρόφασις with respect to its effect, though in his 1972 Pearson objects that 'one would have expected that if πρόφασις means τὸ πρφαινόμενον the medical writers would use the verb προφαίνεσθαι to describe how a symptom 'revealed itself in advance' … but I have not found a single instance of προφαίνεσθαι.' (392). However, Pearson may be refuted by a passage in *Dieb. Judic.* (9.276.18). Hankinson (1987) illuminates the ways in which evidence, antecedence and externality were combined in the Galenic notion of an antecedent cause, and it is suggestive that Galen himself saw the Hippocratic term as the forerunner of his αἴτιον προκαταρκτικόν (*De Causis Procatarcticus* 1.6–7). References to diseases or conditions that arise without a πρόφασις include, among others, *Aph.* 4.548.1–4 and *Morb. Sacr.* 3.9 = L. 6.354.

spontaneity, according to which an event has known causes, though these causes cannot be systematically understood so as to make them subject to intentional intervention. When I take an aspirin for the sudden sharp pain radiating down my left arm and notice that the pain disappears, I know (let us suppose) that the aspirin caused my recovery. Nonetheless, no one would say that I now have the capacity to exercise rational control over the health of those suffering a heart attack. The proper treatment for a heart attack remains, at least in relation to my understanding of the subject, 'on its own.' Moreover, if aspirin therapy found no place in the canon of standard medical interventions appropriate to heart attacks, this would suggest that medical science, at least in its current state, also lacked a detailed and comprehensive understanding of the subject. It is also consistent with the skeptical charge that medicine *could not* ever come by such an understanding. Against this sort of objection, our author responds that 'nothing is useless for good doctors or for medicine itself,' a direct, if unsupported, denial of explanatory spontaneity. But if nothing is categorically explanatorily spontaneous, then, *ipso facto*, nothing will be metaphysically spontaneous, since the explanation of an event is knowable just in case it has causes. Thus, he concludes, 'not a single person who has recovered without a doctor can still give the credit to spontaneity,' by which he means metaphysical spontaneity, or, in the language of *Alim.*, spontaneity 'as far as the cause is concerned.'

**6.3** ὀρθῷ λόγῳ, 'by a correct account': the phrase has sophistic origins, though it penetrated philosophical vernacular deeply enough so that Aristotle was comfortable using it as a term of art (e.g., *EN* 1119a20). Protagoras is reported to have employed it in a conversation with Pericles.

> When an athlete unintentionally struck Epitimus the Pharsalian with a javelin and killed him, Pericles spent an entire day with Protagoras puzzling over whether one should believe that the javelin or the javelin-thrower or those who arranged the contest were more to blame [αἴτιος], according to the most correct account [κατὰ τὸν ὀρθότατον λόγον].
>
> (Plutarch, *Pericles* 36.3, trans. Woodruff and Gagarin 1995)

Gorgias uses the expression ὀρθῶς λέξαι in his defense of Helen (DK 82 B11 §1), and Plato has him utter the phrase ὀρθῶς λέγων at *Gorgias* 450b. An exact parallel to *de Arte* is found in Antiphon's *Truth*: 'painful things do not, on a correct account [ὀρθῷ λόγῳ] benefit nature more than those that bring joy' (F44(a)IV.7–13). A correct account is an explanation or description that is proper to the *explanandum*, and we can say at least that the author means to contrast his own account with other, incorrect ones.

**6.4** τὸ μὲν γὰρ αὐτόματον οὐδὲν φαίνεται ἐὸν, 'for it is evident that spontaneity is nothing at all': our author presents another and yet stronger reason for rejecting claims of metaphysically spontaneous recovery: there is no such thing as spontaneity. Some readers may share Gomperz' worries (1910, 19–20) over the apparent incongruity of 6.4 with c. 2, where our author argued that the critics of medicine cannot say of *technē* that it 'is not' without involving themselves in some sort of absurdity. Should the same not go for τὸ αὐτόματον? Gomperz displays genuine alarm at the problem, but he is at the same time confident that our author possesses too subtle a mind to commit such an obvious blunder. Instead, he concludes, 'the doctrine that leads to such contradictory consequences in the mind of its author was accompanied by restrictions and qualifications that are unknown to us' (1910, 20). In a footnote, he conjectures that for the author of *de Arte* τὸ αὐτόματον is a relational concept and not therefore subject to the same criteria as substantive concepts like *technē* (1910, 161 n. 20.1). Gomperz is right to look for an explanation, but his strikes me as an *ad hoc* solution to a problem that poses only a minor threat once we appreciate his qualification of the claim (see additional notes on 6.4 below).

**6.4** ἐλεγχόμενον, 'upon examination': the verb ἐλέγχειν is yet another legal term (it occurs eighteen times in Antiphon's tetralogies) loosely equivalent to our modern legal idea of cross-examination. In a law court, a defendant might cross-examine a witness or accuser. Or he might examine testimony. The point of cross-examining a witness is of course to de-legitimize the damaging parts of his testimony by showing them to be inconsistent, either with other parts of the witness's own testimony, or with established fact. The cognate ἔλεγχος is the name given to Socrates' method of examining the beliefs of his interlocutors to expose inconsistencies, and *de Arte* undertakes to demonstrate that belief in the spontaneous is inconsistent with our experience of the world.

**6.4** πᾶν γαρ τὸ γινόμενον διά τι εὑρίσκοιτ' ἂν γινόμενον, 'since everything that comes to be would be discovered to do so because of something': the principle of universal causation invoked—that everything comes to be because of something else—indicates a turn to the topic of metaphysical spontaneity. But as will become clear, he will deny that spontaneity exists in any of its forms. The world is fundamentally intelligible in terms of explanatory relationships between events. (That this intelligibility is expressed with the formula τὸ διά τι, instead of, for instance, τὸ ἐκ τίνος, may be significant in that it reveals an intuitive awareness of the distinction between intensional and extensional contexts.) This being the case, there will be no event whose cause or explanation is a brute unknown. An event may be inexplicable relative to a certain person at a certain time—that is, as the Hippocratics recognized, we cannot explain everything all the time—but it does not follow that such events are categorically spontaneous. Thus, by taking on the issue of metaphysical spontaneity, our author hopes to undermine an argument for spontaneity in any of its pernicious aspects.

The optative verb εὑρίσκοιτ' perhaps suggests an inductive argument for the principle of universal causation articulated here. Surely not everything that has or will come to be can be examined, but, if it could, it *would be* discovered to have come to be because of something. Presumably, then, what has already been examined has been discovered to have been caused, and this warrants the inductive generalization to all things. In short, everything so far experienced functions as part of the chain of causes and effects. Hence, if we could examine every phenomenon, we would find out that they all had causes. If everything has a cause, then uncaused, that is, spontaneous, phenomena, do not exist.

**6.4** τὸ αὐτόματον οὐ φαίνεται οὐσίην ἔχον οὐδεμίαν ἀλλ' ἢ ὄνομα, 'spontaneity evidently has no being other than a name': our author's claim is not that the spontaneous is not, but rather that it has no being (that is, no property that would justify the application of a linguistic predicate; see notes on 2.1) other than a name. He takes advantage of what is now commonly called the 'use-mention distinction' in language to sidestep any statement about spontaneity as such. The term 'spontaneous' has being; it is a name. But, since the set of spontaneous events is empty, it is a mere name that fails to refer to anything. Indeed, consistent with the principle voiced at 2.2 that the things-that-are-always are always seen, his claim is open to empirical verification. Speakers of Greek regularly use the word αὐτόματον. Further, there is nothing in the world that happens without a cause. These two empirical facts are enough both to justify his conclusion that 'the spontaneous' is a mere name and to avoid the trap into which the critics fall by alleging that medicine or *technē* is not. (See also my comments on the author's theory of the correctness of names at 2.3.)

The author's use of οὐσίη betrays its relation to an originally literary antithesis wherein οὐσίη was contrasted with ὄνομα. Consider a case from Euripides' *Heracles*, line 337 and following:

> O children, follow on foot your miserable mother
> to your paternal hall, where the property (οὐσίη)
> is controlled by others, but the name (ὄνομα) is yet ours.

We can begin to understand how the tragic antithesis could lead to a philosophical distinction of use to our author. Estate property gives importance to the man who owns it, turns him into a 'man of substance.' His name becomes associated with this property and, thus, with his political and economic power. In the lines from Euripides, the family name has become separated from the family property, just as in *de Arte* 'spontaneity' retains its name though it lacks a corresponding natural property. We see that οὐσίη maintains the tie to its literary origins while moving toward a decisively more abstract sense capable of taking on an increasingly theoretical role. A thing's οὐσίη is what belongs to it; it is the property that gives it significance. But here the significance in question is no longer political or economic, but ontological.

**6.4** ἐν τοῖσι διά τι, 'in virtue of things that come to be 'because of something'': the abstract phrase τὰ διά τι has about it an Aristotelian air that may prompt some to propose a post-Aristotelian date for *de Arte*. However, Gomperz is quick to point out first that comparable articular constructions are present already in Herodotus (τὰ κατὰ τὸν Τέλλον, 1.31) and Thucydides (ἐς τὸ πρὸς Σκιώνης, 4.130; ἀφεὶς τὸ ἐς τὴν Χῖον, 8.41), second that the harshness of τὰ διά τι is mitigated by the preceding διά τι. Thus, τὰ διά τι is just an expedient way for our author to refer back to this quality of occurring 'through something.' *De Arte* contains similar articular prepositional formulations elsewhere (τὰ κατὰ τὰς ἄλλας τέχνας ... τὰ κατὰ τὴν ἰητρικήν, 9.1), though these tend not to provoke as much controversy, presumably due to the fact that they do not as closely resemble Aristotelian formulations.

**6.4** ἐν τοῖσι προνοευμένοισι, 'in virtue of things known in advance': accurate prognosis was a central aim of medicine according to many Hippocratics, an aim that was for obvious reasons closely connected to the doctor's knowledge of how to correctly treat patients (see Introduction 1). Prognosis was usually grounded in the doctor's knowledge of a disease's causes, and so the juxtaposition of ἐν τοῖσι προνοευμένοισι alongside ἐν τοῖσι διά τι is not adventitious. The author means to contrast the prospective, explanatory understanding of the doctor, who knows in advance what will happen when certain treatments are applied, with the retrospective, causal knowledge of the layperson, to whom unexpected success seems spontaneous.

## 7

The questions concerning chance have been settled to our author's satisfaction, but the question of responsibility lingers, though its dynamic is reversed. Whereas in the previous three chapters our author argues that medicine is responsible for patient recoveries, here he is pressed to deny the doctor's responsibility for patient deaths. Our author knows the critics' complaint is unfounded; he dispatches it quickly with the observation that a patient's recovery is dependent on more than just the correctness of the doctor's prescription (7.1). But as in cc. 4 and 5, he quickly turns his attention to a second, more practical, *pistis*. Again, it is a question of who is αἴτιος, and our author proceeds as though defending medicine in a homicide case against the charge that medicine kills its patients, casting doubt on the adequacy of the prosecutor's λόγος. In essence, we, the jury, are to decide the guilt and innocence of two prime suspects, the doctor and the patient. The rhetoric escalates proportionally: witness his reliance on dubious εἰκός reasoning, his hyperbolic astonishment (θαυμάζω), calculated for dramatic effect, not to mention the preponderance of rhetorical questions, as well as the sudden surge in euphonic and metrical affectation, especially in the form of isocolon and paromoiosis (e.g., τοὺς μὲν δεόντως ἐπιτάσσειν, τοὺς δὲ εἰκότως ἀδυνατεῖν in 7.5).

Our author is perhaps counting on the religious echoes of ὑπουργεῖν (see introductory notes to c. 4) to serve as a subtle comparison of the sick man to the impious. The analogy works out well for the doctor. By implication, he is compared to a god. The obedience theme gives the first hint of a new military conceit that will expand in later chapters, especially cc. 11 and 12: the disease is the enemy against which the patient, as soldier, must fight by executing the commands of his general, the doctor.

**7.1** τοῖσι μὲν οὖν τῇ τύχῃ τὴν ὑγιείην προστιθεῖσι, τὴν δὲ τέχνην ἀφαιρέουσι, τοιαῦτ' ἄν τις λέγοι, 'someone could make such arguments against those who attribute health to chance and discredit the art': the recapitulation of the preceding chapters signals a transition to a new topic. In cc. 4–6, our author is preoccupied with challenges to medicine's role in bringing about recovery, both in cases where the sick person underwent medical treatment (c. 4) and in cases where he did not (c. 5–6). Here in c. 7, he returns to the question, originally broached at 4.1, of whether and to what extent the failure of medical treatment to contain or defeat a disease damages the credibility of the art.

7.1 ἐν τῇσι τῶν ἀποθνῃσκόντων συμφορῇσι, 'on the misfortunes of those who died': though our author claims to have closed the door on the arguments from chance, he reopens it a crack with the word συμφορή, which could mean simply 'outcome' but connotes also misfortune or bad luck, thereby foreshadowing his argument that patient recovery is determined not just by the actions of the doctor but also by various extrinsic circumstances for which the doctor cannot reasonably be held accountable.

7.1 τὴν τέχνην ἀφανίζοντας, 'denial of the art': the Greek verb ἀφανίζειν has no suitable English translation in this context. As a term of logical discourse, it indicates a rejection or denial, in this case the denial of medicine's existence, or at least of its efficacy in cases where a treated patient dies. It also echoes the verb φαίνεσθαι and its cognates, which are used throughout *de Arte* to emphasize the phenomenal evidence of a thing or fact, especially the art of medicine, whose existence is demonstrated through its visibility, in keeping with the principle articulated at 2.2. Medicine's existence is apparent to anyone with the eyes to see it. Denial of that fact would require one to obscure or conceal the obvious evidence for it.

7.1 τὴν μὲν τῶν ἀποθνῃσκόντων ἀκρασίην ἀναιτίην … τὴν δὲ τῶν τὴν ἰητρικὴν μελετησάντων σύνεσιν αἰτίην, 'the weakness of those who died … the intellect of medical practitioners': shall we read ἀκρασίην with M or ἀτυχίην with A? Most editors, including Jouanna, prefer ἀκρασίην, which can indicate a debility or weakness of some kind as well as a lack of self-control, both of which our author emphasizes as attributes of the sick patient. At 7.2 he writes that they are ἀδυνατεῖν, powerless, and he describes their loss of will to fight against the disease. Moreover, ἀκρασίη is blamed for various conditions elsewhere in the *Corpus* (it occurs 29 times throughout, with cognate forms occurring 154 times). So in the appendix to *Acut.*: 'one ought to give hellebore to those who flow from the head. But do not give it to those who suppurate internally from abscesses are a burst vessel, or because of weakness (ἀκρασίη) or some other strong cause (αἰτία)' (87.3–7 = L. 2.474–476; cf. *VM* 126.8–14 = L. 1.584, *Int.* 7.190.12–14, *Loc. Hom.* 66.5–8 = L. 6.316.15–18). By contrast, ἀτυχίη occurs only 4 times (its cognate forms 5 times), though one instance is promising as a parallel to *de Arte*: 'for they don't think that the external bandaging and exposure of the wound is responsible (αἴτιος), but rather some other mischance (ἀτυχίη)' (*Fract.* 3.500.9–11). The juridical language of c. 7 might argue for ἀτυχίη, which figures in legal arguments over responsibility for injury: 'again, while the victim suffered the misfortune (συμφορά), it is the striker who suffered the mischance (ἀτυχία) itself' (Antiphon 4.3.4; see also 3.4.10). Our author might have written ἀτυχίῃ as an attempt to turn the tables on those who credited chance with patient recovery: chance does deserve some credit after all—for patient mortality. However, the main argument of c. 7 will turn on the patient's inability to follow the doctor's prescriptions, and Jouanna is correct that one expects the author to point to some quality in the patient (1988, 254 n. 2). The patient's weakness of will is held responsible for his decline, and ἀκρασίην sets the agenda for the chapter.

Reading ἀκρασίην also yields a sophisticated polysemy. The word will encompass the patient's weakness on various levels, including the physical, intellectual and psychological. These forms of weakness will stand in contrast to the doctor's σύνεσις—his intellect (see 1.2), but also his self-discipline and presence of mind (cf. Plato, *Cratylus* 411a, where σύνεσις is grouped in the family of rational virtues that includes also φρόνησις and δικαιοσύνη). It may be that our author means to posit a necessary connection between intellectual virtue and ethical action: intelligence and self-control go hand-in-hand (see also my notes on 11.4). Moreover, reading ἀκρασίην results in near-homonymy with ἀκρησίην, 'bad mixture,' e.g. of humors (cf. *VM* 143.3–6 = L. 1.616). (In the Attic dialect, the homonymy would be perfect: ἀκρασίαν. Perhaps it is significant that A gives also the Attic form ξύνεσιν.) Consistent with his metric principle of therapeutics, which depends on achieving a dietetic balance between excess and deficiency, our author would appear to endorse some version of the theory that disease is due to an imbalance of factors within the body. Yet more intriguing is the fact that he holds both the patient's psychological and physical states responsible for his death. This raises the possibility of some further non-trivial relationship between the psychological and physical. If weakness of will is attributable to all who are sick, as it must be if the argument in c. 7 is to find broad application, then it stands to reason that self-control, or 'psychological health,' if you will, has physical health as a necessary condition. Indeed, our author will stress that the doctor is of healthy mind *and* body (7.3), though perhaps this is already encapsulated here in the word σύνεσις, which in its root meaning of 'unity' or 'union' might refer to the physical harmony of the healthy doctor in contrast to the sick person's imbalance.

We are left with a complete theory neither of disease nor of mind. We do not learn the author's views, if indeed he has views at all, on the basic causal mechanisms or powers that are out of balance when a person is sick (see also notes on cc. 10 and 12, as well as Introduction 4). Further, his incidental remarks on the relation between psychological and physical weakness are compatible with a range of views in the philosophy of mind, though it may rule out the sort of naïve dualism that Plato would have his Socrates defend in dialogues such as the *Phaedo*.

**7.1 τὰ μὴ δέοντα ἐπιτάξαι**, 'to give the wrong orders': literally, 'to order the things that are not appropriate,' i.e., to the situation, in view of the aims of the art. The phrase is common in technical contexts, including medical contexts. Comparable articular constructions occur 40 times in the *Corpus*, usually in the scope of verbs of doing (e.g., ποιεῖν) or applying (e.g., προσφέρειν).

Our author is addressing the possibility not that the doctor prescribed a treatment that harmed the patient and thereby caused his death, but rather that he did not prescribe what was required to return the patient to health. If indeed the critics are charging the doctor with giving the wrong orders, this is an implicit recognition that there are right orders (cf. 5.5–6). The question is whether the doctor has the means to discover them.

**7.1 [ὡς] τοῖσι δὲ νοσέουσιν οὐκ ἔστι τὰ προσταχθέντα παραβῆναι**, '[as though it were] impossible for the sick to deviate from the orders they are given': here lies the substantive premise of what the author will develop into an argument from εἰκός, or probability, in the remainder of the chapter. The death of a treated patient does not necessarily demonstrate the incompetence of the doctor or the inefficacy of standard medical procedure. Other factors, too, will determine whether a patient lives or dies, including at least the following:[63]

1. the accuracy of the doctor's knowledge, either general (e.g., the theoretical propositions on which standard medical procedure is based, or procedure *per se*) or specific (e.g., the particular patient's diagnosis);
2. the doctor's ability to formulate and articulate a prescribed treatment on the basis of his knowledge;
3. the patient's ability to understand the prescribed treatment; and
4. the patient's ability to follow the prescribed treatment.

Factors 1 and 2 will affect the doctor's ability to implement standard medical procedure, while 3 and 4 will affect the patient's ability to implement standard medical procedure as outlined by the doctor. Roughly, these two categories of factor correspond respectively to those intrinsic to the practice of the *technē* and those that are extrinsic. It should be noted that prima

[63] This is the force of Jori's observation that the failure to return to health implies either the doctor's failure to prescribe a cure or the patient's failure to carry it out, or in his logical notation: $\neg\gamma \rightarrow \neg\alpha_1 \vee \neg\alpha_2$ (1996, 195).

facie extrinsic factors such as the seriousness or strength of the disease are disqualified by definition, since in 3.2 our author stipulates that non-intervention is the proper response in such cases. The definition explains, too, the special role of patient mortality in the debate over medicine's existence: it cannot be assimilated under any medical *telos*. It is a clear-cut case of failure.

Of course, the intrinsic-extrinsic dichotomy itself does not guarantee that the doctor could not have made a mistake in a particular case. But surely the author's larger point is well taken: to argue convincingly that the doctor did indeed make such a mistake, more evidence will have to be presented than just the fact that the patient was under the doctor's care when he died. If this is all we know, we do not know enough to convict the doctor.

7.2 καὶ μὴν πολύ γε εὐλογώτερον τοῖσι κάμνουσιν ἀδυνατεῖν τὰ προστασσόμενα ὑπουργεῖν ἢ τοῖσιν ἰητροῖσι τὰ μὴ δέοντα ἐπιτάσσειν, 'in actual fact, it is far more probable that the sick are powerless to follow the orders they are given than it is that doctors give the wrong orders': the adjective εὐλογώτερον signals a sophistic argument from εἰκός, 'probability,' and it anticipates the literal εἰκός claim that will be made later at 7.5. (For more on εἰκός argumentation, see Introduction 2). Our author establishes in the preceding his major premise, namely, a disjunction between intrinsic and extrinsic factors as possible explanations for the patient's death. Here he gives the conclusion: extrinsic factors are the more likely explanation. It is important to understand what does not follow from this conclusion, even if it is justified (to the extent that we may speak of justification with respect to non-deductive inferences). It does not follow that the patient really is responsible for his own death, much less that no doctor is ever responsible for the death of his patient. At best, the conclusion gives some direction to those who, like a jury, are compelled to make a judgment without the benefit of all the relevant facts. Certainty is not, nor can it be, the standard. Accordingly, certainty was not the standard in Greek law courts. Even today, malpractice claims are tried in civil courts, where the standard is likelihood: whoever's story is the more probable, the more believable, the more likely to be true, wins the case. Investigations into fact for the purpose of attaining certainty have limited value in such courts, whether ancient or modern.

7.3 οἱ μὲν γὰρ ὑγιαινούσῃ γνώμῃ μεθ' ὑγιαίνοντος σώματος ἐγχειρέουσι, 'for the latter handle the situation with healthy mind and body': is there a necessary connection between practicing medicine and possessing a healthy mind? Our author may mean nothing more than that one may safely infer of a practicing physician that he is of sound mind simply in virtue of the fact that he is practicing. However, if, as I suggest above in my notes on 7.1, the mental is dependent upon—perhaps even determined by—the physical, then the doctor's healthy mind may be attributable on some level to his healthy body. Perhaps such a relation is subtly implied by using the same word, 'healthy,' to qualify both the doctor's body and mind, though certainly one might talk about the health of the mind without committing himself to some dependence of the mental on the physical (cf. Plato, *Gorgias*, 477bff.). In any case, the question returns: is there a necessary connection between practicing medicine and possessing a healthy body? Here it will help to look ahead to 11.4, where our author claims that, if a sick person knew the causes of his disease, he would not have fallen prey to it in the first place. Health, then, would be a mark of the truly expert doctor with adequate knowledge of diseases and their causes.

7.3 λογισάμενοι τά τε παρεόντα τῶν τε παροιχομένων τὰ ὁμοίως διατεθέντα τοῖσι παρεοῦσιν ὥστε ποτὲ θεραπευθέντα εἰπεῖν ὡς ἀπήλλαξαν, 'reasoning about the present condition as well as conditions in the past similar to those in the present, so that they can tell how they were cured once they were treated': the doctor's task is described as primarily intellectual (hence λογισάμενοι) and involves four distinct mental acts: the consideration of present circumstances; the comparison of the patient's present condition to past patient conditions (implied by the ὁμοίως construction); the consideration of these past conditions; and the inference regarding cures in past cases, which, one presumes, will be applicable to the present. Gomperz, not inaptly, compares *de Arte* to a passage from Plato's *Laches*: 'for instance, in the case of health, there is no other art related to the past, the present, and the future except that of medicine, which, although it is a single art, surveys what is, what was, and what is likely to be in the future' (198d, trans. Sprague in Cooper 1997). This seems to accord well with certain treatises in the *Corpus*.

> State what has happened before, know what is currently the case, predict what will happen. Practice these things. (*Epid. 1* 2.634.6–8)

> It seems to me best for a physician to try to know things in advance. For if he prognosticates and predicts in the presence of his patients what is happening, what has happened, and what will happen (to the extent that any of these things were left out of the patient's original account), the more he will be believed to know his patients' real situations, so that people will dare to place themselves in the doctor's hands. What's more, he will give the best treatment if he knows in advance what will happen on the basis of present symptoms. (*Prog.* 110.1–8)

In these particular examples, 'knowing the past' probably refers to reconstructing a detailed account of the patient's recent medical history and not to past cases. However, past cases are the source of the accounts given in *Prog.* and *Epid. 1*, and their function is obvious enough: to provide future physicians the means of predicting patient outcomes by comparing symptoms to similar cases in the past.

*De Arte* follows the Hippocratic model, which uses past experience as a guide to future results. Unlike *Prog.* and *Epid. 1*, however, it is concerned primarily with how things are really disposed (τὰ διατεθέντα); the physician must recollect not just the symptoms of past conditions, but also their causes, the manner of their treatment and the outcomes of that treatment. Our author's remarks here at 7.3 require the context of his implicit distinction at 5.5 between knowing *that* and knowing *why* along with the connection he makes at 6.4 between knowing why (τὰ διά τι) and knowing the future. Anyone is capable of knowing after the fact what it was that *caused* a sick person to recover his health. But the recovery has been *explained* only once some feature of the cause is related to the recovery by a more general law or universal proposition. Since explanations involve laws or law-like structures, they give the physician a predictive capacity. In the current passage, our author gives an account of just how the physician, in contrast to the layperson, comes by explanations and thus his ability to predict and treat. In a word, he has experience, namely, experience of a variety of relevant cases. By canvassing his memory of the diseases in each case, as well as *what* it was that cured them, he is able to identify similarities and discard dissimilarities as intrinsic or extraneous to the causal process. The intrinsic similarities figure in generalizations about the disease and its cure, and these generalizations allow the physician to predict which procedures will prove effective in the present case.[64]

If one assumes that 1) this method is sound and that 2) the doctor who employs it is sufficiently intelligent and 3) mentally alert, then the possibility of medical error will be relatively slim. We have already seen why our author helps himself to 3. With respect to 1 and 2, however, he begs the question. Indeed, it is the doctor's methods and intelligence (as opposed to medicine's efficacy *per se*) that the critic's objection brings under scrutiny;

64 Our author may use the language of similarity, as well as that of past, present, and future circumstances, to make contact with Gorgias' *Helen* (DK 82 B11 § 11), which has been interpreted by some commentators as a component of the attack on *technē* (see Introduction 5).

they cannot be merely assumed. At least, insofar as they are assumed, the strength of the argument from probability is compromised.

7.3 οἱ δ' οὔτε ἃ κάμνουσιν οὔτε δι' ἃ κάμνουσιν, οὐδ' ὅ τι ἐκ τῶν παρεόντων ἔσται οὐδ' ὅ τι ἐκ τῶν τούτοισιν ὁμοίων γίνεται εἰδότες ἐπιτάσσονται, 'the former, however, while knowing neither what they suffer nor because of what they suffer, nor what will come of their present condition, nor what comes of similar conditions, are given orders': our author emphasizes the patient's ignorance—in contradistinction to the doctor's knowledge—of the past, present and future, and thus of the nature of the disease itself, including its causes. This is also the first trace of a developing martial metaphor: the patient is likened to a soldier who takes orders (ἐπιτάσσονται) from his general without knowing the overall situation or strategy that informs them.

7.3 ἀλγέοντες μὲν ἐν τῷ παρεόντι, φοβεύμενοι δὲ τὸ μέλλον, 'pained in the present and fearing for the future': the patient is described as having not an intellectual but a sensual and affective relationship to the present and future. He does not think; he feels, and his feelings have both physical (ἀλγέοντες) and psychological (φοβεύμενοι) dimensions. Specifically, he fears for the future, which he would not do if he knew (on a suitably robust construal of the term 'know') that his condition were curable. (Assuming that it is, as a matter of human psychology, impossible to fear a good *qua* good.)

7.3 πλήρεις μὲν τῆς νούσου, κενεοὶ δὲ σιτίων, 'they are full of disease but empty of food': the two adjectives πλήρης and κενός constitute a regular antithesis in Greek. Here they recall the theoretical commitment to health as balance. The patient, being ill, is not in a state of measured balance, and our author represents this symbolically by attributing to him the two extremes of fullness (or excess) and emptiness (or deficiency). There is little to no special medical significance, however. The phrase πλήρεις μὲν τῆς νούσου echoes literary descriptions of illness in tragedy (e.g., Sophocles, *Ant.* 1052). At most, it refers to the mastery of the body by the excessive factor, a nosological commonplace in early Greek medical theory (see Introduction 4). With the phrase κενεοὶ δὲ σιτίων our author cannot mean that lack of food is a typical cause of disease, since he has already included fasting as a potential curative at 5.4; if anything, he is referring to the general tendency of the sick to avoid eating. Moreover, he may be trying, in preparation for the impending introduction of a key metaphor, to evoke the image of a starving, undersupplied army or city-state (see following note).

7.3 ἐθέλοντες δὲ τὰ πρὸς τὴν νοῦσον ἤδη μᾶλλον ἢ τὰ πρὸς τὴν ὑγιείην προσδέχεσθαι, 'consenting at last to admit those things that promote disease rather than those that promote health': the verb ἐθέλειν connotes consent, i.e., to external proposals or desires, sometimes reluctantly; προσδέχεσθαι is often used of the admittance of outsiders into a city, including the reception of foreign emissaries. The resulting metaphor is elaborate, comparing patients to the soldiers and citizens of a besieged city-state who, tired of resisting, stop listening to their generals and refuse their allies, instead admitting into their midst the diplomatic representatives of the enemy with the intention of negotiating a complete surrender.[65] By analogy, the patient's weakened condition leads him to choose measures that offer temporary relief, though they are expedient to the disease in the long term. The drama of the struggle is heightened by the adverb ἤδη ('at last'), which tells us that this consent was granted all at once, only then and not before, and with irrevocable results.

7.3 οὐκ ἀποθανεῖν ἐρῶντες ἀλλὰ καρτερεῖν ἀδυνατέοντες, 'not because they desire death, but because they are powerless to endure': that the patient is 'powerless' to endure suggests a failure of motivation. He, or at least the part of him motivated by rational considerations, is overpowered by his fear, his desire to be released from pain, etc. The author's interjection, 'not because they desire death,' is important. He does not mean that the patient desires what he believes to be an evil. Rather, he is the site of a battle between competing desires: a desire for cure and a desire for the immediate alleviation of pain. Both are desires for a good, but they are incompatible under the circumstances. The sick person, unable to sustain the psychological effort required, succumbs to his desire for comfort. All this is described in dramatic language, as Jouanna recognizes, noting that θανεῖν ἐρᾶν hails from tragedy (Sophocles, *Ant.* 220; Euripides, *Hec.* 358 and *Hel.* 1639).

7.4 πότερον εἰκὸς, 'which is more likely': our author is not directly comparing the likelihood of physician error to that of patient error, but rather he is comparing the likelihood of patient error to non-error and, likewise, that of physician error to non-error.

7.5 ἆρ' οὐ πολὺ μᾶλλον τοὺς μὲν δεόντως ἐπιτάσσειν, τοὺς δὲ εἰκότως ἀδυνατεῖν πείθεσθαι, μὴ πειθομένους δὲ περιπίμπτειν τοῖσι θανάτοισιν, 'isn't it much more

---

[65] Jouanna senses a comparison between the patient and the soldier but takes the analogy no farther (1988, 255 n. 2).

likely that doctors give the right orders, but that in all probability the sick are powerless to obey them, and by not obeying them meet their deaths?': so concludes the nested argument from probability begun at 7.1.

1. If patient P dies, then the death is attributable either to intrinsic factors or to extrinsic factors (7.1).
2. Suppose P dies.
3. *P*'s death is attributable either to intrinsic factors (physician error) or to extrinsic factors (patient error).
4. The doctor was physically healthy, psychologically sound (i.e., in control of his rational faculties and responsive to their dictates), and had full knowledge of the situation (7.3).
5. Thus, it is more likely that he made no error than that he did (7.4).
6. The patient was physically ill, psychologically weak (i.e., susceptible to pressure from immoderate desires), and had no knowledge of the situation (7.3).
7. Thus, it is more likely that he made an error than that he did not (7.4).
8. Therefore, the likeliest scenario is that the patient erred while the doctor did not (7.5).

Steps 4 through 7 are required because the disjunction in 3 is inclusive. Whether or not patient error is more likely relative to physician error, it could be that both are likely in an absolute sense, so that the likeliest scenario would be one in which the physician and patient are jointly responsible. This of course, would not suit our author's purpose, and so he is compelled to argue that physician error is in itself unlikely.

## 8

Whereas in c. 7 medicine was blamed for the deaths of patients it treated, here in c. 8 it is blamed for the death of patients it refused to treat. Our author's explicit response comes in the form of two closely related *pisteis*. The first is a theoretical defense of non-intervention in cases of terminal illness on the grounds that medicine is constrained by physical necessity (8.1–4). The second is a piece of practical advice to any doctor who finds that none of his usual remedies are working: blame the strength of the disease (8.5).

The language of the chapter sustains the military metaphor—the term ἐπικουρίη ('help,' 8.1) is often used for aid in battle, and τὰ ὄργανα ('instruments'), which are said to be 'allied with' medicine (8.5), could also denote weaponry (Plato, *Republic* 374d; *Laws* 956a). More striking, however, is the ambiguously religious language, which in this chapter is not metaphorical. Through a string of litotes our author makes veiled allusions to the Greek religious concept of pollution and related practices. The physician's desire not to touch a disease (μὴ θέλοντας ἐγχειρεῖν, 8.1) evokes the shunning of the polluted, while the critics' call for the physician to touch what is unfit (ὧν μὴ προσήκει ἅπτεσθαι, 8.6) reads as a violation of religious prescription. Finally, there is the suspicious reference to an art capable of treating the physically incurable, an 'art other than the one of which fire is an instrument' (8.4), and which is potentially even more powerful than medicine.

Indeed, if anything is more striking than the implicitly religious content of the chapter, it would be the vicious hilarity of our author's *ad hominem* assault on the critics within the first several lines, which suggests that the critics' complaint about non-intervention is a reaction to the doctor's refusal to attempt a cure for their delusions.

**8.1** εἰσὶ δέ τινες, οἳ καὶ διὰ τοὺς μὴ θέλοντας ἐγχειρεῖν τοῖσι κεκρατημένοισιν ὑπὸ τῶν νοσημάτων μέμφονται τὴν ἰητρικήν, 'there are some, too, who criticize medicine on account of those who do not consent to handle people who have been overcome by their diseases': our author continues to counter objections based on patient mortality. This particular objection appears to challenge the third condition of the tripartite definition of medicine (3.2), though our author formulates his response not as though he were justifying a subsidiary *telos* of medicine so much as defending the rationality of a common medical practice. He does not point out, for example, that intervention in hopeless cases gratuitously multiplies risk or discomfort. Instead, he will argue simply that intervention in such cases is pointless; thus, it is unreasonable to require that doctors take them on. Furthermore, it is perfectly reasonable to expect the doctor to avoid such cases, since, as the objection from the immediately preceding c. 7 shows, he will be held responsible for the death of patients whom he has treated.

**8.1** ὡς ταῦτα μὲν καὶ αὐτὰ ὑφ' ἑωυτῶν ἂν ἐξυγιάζοιτο ἃ ἐγχειρέουσιν ἰᾶσθαι, ἃ δ' ἐπικουρίης δεῖται μεγάλης οὐχ ἅπτονται, 'they say that doctors make an attempt to heal diseases that would resolve themselves on their own but do not touch those in great need of help': the objection gets personal. Not only do doctors fail to have any of the knowledge they claim to have, but they know it. Their refusal of hopeless cases is essential to the ruse they perpetrate on credulous and unsuspecting patients (see notes on the following lemma and 8.5).

The premise that some diseases would clear up on their own is rejected by our author already in his argument against spontaneous recovery in c. 5 and is not mentioned hereafter.

**8.1** δεῖν δέ, εἴπερ ἦν ἡ τέχνη, πάνθ' ὁμοίως ἰᾶσθαι, 'but if indeed medicine is, it ought to try to heal all alike': here ἰᾶσθαι is conative, continuous with the sense of ἐγχειρέουσιν ἰᾶσθαι in the preceding. The expectation is not that medicine should cure all those in its care (though the critic may believe that as well), but that a doctor should never be at a loss when faced with a disease. He ought in every case to attempt a cure. Therapeutic *aporia* in a particular case implies a defect in the doctor's knowledge of how such cases are to be treated. Again, our author follows his familiar formula of conceding the critic's minor premise (in this chapter, that doctors refuse to intervene in terminal cases) while rejecting the major premise (given here).

Two distinct allegations are in play. The first, and more mundane, is that doctors are utterly corrupt in their profession of technical expertise, when in reality they know nothing at all about the business of curing diseases. Patients are 'treated,' and those who recover are said to have been 'cured,' though the doctor's ministrations were causally irrelevant to their recovery. 'Non-intervention' is nothing more than the quack's excuse for washing his hands of those who show no improvement. Accordingly, I suggest that the phrase μὴ ἐγχειρεῖν in its various forms (but especially in cc. 3 and 8; see notes on 3.2) means not just 'refuse' or 'not attempt' but rather must make room for the possibility that the doctor will 'leave off' or 'discontinue' treatment already begun. (The phrase may also mean, quite literally, 'not take in hand,' i.e., 'not touch,' potentially a nod to the notion of religious pollution by contact. Cf. Antiphon 5.82: οἶμαι γὰρ ὑμᾶς ἐπίστασθαι ὅτι πολλοὶ ἤδη ἄνθρωποι μὴ καθαροὶ χεῖρας ἢ ἄλλο τι μίασμα ἔχοντες. See also notes on 8.6 below.) The second, more theoretical, allegation is that expert knowledge of a domain ought to be exhaustive, so that any failure to know how to treat a patient calls that knowledge into question. Since our author has already dealt in c. 4 with the accusation that the doctor's treatment is causally irrelevant to his patient's recovery, it remains to justify the practice of non-intervention.

**8.2** εἰ ἐμέμφοντο τοῖσιν ἰητροῖσιν ὅτι αὐτῶν τοιαῦτα λεγόντων οὐκ ἐπιμέλονται ὡς παραφρονεύντων, εἰκότως ἂν ἐμέμφοντο μᾶλλον ἢ κεῖνα μεμφόμενοι, 'if such people criticized doctors for ignoring them because they were delirious, then their criticism would be more plausible than it is': once again our author indulges in probability arguments, this time to level an *ad hominem* attack on the mental competence of the detractors. The joke is not without a serious point. It adumbrates the substantive argument to follow, namely that, in demanding of the art that it cure every disease, the detractors are expecting the impossible, which is fundamentally irrational.

The phrase οὐκ ἐπιμέλονται indicates that doctors do not take such criticisms seriously, facetiously echoing the original objection that doctors fail to provide care where they ought to. It is understandable that doctors would not care about what such critics have to say, and it is likewise understandable that doctors would not provide care to patients who could not benefit therefrom. The sarcasm is sharpened by παραφρονεύντων, which, along with its cognates, is used in the *Corpus* to denote delirium in a patient (e.g., *Prog.* 2.120.5–6). The critics are diagnosed as being sick in the head. As such, they ought to be entreating doctors for help, not mistreating them for personal gain.

**8.2** εἰ γάρ τις ἢ τέχνην, ἐς ἃ μὴ τέχνη, ἢ φύσιν, ἐς ἃ μὴ φύσις πέφυκεν, ἀξιώσειε δύνασθαι, 'for if a person expects art to have power in matters where art is not, or expects nature to have power in matters where it is not present': the τέχνη-φύσις antithesis is not strictly exclusive. Art depends on or cooperates with nature in various ways, but especially insofar as it operates within its causal framework, matching means to ends (cf. 6.3–4). Thus, physical possibility (as distinguished, for example, from logical possibility) places obvious limits on technical possibility, as our author will illustrate.

**8.2** ἀγνοεῖ μανίῃ ἁρμόζουσαν ἄγνοιαν μᾶλλον ἢ ἀμαθίῃ, 'he is ignorant of an ignorance more in tune with madness than with lack of learning': it suits the rhetorical playfulness of the text to translate the cognate accusative into English. Indeed, it may be more than a mere flourish. Surely it is no mere flourish when Socrates in the *Apology* distinguishes himself from others on the grounds that he knows that he knows nothing, whereas most know not even this (21d). The distinction could be applied here in *de Arte*, since the gist of our author's defense is that cases in which a physician does not know how to cure a disease are special cases of ignorance. It is not that the physician simply does not know what to do to cure the disease. Rather, there is nothing that can be done, and *this* he knows, that is, he can give a reasonable explanation of his *aporia*. Medicine should not be criticized on this account, objects our author, and he is right. The critics' allegations, by contrast, do not qualify as knowledge (in virtue of their being false and thus unknowable); moreover, they are falsely believed to be true by those who make them.

Jouanna is correct that μανίη recalls the phrase κακαγγελίη φύσιος at 1.2, but his idiosyncratic interpretation of the earlier passage prevents him from noticing the connection also between ἀμαθίη and ἀτεχνίη (1988, 256 n. 1; see my notes on 1.2). The critics suffer from an intellectual defect—madness—that prevents them from understanding the rational principles that form the basis of all technical activity. They are not merely unlearned or untrained in the art; they are hopelessly uneducable. Etymologically akin to μαντικῄ, soothsaying, μανίη is often a frenzy of divine origin (Euripides, *Ba.* 33, 305; Sophocles, *Aj.* 611; Plato, *Phaedrus* 256b). It is therefore not susceptible to cure by human means; relief follows instead upon placation of the proper god (Euripides, *IT* 83, 981). In tragedy, μανίη may be a character's unwillingness to listen to reason, his obstinate perseverance against impossible odds (Aeschylus, *Pr.* 1057). The same idea surfaces in legal contexts, and Demosthenes states unequivocally that 'it is madness to do something beyond one's power' (μανία γὰρ ἴσως ἐστὶν ὑπὲρ δύναμίν τι ποιεῖν, 21.69; see also Lysias, 3.29). Likewise, the critics of medicine are mad to expect doctors to attempt impossible cures, which would include, ironically enough, curing the critics of just such madness.

**8.3** ὧν γὰρ ἔστιν ἡμῖν τοῖσί τε τῶν φυσίων τοῖσι τε τῶν τεχνέων ὀργάνοισιν επικρατεῖν, τούτων ἔστιν ἡμῖν δημιουργοῖς εἶναι, ἄλλων δὲ οὐκ ἔστιν, 'for of those things that we can master using the instruments of art and nature, we can be craftsmen. Of other things, we cannot': the plural τῶν φυσίων where one would more naturally expect the singular, τῆς φύσιος, has given commentators pause. Part of our author's motivation is aesthetic. He wants the same number of syllables as and homoioteleuton with τῶν τεχνέων. Still, we must explain what he means, and this explanation should take into account the singular use in the previous sentence.

I keep with tradition in translating these phrases as singular, despite Ducatillon's protest that this fails to respect the plural (1977a, 55). Following Gomperz ('durch die Kräfte der Körper und durch die Hilfsmittel der Künste,' 1910, 202–203 n. 1), Jones decides that the natures in question are individual (i.e., physiological) natures, what he terms 'the natural powers of the human constitution,' and that the organs of these natures are the bodily organs (1910, 202 n. 1). The bodily organs are what the doctor manipulates using the tools of his trade in order to effect health.

Jones' interpretation seems strained (Aristotle does refer at *de An.* 432a2 to the hand as the ὄργανον ὀργάνων, but he seems to be likening the hand to a tool, not tools to hands), and Ducatillon understandably rejects it (1977a, 55). She proposes instead that 'natures' refers to the innate capacity that, in addition to sufficient training, is articulated at the close of c. 9 as a requirement of good physicians. The instruments of nature are thus 'the natural talents' (1977a, 55). Ingenious as this may be, it expects too much of the Greek word ὄργανον. In addition, we are left with no sense for the contribution this pronouncement makes to the overall argument of c. 8.

The only instrument used to illustrate the point is fire, of which our author writes that it is the most extreme of the caustics employed in medicine (see notes below). Fire (by which is meant the tools of cautery, cf. *Aph.* 4.609.1–3, excerpted below) is an instrument. It is an instrument of the art insofar as a craftsman employs it toward a certain end, and it is an instrument of nature insofar as fire has a form or nature comprising various causal powers (cf. 6.3), including the power to burn (hence its characterization at 8.4 not as the hottest thing, but as the most extreme τῶν καιόντων, literally, of the things that burn). Art depends in its operations on the powers, and thus on the natures, that exist in the world; by manipulating natural things in response to particular circumstances, the physician brings about the state of health in his patient, which is itself a natural result. Medicine has a nature and a form in virtue of the fact that its treatments amount to the calculated application *of* things with powers *to* things with powers. As natural things possessing certain causal powers, medical instruments such as fire exhibit regular, necessary behavior. Fire burns *by nature* at such and such an intensity; thus, it *must* burn at this intensity. Here is where the modal claims of 8.3 gather force. If we expect fire to burn at a different intensity, we are requiring of it something that exceeds its nature; we are asking the impossible of nature. In that we are demanding of medicine that it somehow make fire burn at a different intensity (for this is what would be required to cure the disease), we are asking the impossible of the art. The art cannot be justly criticized for failing to achieve the impossible (cf. *Alim.* 141.22–23 = L. 9.102).

In fact, it is wrong to criticize any art on these grounds. Jouanna perceives in the general references to τέχνη and δημιουργοί, as opposed to medicine and doctors specifically, an argument that is conceived not only as a defense of medicine but of any art under similar attack, and he takes the relative rarity of the term δημιουργός in the *Corpus* as evidence that it was unusual for physicians of the period to apply the latter term to themselves (1988, 256 n. 2). However, I see the diction in this passage not as a feature of some general defense of all arts, but rather as part of a second, dialectical line of argument in defense of medicine. In demanding of medicine that it succeed even in the face of physical impossibility, the critics are holding medicine to a standard to which they would not hold other arts (unless they were out of their minds). This anticipates our author's move at 11.7, where he opts again for the term δημιουργίη, probably in an attempt to assimilate medicine to productive handicrafts like shoemaking and metalworking in contradistinction to edifying arts like astronomy. The same motive may be in play here.

8.3 ὅταν οὖν τι πάθῃ ὥνθρωπος κακὸν ὃ κρέσσον ἐστὶν τῶν ἐν ἰητρικῇ ὀργάνων, 'thus, whenever a person suffers some evil that is stronger than the instruments of medicine': the inferential particle οὖν flags a logical consequence of the preceding, which amounts to a reiteration, specially tailored to medicine, of the conclusion articulated at 8.2.

Our author speaks here (and in the remainder of c. 8) not of disease but more ambiguously of κακὸν ὃ κρέσσον, 'some evil that is stronger.' Since craftsmen have already been described as availing themselves of the instruments of both art and nature, one might reasonably ask what could be stronger than nature. The adjective κακόν would leave open the possibility that a malevolent supernatural factor is involved.

8.4 αὐτίκα γὰρ τῶν ἐν ἰητρικῇ καιόντων τὸ πῦρ ἐσχάτως καίει, 'for example fire burns the most intensely of all the caustics used in medicine': the adverbial phrase αὐτίκα γὰρ introduces an illustration, in concrete terms, of the argument's general thesis (see notes on 8.3). Fire refers not only to the natural phenomenon or substance but probably also to cauterization as a medical procedure. If so, it is the only explicit reference to surgery in *de Arte*, which otherwise limits the physician to diet and drugs. The example is chosen perhaps in part for its symbolic power. In mythology, fire is identified, through Prometheus, with the very idea and origins of *technē*. Thus, by imagining an evil that is stronger even than fire, he imagines something that, on common cultural conceptions, lies outside the power not just of medicine but of any *technē* whatsoever.

In stating that 'fire burns the most intensely of all the caustics,' our author recognizes a scalar structure to the strength or intensity of causal powers such that the same power can be present in different objects to different degrees. Likewise, only certain objects have the potential to be affected by a certain power, and these conform to a scalar distribution of activation thresholds so that it makes sense to say of such an object that it is susceptible to being affected by a certain power at or above a certain level of intensity.[66] Given the wide range of combustive power and combustion

[66] Jori labels these the art's qualitative and quantitative limiting factors, respectively (1996, 218), which is acceptable so long as one is careful not to suppose that all powers have

thresholds of objects used in the maintenance of civilized life, fire is a convenient example. Straw will start to burn from the friction of two sticks, while other things—stones, for example—appear relatively unaffected by even the hottest fires. Logically speaking, there is nothing that prevents the same principles from applying to diseases, so long as this is permitted by the underlying physics, of which we are told little in *de Arte*.

There is the further question of whether the qualification ἐν ἰητρικῇ ('used in medicine') would strike the ancient Greek audience as otiose. Would fire have been regarded as the hottest natural thing or at least as the upper limit of a range of caustic agents? Pre-Socratic theories of nature like that of Empedocles, which gave to fire the status of a basic element, suggests that it was, as does the LSJ, which notes that fire is used in epic as a poetic symbol of irresistibility (*Il.* 6.182, 11.596, 17.565, 20.371).

**8.4** τῶν μὲν οὖν ἡσσόνων τὰ κρέσσω οὔπω δῆλον ὅτι ἀνίητα, τῶν δὲ κρατίστων τὰ κρέσσω πῶς οὐ δῆλον ὅτι ἀνίητα, 'clearly, then, things that are stronger than the lesser caustics are by no means untreatable. But isn't it clear, too, that things stronger than the most powerful caustics are untreatable?': our author's mastery of balance in the form of parisosis and paromoiosis is on display. By simply replacing ἡσσόνων with κρατίστων and reversing the syllables of οὔπω to yield πῶς οὐ, he achieves a world of difference in meaning.

The phrase τῶν δὲ κρατίστων τὰ κρέσσω ('things stronger than the most powerful') has a paradoxical flavor, but the larger point makes perfect sense. Logically speaking, nothing prevents a disease (or other evil) from exceeding the physical limits of fire as a curative. To use an example from modern medicine, various strains of a bacterium may be vulnerable to our most potent antibiotic, though other strains may prove resistant and thus will be untreatable. Still, the modern example highlights the shortcomings of our author's argument. Even if it is possible, in principle, that some evils exceed the caustic power of fire, the doctor's practice of refusing hopeless cases is justified only if such evils actually exist. That some patients are not cured does not show that they could not be.

**8.4** ἃ γὰρ πῦρ οὐ δημιουργεῖ, 'as for the things that fire does not work on': an odd expression complicated by a contested reading in the MSS, M giving οὐ after πῦρ while A does not. Either way, the sentence illustrates our author's

---

a numerically determinable or measureable absolute value. There is no evidence that our author believes this to be true.

penchant for personification (cf. 1.3, 9.1), but the poetic device has a purpose. By elevating fire from instrument to agent, our author seeks to deflect blame. If fire fails to cure, this is nature's fault, not the physician's.

**8.4** ἄλλης τέχνης δεῖται καὶ οὐ ταύτης ἐν ᾗ τὸ πῦρ ὄργανον, 'they require an art other than the one of which fire is an instrument': what does our author mean by 'another art?' He may be alluding to prayer, magic, or some other form of religious healing. Though he does not elsewhere indicate that he puts stock in such methods, this would be consistent with the religious imagery in the preceding chapters. If, as I suggest above, fire is to be generally identified with technical mastery of the world by natural means, then our author might well be understood as recommending a supernatural solution to the incurable affliction. In a very real sense, this would be to abandon a technical approach altogether, and it may be that ἄλλης τέχνης refers to nothing at all: 'if medicine can't cure you, no *technē* can. Start praying.'

**8.5** ὧν ἁπάντων φημὶ δεῖν ἑκάστου οὐ κατατυχόντα τὸν ἰητρὸν, 'I claim that if the doctor is unsuccessful with each of all these': the verb κατατυγχάνειν with genitive object means to 'reach the object of' or 'succeed in respect of.' But our author is discussing cases in which medicine's instruments are ineffective, prompting Diels (1914, 396–397) to compare this passage to the final entry in *Aph.*: 'whatever sorts of things drugs do not cure, iron cures; whatever iron does not cure, fire cures; whatever fire does not cure, these one must believe incurable' (4.609.1–3; cf. also *Loc. Hom.* 52.9–10 = L. 6.298, where the author advises doctors to modify the course of treatment whenever the disease is unresponsive). The genitive construction ὧν ἁπάντων ... ἑκάστου must refer to the doctor who has exhausted all the tools at his disposal with no success. Accordingly, most editors have emended the text to include a negative particle, though none is retained in the MSS. I follow Gomperz in printing ἑκάστου οὐ κατατυχόντα. Jouanna is the only editor to retain the original MS reading here. In defense, he suggests that to be successful with respect to some instrument is to use that instrument correctly according to the rules of the art. This stretches κατατυγχάνειν, however, and leaves the salient condition unspoken, namely, that the patient does not recover.

Either way, there can be no doubt that our author here shifts his focus from the theoretical allegation to the practical (see notes on 8.1). Our author is constructing a defense for doctors against the complaint that they begin by treating patients but, when the patients' conditions do not improve, stop the treatment. It is not just that medicine is ineffectual (the charge aired in c. 4), but that doctors are dishonest. They treat their patients and then wait to see what happens. If the patient seems to be recovering, they continue treatment. If the patient takes a turn for the worse, they stop treatment so that they will not incur blame for his death. This trick requires no medical knowledge; anyone could do it, but few would. The physician is extraordinary only in his lack of scruple.

**8.5** δεῖν ... τὸν ἰητρὸν τὴν δύναμιν αἰτιᾶσθαι τοῦ πάθεος '[the doctor] ought to hold responsible the power of the affliction, not the art': given the ethical and personal dimensions of the allegation, it is no surprise that this sentence reads like a memo from legal counsel. Strictly speaking, our author does not assert that when doctors fail, the strength of the disease really is to blame. (Perhaps he perceives the fallacy inherent in parlaying a sound defense of non-intervention as a general practice into defenses of particular cases of non-intervention.) Instead, he merely instructs failed physicians to blame the strength of the disease. The strategy is to shift the burden of proof to the 'prosecution.' Having firmly established that it's at least possible for a disease to be incurable, our author now demands that the prosecution show that it was physician error or ignorance, not incurable disease, that was responsible for the outcome.

**8.6** παρακελεύονται καὶ ὧν μὴ προσήκει ἅπτεσθαι οὐδὲν ἧσσον ἢ ὧν προσήκει, '[they] are demanding that they touch what is improper no less than what is proper': another iteration of our author's countercharge that the critics of medicine are expecting the impossible, this version trades on the potential religious associations of the phrase ὧν μὴ προσήκει ἅπτεσθαι. 'Touching what is improper,' literally means to handle or become involved with something with respect to which one has neither right nor obligation (cf. Demosthenes, *Against Evergus and Mnesibulus* 47.53; Plato, *Republic* 474c). I suspect, however, that here it serves also as a subtle allusion to pollution (μίασμα), or rather to the fact that one was advised to avoid contact with a polluted person for fear of disrespecting the gods or becoming contaminated oneself.[67] This would unleash the full rhetorical force of our author's earlier remark at 8.4: the other 'art' required when fire fails would be some sort of religious purification. This is not the doctor's domain, and, moreover, to insist that

[67] For a general study of the Greek concept of pollution, see Parker (1983). Hankinson (1995b) comments on the lack of interest in pollution in the Hippocratic *Corpus*. An illuminating study of some Hippocratic attitudes toward religious purification is found in van der Eijk (1990).

he treat the polluted is itself impious. This in turn opens up another avenue for an *ad hominem* attack on the patients themselves. Incurable patients are reprehensible, untouchable, cursed as a result of some crime. They have no one to blame but themselves for bringing the gods' wrath down upon them. Surely doctors cannot be expected to prevent their punishment.

**8.6** ὑπὸ μὲν τῶν ὀνόματι ἰητρῶν θαυμάζονται, ὑπὸ δὲ τῶν καὶ τέχνῃ καταγελῶνται, '[while] they gain the admiration of those who are doctors in name, they are ridiculed by those who are doctors also in virtue of their art': the contrast between ὄνομα and τέχνη is a reprise of that between ὄνομα and οὐσία at 6.4, the difference being that between the word (e.g., 'spontaneity') as it applies to a nonexistent natural kind and the word (e.g., 'doctor') as it applies to particular things eligible for membership in an existent kind. The word 'doctor' is applied to a range of people, only a subset of whom actually belong to the class of those with medical expertise. Those who do not belong are doctors only in an attenuated sense, which is to say they are not *really* doctors (see notes on 2.3).

**8.7** οὕτως ἀφρόνων ... οὔτε μωμητέων οὔτ' αἰνετέων δέονται, 'have no need for criticism or praise that is so senseless': our author revives the theme of madness introduced by παραφρονεῖν and μανία at 8.2. The reference to praise and blame is perhaps meant as an allusion to the two most common modes of rhetoric (see Introduction 2). Rhetoric as practiced by the critics is useless to medicine, which is not to say that all rhetoric, properly conceived and practiced, is useless. Certainly the doctor has an interest in rhetoric that correctly identifies and condemns the causes of failure while praising the genuine successes of the art.

**8.7** οἱ ταύτης τῆς δημιουργίης ἔμπειροι, 'those experienced in this craft': it is tempting to make a connection between the emphasis on experienced (ἔμπειροι) craftsmen and the tripartite theory of *technē*, which stressed nature, education and experience (ἐμπειρία) as the decisive factors in cultivating any art (Hutchinson 1988, 29–33). But while our author will cite nature and education as prerequisites for any skilled practitioner, this is his only overt reference to experience. Still, his description of method at 7.3 suggests that experience with particular cases is crucial to a doctor's competence at diagnosing and treating disease, and the present context makes ἐμπειρία at least a necessary condition of genuine expertise. (Note that the difference between genuine doctors and doctors in name only is their level of experience, not a mental defect such as μανίη, which is reserved for the critics alone.) Even so, here our author appeals to experience with an eye to its rhetorical impact, not its theoretical significance. To call certain physicians experienced means just that they have experience in actually healing patients rather than merely talking about medicine.

**8.7** λελογισμένων, 'people who have rationally considered': time and again, our author opposes reason to unreason in the form of weakness (7.3) or, as here, madness. In *de Arte*, the verb λογίζεσθαι and its cognates are often predicated of physicians (7.3, 11.3; but see 7.5), though here it is used of those from outside the art who have a reasonable conception of its aims and limits. This, among other considerations, seems to count against Vegetti's conclusion that such outsiders have a privileged perspective from which the *technitēs* himself is excluded, since his inquiry is confined to what is correct in the art, while the outsider is an expert in οὐσία and λογισμός (1964, 359; see also Introduction 5 and the following note). Rather, the outsider is likely someone skilled in the art of praise and blame (i.e., rhetoric) who is educated enough in the basic principles of the art so as to form a set of reasonable expectations for its success.

**8.7** πρὸς ὅ τι αἱ ἐργασίαι τῶν δημιουργῶν τελευτώμεναι πλήρεις εἰσί, καὶ ὅτευ ὑπολειπόμεναι ἐνδεεῖς, 'in relation to what the products of craftsmen are fully finished; in what respect imperfect products are deficient': the success or failure of the craftsman must be measured against a clear conception of the *telos* of the *technē*, so that it is clear *whether* and *how* alleged failures are such. Apparently, even non-experts may lay claim to such knowledge, though our author, rather conspicuously, does not credit them with knowing *why* (that is, by what specific causal mechanisms) the failures occur. Sextus Empiricus reports that Anacharsis of Scythia attacked *technē* on the grounds that neither experts nor non-experts were competent to judge the quality of technical products (M 7.55–59), and it may be that 8.7 is framed partly in response to that or similar criticisms (see Introduction 5): both experts and non-experts are competent to judge the products of a *technē*, so long as they have a correct conception of its *telos* and are capable of understanding the limits that physical impossibility places on technical possibility, which would seem to be available to anyone who is not mad (cf. 8.2) and can reason (λογίζεσθαι; see earlier note).

**8.7** τῶν ἐνδειῶν ἅς τε τοῖσι δημιουργεῦσιν ἀναθετέον, ἅς τε τοῖσι δημιουργεομένοισι, 'concerning these deficiencies, which are to be attributed to the craftsmen and which to the things being crafted': our author shifts back to the generic language of craft and technical production here as though discussing *technē per se*, which results in strange turns of phrase, most notably the reference to τοῖσι δημιουργεομένοισι, literally 'the things worked by craft,' which in a medical context might refer to the overpowering diseases or the inadequate instruments, since both play a role in medical failure, though the phrase might refer also to the patients themselves, since it is to them that he directly applies his treatments. Probably our author means to include all of the above, which indicates an implicit recognition of the distinction between intrinsic and extrinsic factors responsible for technical failure (see notes on 7.1).

## 9

Though it may not technically qualify as anacolouthon, the compressed syntax and extended articular constructions, as well as the parenthetical quality of the relative clauses, certainly lend this passage a casual, disjointed feel. Not only does it recall 3.2 in style and function, but, in rhetorical terms, this constitutes a third *prothesis*, a reiteration of the goal of the speech (cf. 1.3 and 3.1). Here our author shifts from arguments to facts, and as he goes on to construct a disinterested narrative account (*diēgēsis*) of medical procedure, the personal and polemical tone of the treatise relaxes considerably. First-person references drop out. *Ad hominem* attacks and probability arguments fall by the wayside. The particle γάρ becomes rarer, and its occurrences link sentences whose logical connection is less rigid. But though *de Arte* from this point forward is less polemical and argumentative, it is no less rhetorical insofar as our author continues to showcase his stylistic talents. Note especially the metrical symmetry and euphony of quasi-antitheses in 9.3, not to mention the parisosis, paromoiosis, and pseudo-antistrophe in 9.4.

**9.1** τὰ μὲν οὖν κατὰ τὰς ἄλλας τέχνας ἄλλος χρόνος μετ' ἄλλου λόγου δείξει, 'demonstrations concerning the other arts will take place at another time and with another discourse': but, literally, 'another time will demonstrate the things concerning the other arts with another discourse.' Again, a case of personification (cf. 1.3, 8.4), not just of χρόνος but also of λόγος, since the preposition μετά does not serve an instrumental function but rather indicates alliance or cooperation: 'working together with another discourse.' It is unclear why our author employs the device here, though its effect is to render his connection to the other discourse or discourses more remote. Thus it is that this passage has traditionally come under special scrutiny by commentators debating the question of the treatise's authorship (see further Introduction 5).

**9.1** οἷά τέ ἐστιν ὥς τε κριτέα, 'what sorts of things it involves and how they are to be judged': our author does not use κριτέα as a technical epistemological term. He will claim in c. 9 that the art has judged (κρινεῖν) certain diseases to be non-evident, by which he means only that the art has identified a special category of diseases. But he no doubt has in mind also judgments as to whether medicine or chance is responsible for recovery, and whether doctors or patients are responsible for patient mortality, etc. There is never any sustained discussion of a criterion for knowledge or judgment as such (which is not to say that our author does not employ one). The judgments in question are most likely evaluations of an art's success or failure—and, ultimately, existence—that should be sensitive to the unique challenges facing the particular *technē*. (Again, this may signal our author's engagement with the criticism leveled by Anacharsis of Scythia; see notes on 8.7, but especially Introduction 5.) Thus, our author will shortly introduce the distinction between evident and non-evident diseases. One might justifiably expect of the doctor a high degree of speed and accuracy in the diagnosis and treatment of the former, while such expectations should be adjusted in proportion to the non-evidence of the latter.

**9.2** τοῖσι ταύτην τὴν τέχνην ἱκανῶς εἰδόσι, 'according to those with sufficient knowledge of this art': the first of many appeals to the authority of those with medical expertise (see especially 10.2 and 11.3). However, there is no evidence from the *Corpus* to indicate that Greek physicians regarded the evident and non-evident as especially useful categories from the standpoint of therapy. To wit, the various special terms that might be used of non-evident diseases do not exhibit a high frequency. The adjective ἄδηλον occurs a mere twenty times, three of which belong to *de Arte*, three to the epistles. Otherwise, it occurs in treatises clearly under the influence of philosophy, and, within these treatises, in highly philosophical contexts: *Vict.* 136.5–14 = L. 6.488; *Alim.* 141.23–24 = L. 9.102 and 142.6 = L. 9.104; *Praec.* 31.26 = L. 9.256; and *Morb. Sacr.* 20.2 = L. 6.380. The adjectives φάνερος and ἀφανής are also rare in the *Corpus* and again are found in more 'philosophical' treatises, e.g., *VM* 119.5 = L. 1.572; *Flat.* 103.10–11 = L. 6.90, 106.9–10 = L. 6.94; and *Nat. Hom.* 164.7 = L. 6.32 and 178.6 = L. 6.42. An interesting exception to the rule is the treatise *VC*, chapters 9 through 14 (3.210–242), where in the course of a detailed medical discussion of the diagnosis and treatment of various skull fractures, the author makes a firm distinction, for methodological purposes, between the evident and non-evident.

**9.2** τὰ μὲν τῶν νοσημάτων οὐκ ἐν δυσόπτῳ κείμενα, καὶ οὐ πολλά, τὰ δὲ οὐκ ἐν εὐδήλῳ, καὶ πολλά, 'some diseases are located where they are not hard to see—though these are few—while others are located where they are not very evident, and these are many': our author makes the distinction between diseases in places open to inspection and those that are not. His main concern for the remainder of the treatise will be to show that doctors are able to make discoveries about and diagnose 'hidden' diseases. This is crucial, since, by his account, the great majority of diseases fall into this category. His motivation for the discussion may be at least partly philosophical in nature, an attempt to make contact with fifth-century epistemological debates over the status of the non-evident. In fact, our author will transition into explicitly philosophical terminology in c. 11 where he will refer to hidden diseases as ἄδηλον, a term of undeniable philosophical provenance (see Introduction 3).

For now, he restricts himself to the terms δύσοπτον and εὔδηλον, neither of which find special application in the philosophical literature, though the latter is etymologically related to ἄδηλον. The former is especially uncommon and does not appear again until Polybius (18.4.2), from which Jouanna infers that it is of Ionic origin (1988, 257 n. 5). That may be, but it is more interesting to ask why our author avails himself of this obscure term. The answer lies in the calculated antithesis of δύσοπτον and εὔδηλον. He opposes to the 'manifestly evident' not what is non-evident (ἄδηλον) or invisible (ἀόρατος, which itself has a philosophical pedigree: the Pythagoreans DK 58 B1a; Empedocles DK 31 B110), but rather what is not well seen. But what is difficult to see is not therefore impossible to see, suggesting even that non-evidence comes in degrees.

**9.3** τὰ μὲν ἐξανθεῦντα ἐς τὴν χροιὴν 'things that erupt on the skin': the verb ἐξανθεῖν is not widespread in the *Corpus*, though the nominal form ἐξάνθημα occurs some 16 times, mostly in the *Epidemics*. Our author uses the attributive participle instead of a specific disease name or nosological term probably because he is concerned with epistemological, not biological or medical, categories. His point is that evident diseases are such in virtue not of some special intrinsic quality but rather because they affect an exterior part of the body. We may infer that non-evident diseases are such in virtue simply of their affecting internal parts of the body (see 10.1).

**9.3** παρέχει γὰρ ἑωυτῶν τῇ τε ὄψει τῷ τε ψαῦσαι τὴν στερεότητα καὶ τὴν ὑγρότητα αἰσθάνεσθαι, καὶ ἅ τε αὐτῶν θερμὰ ἅ τε ψυχρά, 'they offer us the opportunity to perceive their solidity and liquidity by our senses of sight and touch, as well as which of them are hot and cold': this is the first clear evidence that our author's repeated references to the visibility of objects, as well as to the human visual faculty, are symbolic of perception generally, including all the senses.

The sudden intrusion of the first-person plural is meant to emphasize the universality of the facts presented: anyone (not just the doctor) with a functioning perceptual apparatus can identify and describe skin eruptions. This will be immediately contrasted with experts, who know how to treat such diseases (9.4), and who are also capable of identifying internal, non-evident diseases (cc. 11 and 12).

Our author comes very near to naming the four classic qualities or powers of Greek medical theory: the hot, the cold, the wet, and the dry (see Introduction 4). For dryness, however, he has substituted στερεότης, solidity. It may well be that, for him, dryness and solidity amount to the same thing, since both are exclusive of liquidity. Certainly, his word for liquidity, ὑγρότης, also connotes softness or suppleness. From a practical diagnostic perspective, 'liquidity' may refer to the weeping of fluid from a wound (cf. *Loc. Hom.* 68.28–70.5 = L. 6.322), while 'solidity' may refer to a scab.

**9.3** ὧν τε ἑκάστου ἢ παρουσίῃ ἢ ἀπουσίῃ τοιαῦτ' ἐστίν, 'these diseases being the sorts of things they are through the presence or absence of each of these': it is not clear whether 'each of these' refers to hot and cold, or also to solidity and liquidity, or perhaps includes also color and swelling. These last two are doubtful since, first, they occur in the preceding sentence, and, second, there would be no sense to the idea of skin eruptions absent of color. Whichever combination of qualities is meant, they are constitutive of the forms of skin eruptions and perhaps of all diseases. It is their presence or absence (probably in varying degrees; see 8.4) at the site that makes a disease the kind of disease it is, but, more importantly for the argument, their phenomenal character closes the diagnostic gap between symptom and underlying cause. There is nothing to the disease over and above (or, better, under and below) the observed qualities, making diagnosis efficient and accurate.

**9.4** ἀναμαρτήτους, 'free from error': literally, there should be 'no missing the mark' in such cases. Our author does not mean that it is reasonable to expect treatment in all cases to be successful (the patient could still disobey his orders, after all), but rather that intrinsic factors ought to play no role in cases of failure (see notes on 7.1), since there is general knowledge of the diseases and their cures. The immediate implication is that any failure resulting from intrinsic factors is to be attributed to the doctor's ignorance or misapplication of technical knowledge, not to the art itself (cf. 5.5).

**9.4** οὐχ ὡς ῥηϊδίας, ἀλλ' ὅτι ἐξεύρηνται, 'not because they are easy, but rather because they are fully discovered': that is, curing such conditions is not something an untrained layperson could do. Finding a cure still requires research (perhaps according to the method described at 7.3) into causes and effects and, ultimately, a genuine explanation, even if the process is made somewhat easier (but not easy) by the fact that the phenomena are external and thus more readily observed. By contrast, one may infer that research into and diagnosis of non-evident diseases will involve substantial obstacles that will mitigate the doctor's failure to formulate a timely diagnosis and treatment plan. Since the majority of diseases are non-evident, much of the doctor's work would benefit from such a lowering of expectations.

**9.4** ἐξεύρηνταί γε μὴν οὐ τοῖσι βουληθεῖσιν, ἀλλὰ τούτων τοῖσι δυνηθεῖσιν, 'such discoveries being made not by those who have merely the desire, but by those who have also the power': again the βούλησις-δύναμις antithesis rears its head, recalling the 'mediocrity of those with ambition but utterly without power' of 1.2 and the 'doctors in name' of 8.6.

**9.4** δύνανται δὲ οἷσι τά τε τῆς παιδείης μὴ ἐκποδών, τά τε τῆς φύσιος μὴ ἀταλαίπωρα, 'and power is available to those whose training is not lacking and whose natures are not indolent': the modified anastrophe with δύνανται and the parallelism of phrasing indicate that παιδεία and φύσις are to be regarded as an antithesis (cf. *Alim.* 145.12 = L. 9.112, as well as 1.2 and my notes). Here our author emphasizes natural ability and education as the jointly sufficient conditions of expertise, leaving out the third member of the traditional triad, experience. (However, see my notes on 8.6 and 7.3. Concerning Pre-Socratic and sophistic theories of technical education, see Heinimann 1961 and Hutchinson 1988.) Even the role of nature is minimized.[68] The technical student does not need any special aptitude or superlative intellect to succeed; he simply must not be lazy. Education can turn anyone into an expert so long as he puts his mind to it.

---

[68] This would be true even on the best interpretations of the alternative reading given by M, ταλαίπωρα, preferred by most editors prior to Jouanna.

## 10

Our author's objective in this chapter is first and foremost to give an account of the *spatial* constraints on the doctor's knowledge of internal diseases. To that end, he depicts the body as an organic container holding organs that are themselves containers of other things. This picture shows why knowledge of hidden diseases is more difficult to attain than 'open' diseases.

None of this proves anything about disease as such—the physician can still have everything wrong when it comes to internal diseases. But it does inspire the hope that physicians can succeed in knowing things that are at first sight hidden from them. Our author is concerned to sketch the structure of the body—quite generally—to account for this 'discoverable obscurity.' At the same time, his actual knowledge of anatomy seems hardly more detailed than that of the audience for whom he is presumably writing. While he introduces technical terminology for familiar parts of the body, rarely if ever does the discussion turn toward organs that would have been utterly unknown to a lay audience—when the opportunity arises, he waves his hands and assures us that doctors know all about the more complicated matters. Perhaps more perplexing, we get very little sense for the physiology of the human body. The author never tells us in any great detail what any one of the organs does nor how it functions within the overall system.[69] Instead, organs are identified mainly by their extrinsic spatial relations to other organs.

The style, too, seems ill suited to serious anatomical exposition. The affectation of the phrases τῆς κεφαλῆς κύκλος in 10.4 is awkward and off-putting. To my knowledge, nothing comparable is found elsewhere in the *Corpus*. Likewise, Gomperz complains that the anastrophe of ἔχουσι μὲν τοίνυν οἱ βραχίονες σάρκα τοιαύτην, ἔχουσι δ' οἱ μηροί, ἔχουσι δ' αἱ κνῆμαι at 10.3 borders on the ridiculous (1910, 130), and we might add to these the repetition of ἔτι δὲ καὶ at 10.4–5.

**10.1** πρὸς μὲν οὖν τὰ φανερὰ τῶν νοσημάτων οὕτω δεῖ εὐπορεῖν τὴν τέχνην· δεῖ γε μὴν αὐτὴν οὐδὲ πρὸς τὰ ἧσσον φανερὰ ἀπορεῖν, 'with respect to evident

[69] So Jori writes of a gradual initiation, without trauma, of the audience into the world of technical medicine (1996, 235), but our author's objective is more to mystify than to initiate. His appeals to authority have a patronizing and pedantic, not gentle, tone, and he leaves his audience with little more anatomical knowledge than they already had, not including his vague promises about harmful fluids and myriad cavities. My analysis is more congenial to recent remarks on *de Arte*'s relation to general trends in Greek medicine made by Holmes (2010, 17–19; 121–122).

diseases, then, the art ought to be thus well equipped. But neither ought it be unequipped with respect to less evident diseases': the verb εὐπορεῖν (already familiar from 1.3) contrasts with ἀπορεῖν to exploit yet another antithesis of philosophical significance. Perhaps the closest parallel comes from a fragment of Archytas (see also Democritus, DK 68 B106; and Cleoboulus, DK 10 3a20).

> It is difficult (ἄπορος) and rare for one who does not conduct an investigation to make full discoveries (ἐξευρεῖν), but if he conducts an investigation, it is accomplishable (εὔπορος) and easy (ῥάϊδιον), while it is impossible for one who does not know how to conduct an investigation. (DK 47 B3 4–6)

It is no accident that our author employs this antithesis in the context of fully discovering cures that are not easy (οὐχ ὡς ῥηϊδίας, ἀλλ' ὅτι ἐξεύρηνται, 9.4)—'to have the means to discover' seems to have been an early way in which Greek thinkers referenced a vague notion of method. One might be ignorant of something for a variety of reasons. To say that he is not equipped to know it, however, is to say that he does not have the tools to make the discovery, that is, he does not grasp the method by which such discoveries are made.

In the Great Speech in Plato's *Protagoras*, the elder sophist speaks of human beings as having εὐπορία (322a) once they have been given technical wisdom by the gods, while before they acquire such knowledge they have ἀπορία (321b–c). In the *Meno*, Socrates says: 'I myself do not have the answer (οὐκ εὐπορεῖν) when I perplex others, but I am more perplexed than anyone when I cause perplexity (ποιεῖν ἀπορεῖν) in others. So now I do not know what virtue is.' (80c–d, trans. Grube in Cooper 1997). The antithesis as employed by Protagoras and Socrates has epistemic import. There is some epistemic aim or goal (knowing how to survive in the Protagorean myth, knowledge of virtue in the Socratic dialogue) with respect to which being well or ill equipped depends not just upon whether or not one actually has such knowledge but also upon whether one has the means of acquiring it. In fact this latter problem becomes the central topic in the *Meno*: what sort of method could there be for escaping a state of ignorance?

By invoking the εὐπορία-ἀπορία antithesis, then, our author signals his intent to focus not on medical discoveries *per se* but rather on the method by which they are made. The remainder of the treatise bears this out. He will not concern himself with regurgitating detailed and accurate medical facts (except insofar as this validates his method), but rather with explaining and justifying the method by which physicians go from a state of complete ignorance about non-evident diseases to having at least some knowledge about them. His goal, it is worth mentioning, is not to show that the doctors have completely discovered (ἐξευρεῖν) the causes and proper treatment of non-evident diseases, but only that they are not at a complete loss when dealing with them (οὐδὲ πρὸς τὰ ἧσσον φανερὰ ἀπορεῖν).

**10.1** ἔστιν δὲ ταῦτα ἃ πρός τε τὰ ὀστέα τέτραπται καὶ τὴν νηδύν, 'namely, those affecting the bones and the bodily cavity': the word νηδύς has been long pondered by commentators because our author seems to employ it in an unusual sense. The LSJ cites the treatise as the authority for the meaning 'any of the cavities in the body.' It is true that the term will be applied subsequently to all bodily cavities generally, while elsewhere in Hippocratic and other literature it means 'stomach,' 'intestines,' or even 'womb.' Often it refers to the internal region of the abdomen and so is sometimes translated as 'belly.' The recognition of the specialized use in *de Arte* goes back to Erotian, who notes: '*nēdus*: this is what he calls the entire cavity' (νηδύν · οὕτω καλεῖ πᾶσαν κοιλότητα κτλ., Nachmanson 63, 3–6).

However, it would seem that our author starts out using νηδύς in the conventional way. Here, he introduces it as the internal cavity that contains the majority of the vital organs, and this accords quite well with traditional usage. It is only in the following sentence that he begins to employ the term idiosyncratically. This is why the clarification 'the body has not one (sc. cavity), but many' is necessary (10.2). The audience would otherwise be confused by its application to other cavities besides the abdominal. At the same time, there is little indication that our author is flagging an unfamiliar or strange technical term (as he does with ἣν μῦν καλέουσι and θώρηξ καλεόμενος later at 9.3–4). Instead, the transition from conventional to unconventional uses of νηδύς is driven by his project of demonstrating that there is no special problem, epistemologically speaking, with supposing one can know things about the body's interior. Surely all would acknowledge that they have bones and an internal cavity, even if they cannot actually see these parts of themselves. Likewise, the physician can speak with confidence of other internal spaces and cavities in the body even though these are not open to casual inspection. Of course, the physician could err in mapping out the internal structure of the human body. The point is not that the physician is infallible, but rather that no sensible person would object on epistemological grounds to the possibility of acquiring at least some knowledge of the body's internal structure.

**10.2** δύο μὲν γὰρ αἵ τὸ σιτίον δεχόμεναί τε καὶ ἀφιεῖσαι, 'there are two that take in and expel food': probably he has in mind the stomach and intestines, though we cannot rule out the possibility that he is referring to the oral and anal cavities, or some combination or fusion (respectively) thereof.

**10.2** ἄλλαι δὲ τούτων πλείους, ἃς ἴσασιν οἷσι τούτων ἐμέλησεν, 'there are many others that are known to those who care about these matters': our author says little about anatomy that would not be plain to any layperson. By appealing to popular knowledge of anatomy, he secures assent to the basic proposition that some of the body's internal structures can be known. The anatomy of more obscure or complicated structures (the 'many other' cavities) is continuous with this popular knowledge, which differs from the knowledge of 'those who care about these matters' (cf. 1.3, 9.2, and 11.3) not in kind but rather in degree. In c. 10, he continually reminds the audience of this difference in degree by employing technical terms and calling attention to the fact that he is simplifying his anatomical presentation. Whether his own anatomical knowledge extends beyond the immediate content of his presentation is impossible to say. Certainly, this is no proof of his medical expertise. (See also Introduction, sections 4 and 5.)

**10.3** ὅσα γὰρ τῶν μελέων ἔχει σάρκα περιφερέα ... πάντα νηδὺν ἔχει, 'for all of the limbs surrounded by flesh ... have a cavity': Jouanna insists that τὰ μέλεα are body parts as opposed to limbs (1988, 235 n. 4). However, our author goes on to name the legs and arms as representative examples, which he then distinguishes from the head and trunk. These examples are what give the causal γάρ its force. Their existence provides a reason for accepting the earlier claim that there are more cavities in the body than just the two that take in and expel food matter.

The structure of the described anatomy is lamentably unclear. Is there a cavity beneath or inside the muscle? Perhaps the author is referring to the larger arteries in the limbs (e.g., the femoral artery in the leg). Alternatively, he may be conceiving of the entire area under the skin and above the bones as a hollow cavity filled with various tissue, including, most conspicuously, muscle tissue. This would fit his philosophical objective—to depict the body as a composite of progressively more concealed 'layers'—and it is suggested, if not implied, by the general proposition, articulated a few lines later in the chapter, that 'everything discontinuous, whether concealed by skin or flesh, is hollow.'

**10.3** ἣν μῦν καλέουσιν, 'so-called 'muscle'': that 'muscle' is a medical term of art does not fully explain the fact that it is singled out for special attention by our author (cf. Jouanna, 1988, 191 n. 5; 236 n. 1). As noted earlier, he uses νηδύς in an unusual way and without comment. The qualification 'so-called' is reserved, here and at 10.4, for technical terms with their origins in metaphor. (The word μῦς means literally 'mouse.') It may be that our author is flagging the conventional element in the correctness of names; nothing prevents transference of the natural kind-name 'mouse' from the miniscule mammal to the muscle (see notes on 2.3).

**10.3** πᾶν γὰρ τὸ ἀσύμφυτον, ἤν τε δέρματι ἤν τε σαρκὶ καλύπτηται, κοῖλόν ἐστι, 'for everything that is not grown together, whether covered by skin or flesh, is hollow': this reads as a definition of κοῖλόν: an enclosed structure is hollow (or has a cavity) if it is not composed throughout of the same *kind* of tissue; the adjective ἀσύμφυτον recalls our author's discussion of φύσις at 2.3 and its association both with growth and with natural kinds (only two tissues of the same kind can grow together). As in c. 2, there is the possibility of an allusion to Empedocles, who used the participle συμφύντα to describe the fusion of his roots (DK 31 B26); see also notes on 10.4 below.

**10.3** πληροῦται τε ὑγιαῖνον μὲν πνεύματος, ἀσθενῆσαν δὲ ἰχῶρος, 'when healthy is full of breath; when weak, of fluid': hollow cavities do not therefore contain nothing at all, since they are full at all times either with breath or fluid. The physiological implications of this last remark remain frustratingly vague. The association of breath with health may ally *de Arte* with treatises like *Flat.* and *Morb. Sacr.* and philosophical theories like that of Diogenes of Apollonia (see also Introduction 4), but only if there is a casual connection between breath and health. Such a connection would be consistent with, but not demanded by, the language here in 10.3. The same holds for the association of morbidity with fluid. Jouanna, following Demont (1981), suggests that ἰχώρ is a serous humor of the kind that flows from sores or ulcers. This would explain its pathological association, and I am willing to consider Jouanna's extension of the term to apply to any humor whatsoever (1988, 236 n. 2), though this does not make clear precisely how ἰχώρ is supposed to be connected to morbidity. Perhaps it obstructs the flow of life-giving breath; but again, this assumes a causal connection between breath and health that is, like the connection between fluid and morbidity, merely suggested by the text, even if the basic scheme does find support in other pneumatic treatises in the *Corpus*. The build-up of fluid in the cavities could, for example, result incidentally from humoral excesses that weaken the body by any one of a number of alternative causal mechanisms. That our author is content to let such questions linger indicates, I think, that his agenda is only incidentally physiological. The essential concerns are epistemological.

**10.4** ὅ τε γὰρ θώρηξ καλεόμενος, ἐν ᾧ το ἧπαρ στεγάζεται ὅ τε τῆς κεφαλῆς κύκλος, ἐν ᾧ ὁ ἐγκέφαλος, τό τε νῶτον πρὸς ᾧ ὁ πλεύμων, 'for the so-called trunk encases the liver and the round part of the head contains the brain; next to the back are the lungs': the technical medical term θώρηξ was taken over from military usage, where it refers to a piece of armor that covers the chest and abdomen. The verb στεγάζειν represents our author's passing nod to its origin (Jouanna 1988, 259 n. 4; see also note on 10.3). The anatomical θώρηξ covers and protects the liver just as the military θώρηξ covers and protects the body. Again, the simile serves our author's purpose by reinforcing his picture of the body as a complex of coverings, as does his alliterative reference to ὅ τε τῆς κεφαλῆς κύκλος, ἐν ᾧ ὁ ἐγκέφαλος. The very names of these parts allude to their relation of concealment to other parts.

**10.4** τούτων οὐδὲν ὅ τι οὐ καὶ αὐτὸ κενόν ἐστιν, πολλῶν διαφυσίων μεστόν, 'none of these is not itself empty, each being full of natural fissures': Jouanna remarks that κενόν and μεστόν form a 'purely formal' antithesis (1988, 259 n. 5), though our author quite clearly is playing with paradox ("being full, they are empty"), a paradox that depends on the conceptual opposition between emptiness and fullness (cf. 7.3).

The other opposition in play is that between διάφυσις and σύμφυσις (contained in τὸ ἀσύμφυτον at 10.3), literally the difference between a 'divided growth' and a 'growing together.' Empedocles may have invented the antithesis; he used the verbal forms to characterize the separation and fusion of his elements (DK 31 B17, B26). The word διάφυσις has been rendered as 'interstice' by most translators, but the particular organs in question—the liver, brain, and lungs—all have in common a lobular structure defined by obvious fissures (e.g., the falciform, right triangular, and coronary ligaments of the liver; the longitudinal cerebral fissure of the brain, not to mention the cerebral sulci generally; and the oblique and horizontal fissures of the lungs) that are evident also in the organs of domesticated animals. Indeed, 'crack' or 'crevice' is the common meaning of διάφυσις, and that is probably what our author has in mind, though other interpretations cannot be ruled out. Craik, for example, believes the reference is to the sponginess of the lungs (2009, 20), which our author would have then projected onto the brain and liver.

**10.4** ἔστι δ' οἷσιν οὐδὲν ἀπέχει πολλῶν ἀγγεῖα εἶναι τῶν μέν τι βλαπτόντων τὸν κεκτημένον, τῶν δὲ καὶ ὠφελεύντων, 'and in these cases nothing prevents the presence of receptacles for many things, some of which are harmful to their possessor, and some of which are beneficial': Heinimann notes that ἀγγεῖον here does not have its fourth-century meaning of 'vessel' (e.g., veins and arteries) but rather its original meaning of 'container' or 'receptacle' (1961, 112 n. 32). The word choice again reflects our author's concern for epistemological, not medical, matters.

The participles βλαπτόντων and ὠφελεύντων recall the same opposition at 5.5, but, more immediately, parallel ὑγιαῖνον and ἀσθενῆσαν at 10.2. The link may be the lungs. It is tempting to draw a connection between the lungs as vessels that may contain harmful or beneficial things and the general principle that fluid weakens while air makes healthy. When the lungs are able to inflate with air, they function well. But when they are filled with fluid, they are sick. The general principle would appear to find confirmation in the sick person's expectoration of mucus. Expectoration of phlegm is cited as an aid to diagnosis at 12.4, and it plays an important role in Hippocratic medicine generally. For example, the author of *Morb. Sacr.* hypothesizes that seizure disorders are caused by the blockage of air by cold phlegm descending from the brain, which is connected to the liver and the lungs by the main channel of a large hepatic vein (11.6–16.23 = L. 6.366–374). The pathological process envisioned is intriguingly consistent with some of the physiological ideas articulated in *de Arte*, but it is difficult to say more given the vagueness of our author's descriptions. In any case, the vagueness here at 10.4 contains an implicit appeal to medical authority. Experts will know which contents harm and which benefit. Laypersons need not trouble with the details.

**10.5** ἔτι δὲ καὶ πρὸς τούτοισι φλέβες πολλαὶ καὶ νεῦρα οὐκ ἐν τῇ σαρκὶ μετέωρα ἀλλὰ πρὸς τοῖσιν ὀστέοισι προστεταμένα ⟨ἃ⟩ σύνδεσμός ἐστι τῶν ἄρθρων, καὶ αὐτὰ τὰ ἄρθρα, 'there are numerous vessels, as well as sinews that are not on the surface of the flesh but rather are stretched out along the bones and form a bond for the joints, and also the joints themselves': the sense is plain, but the syntax was adjusted by Diels to provide a better parallel with the preceding (1914, 397). The anatomical descriptions echo passages in *Loc. Hom.* (cf. 38.24–25 = L. 6.280, 42.3–6 = L. 6.284, and 46.22–27 = L. 6.290; see also following notes).

**10.5** ἐγκυκλέονται, 'circle round': this is the second allusion to circularity (see also τῆς κεφαλῆς κύκλος at 10.4) in c. 10, or perhaps even the third, if one includes περιφερέα at 10.3. This induces Jori to stress the roundish ('tondeggiante') structure of the body on our author's description (1996, 236), though I'm reluctant to read much into this coincidence of circles except insofar as it reinforces the three-dimensionality, and thus the depth, of the body.

**10.5** καὶ τούτων οὐδὲν ὅ τι οὐχ ὕπαφρόν ἐστι, 'none of these does not have a viscous quality': the reading is much disputed (see Jouanna 1988, 204, as well as his account on 260 n. 8, preceded by Diels, 1914, 397–398), though both A and M agree on ὕπαφρόν. The matter is complicated by Erotian, who reports that Heraclides of Tarentium glosses ὕποφρον, giving it a sense equivalent to κρυφαῖον ('hidden'), and by Hesychius, who attributes this same sense to ὕπαφρον. Textually, Jouanna takes the more conservative route, printing ὕπαφρον, and I follow him.[70] Concerning the translation, Jouanna poses a dilemma between emphasizing the root, ἀφρός, 'foam,' or the prefix, ὑπό, which could have the force of 'slightly' or 'secretly,' or perhaps even spatial significance: 'underneath.' He ultimately splits the difference, rendering ὕπαφρον as 'écumeuse à l'intérieur' ('foamy on the inside'; 1988, 236), though this strikes me as too neat. The real dilemma, on my view, lies in the choice between the standard meaning of ὕπαφρον, foamy, viscous, even slimy—the adjective is routinely applied to bodily fluids such as semen and saliva—and the sense introduced by Hesychius ('hidden').

The facts of human anatomy incline us toward the former, as illustrated by a passage from *Loc. Hom.* that resonates with the description here in *de Arte.*

> Mucus (μύξα) occurs naturally in all people, and when this is pure the joints are sound and therefore supple, since they are lubricated against one another. Pain and discomfort arise when moisture flows from the flesh when it has suffered in some way. First, the joint is stiff, for the moisture which has flowed into it from the flesh is not a lubricant.
>
> Then, since moisture has become too copious and is not still being watered by the flesh, it dries up and, since there is too much of it (πολλὴ ἐοῦσα), the joint not being able to contain it, it flows out and, harmfully congealed (κακῶς τε πεπηγυῖα) it swells the cords by which the joint is bound together (συνδέδεται), and makes them free and loose. Through this people become lame; when it happens more severely more so, and when less severely less so.
>
> (*Loc. Hom.* 46.17–27 = L. 6.290; trans. Craik)

Our author, like the author of *Loc. Hom.*, is describing the viscous fluid of the synovial joints, contained in articular capsules, though it is interesting that 1) *Loc. Hom.* does not identify the capsules themselves, though this seems to

---

[70] Dissenting, Craik reads ὕποφρον with Heraclides and Erotian, taking it to mean 'arcane' or 'secret' (2009, 20). This may well be right, and it is tempting to follow Craik's lead, but many have resisted the temptation. The term itself and the sense given by Heraclides is poorly attested, and, though Erotian quotes it in context, he mangles the passage and its logic (οὐθὲν ὅτι καὶ ὕποφρον, Nachmanson 88, 16–89, 2), raising doubts about the accuracy of his source.

be the salient point for our author; and 2) the author of *Loc. Hom.* is keen to provide a physiological account of joint ruptures, while such an account is conspicuously absent from *de Arte*. Instead, our author persists in sketching the body as a system of hidden containers within containers, full of hidden things, and his reference to chambers (θάλαμαι, see following) would seem to explain the joints' concealment more than their viscosity. Thus, while I translate 'viscous,' I do so with apprehension, since it may be that the correct meaning is 'hidden' *vel. sim.* There is always the possibility, too, that the ambiguity is intentional.

**10.5** καὶ ἔχον περὶ αὐτὸ θαλάμας ἃς καταγγέλλει ὁ ἰχώρ, ὅς, ἐκδιοιγομένων αὐτέων, πολλός τε καὶ πολλὰ λυπήσας ἐξέρχεται, 'each being surrounded by chambers that are indicated by fluid, which issues forth copiously when the cells are completely ruptured, causing a great deal of pain': it may be, as Jouanna suggests (1988, 261 n. 1), that ἰχώρ is in excess (πολλός), and this accounts for the attendant rupture, though, once again, the language does not require this interpretation. Even if Jouanna is correct, it is still possible that the fluid in question is not intrinsically pathological, since the description is consistent with (and perhaps demands) the continuous presence of fluid in the articular capsules. Our author's concerns remain epistemological, not physiological, and fluid is important mainly for what it signifies (καταγγέλλει). When fluid is observed flowing from the site of a wound, we are left with two possibilities. Either the fluid is materializing *ex nihilo* at the edge of the wound, or it is coming from some hidden source. The second possibility is clearly preferable. Our author, not unreasonably, thinks he can get a sense for what is inside of the body—what is hidden—by paying attention to what comes out of it. (See also 12.1–3 and Appendix 4).

## 11

After the brief anatomical digression of c. 10, which described the spatial constraints on knowledge of non-evident diseases, our author turns to consider at length the *temporal* constraints. The chapter itself is divisible into three main parts: the problem statement (11.1–3), the therapeutic narrative (or 'narrative proper'; 11.3–6), and the consistency argument (11.7).[71] The

[71] My analyses of chapters in *de Arte* tends to emphasize their divisibility, at least into distinct *pisteis*, but Jori deserves credit for recognizing that the complexity of c. 11 calls for a more complicated schema. It should be added, however, that there was prior to Jouanna's

chapter begins by enumerating a variety of factors that will affect the doctor's ability to diagnose a non-evident disease. By 11.3, it is clear that his main concern is the slowness of diagnosis, which he blames on the disease and the patient. So begins his therapeutic narrative, an account of how non-evident diseases are diagnosed by doctors.[72] The transition to narrative is signaled by tense and aspect markers that establish the precise temporal relations between events in the story (λογισμῷ μετῄει at 11.3; αἰσθομένη at 11.5; οὐ λαμβανόμενοι γὰρ ἀλλ' εἰλημμένοι at 11.6). Examples of narrative in Athenian forensic oratory usually exhibit the same shift in tense (an illustrative but by no means exhaustive list would include Lysias 12.4, and 32.4; Antiphon 1.14), for obvious reasons. To convince a jury, plaintiffs need to tell a plausible story (in the past tense) about what the accused did and why he should be punished. Defendants need to tell an alternative story that minimizes, excuses or distracts from the role they played in the events leading up to the complaint.[73]

The accepted facts are these: the doctor took the patient under his care but was unable to diagnose the disease, and the patient died. This our author does not dispute. In dispute, rather, is the relative culpability of the three characters who play roles in the story, namely, the doctor, the non-evident disease, and the patient. According to our author, the actions (or, in the case of the patient, inaction) of the latter two are ultimately responsible for the patient's death. Again, the issue of responsibility takes center stage, and it is no accident that the language used to describe the doctor's actions suggests an analogy between the diagnosis and treatment of the causes of disease and the prosecution of a criminal in a law court. But there are other metaphors at work, too. Most noticeably, the doctor is compared to

---

work an editorial tradition of isolating 11.7 as a separate chapter of its own. In a sense, then, there has been longstanding consensus that c. 11 was divisible. Jori, for his part, analyzes the chapter into four parts (1996, 240–241): the statement of the problems of effort and slowness through 11.4, the narrowing of the subject to slowness at 11.5, the agonistic account of the doctor's encounter with disease at 11.6, and the comparison to other *technai* at 11.7. As with some of Jori's other structural analyses, I grant its thematic and heuristic value, though I doubt its correspondence to the actual structure of composition.

72 Compare the narrative analysis of this chapter in Holmes (2010, 174ff.).

73 Recent work by Gagarin on narrative and storytelling in Athenian (and, for that matter, American) law shows that in ancient exchanges of forensic rhetoric, 'the defendant's story fits the facts, just as the plaintiff's does' (2003, 201). Following contemporary trends in the 'Law and Literature' movement, Gagarin takes the view that legal reasoning is not simply a process of deducing conclusion from available facts, but rather includes an evaluation of narratives that supply a context for facts. The success of a legal argument sometimes hinges not so much on its logic as on its literary quality.

a military commander pursuing the enemy; but perhaps also to an athlete racing against a competitor; or to a hunter seeking out his prey. These activities have in common two key features: they are all agonistic, a point anticipated already by Ducatillon (1977b, 153), and (with the exception of athletic competition) they require the practitioner to ascertain what is non-evident to him. If non-evidence is not in itself an insurmountable obstacle to the success of these *technai*, why should it pose such a threat to medicine?

As one might expect, the prose in c. 11 is highly stylized. I discuss the more prominent figures in my commentary below, but by far the most conspicuous is the sprawling anacoluthon that afflicts the argument in 11.7, which has incited its share of textual controversies. I do not know whether there is a special motive for the syntactic disruption, though I find it suspicious that the 'speaker's' skill should 'fail' him at the very moment he is discussing the appropriate standards by which to judge technical failure across the various arts.

**11.1** οὐ γὰρ δὴ ὀφθαλμοῖσί γ' ἰδόντι τούτων τῶν εἰρημένων οὐδενὶ οὐδὲν ἔστιν εἰδέναι, 'of course, it is impossible for a person who sees only with his eyes to know any of the things just mentioned': the stressed double negative οὐδενὶ οὐδὲν makes it clear that our author regards the internal structures of the body as completely unavailable to the senses. There is just no possibility of knowing about them if one is using only his eyes—the particle γε tells us that the eyes are insufficient, but perhaps still necessary, to attain this knowledge. We have already seen enough of our author's method to understand why this is so. Internal structures are inferred from what can be seen. The presence of fluid-containing cells within the body is inferred from the effluence of fluid from the body. This effluence is directly observed. It may even be the case that principles such as 'fluids do not simply come out of nowhere' should be regarded as empirical claims.

Thus, we could formulate our author's inference to 'extra-visual' knowledge as an inference of the following kind.

1. Fluid is escaping from point A in this body.
2. As a general rule, fluid does not simply come out of nowhere.
3. The fluid escaping this body at point A is not coming out of nowhere.
4. Therefore, the fluid is coming from somewhere, i.e., there is a reservoir of fluid inside the body.

Premises 1 through 3 may find some confirmation, to greater or lesser degrees, in the evidence of the senses. Regardless of whether our author's inference to 4 is made completely from empirical premises, however, surely it cannot be made without such premises. Thus, perception and observation are crucial to knowledge, even when such knowledge is of things that cannot be directly observed. It is also worth reiterating that 1 through 4 offer very little in the way of knowledge about physiology. The physician needs to know not just that there is fluid inside the body, but also how the fluid acts upon and reacts to other substances and processes in the body. In short, he must hold that observations of external phenomena are relevant to unobserved, internal phenomena. Explaining how they could be so relevant becomes one of our author's tasks over the course of the next few chapters.

**11.1** διὸ καὶ ἄδηλα ἐμοί τε ὠνόμασται καὶ τῇ τέχνῃ κέκριται εἶναι, 'for this reason, I have given them the name 'non-evident,' and so they have been judged by the art': anything whose existence or nature is known through inference and not purely through observation is non-evident. As mentioned earlier (see notes on 9.2), there is no evidence that Greek physicians made a formal therapeutic distinction between evident and non-evident diseases. That is not to say that they did not use such language in talking about disease—it was not meaningless for a doctor to say that a disease was internal and thus non-evident. Surely, the categories are implicit in many discussions of disease in the *Corpus* (e.g., *Flat.* 103.8–12 = L. 6.90). However, the explicit recognition and treatment of the categories in epistemological terms is a philosophical, not strictly medical, matter. This is the point of the contrast between naming and judging. (Again, the relative ease with which names are coined may demonstrate the conventional element in our author's theory of the correctness of names, though it should be noted that the above name is applied for a reason: it marks a very real feature of certain diseases. See notes on 2.3.)

**11.1** οὐ μὴν ὅτι ἄδηλα κεκράτηκεν ἀλλ' ᾗ δυνατὸν κεκράτηται, 'however, they have not prevailed just because they are non-evident; rather, they have been prevailed over where possible': it is difficult to find a consistent English equivalent to the Greek verb κρατεῖν as employed in *de Arte*. Usually it is used of diseases that have overcome the sick person (e.g., 3.2 and 8.1), but here it is intransitive, and its extension is expanded to include the category of the non-evident generally—not just non-evident diseases, but the internal structures and processes of the human body that are not open to direct observation. This signals a shift in the locus of metaphor. The sick person's battle with the disease (cf. 7.3) is referred back to the doctor's epistemic conquest of the non-evident. He wins by knowing and understanding the patient's body; the patient's body wins by remaining unknown and mysterious. It is not difficult to imagine that some critic had declared the war all but over and the non-evident victorious, prompting our author's response in *de Arte*. (See further Introduction 5.)

**11.1** δυνατὸν δὲ ὡς αἵ τε τῶν νοσεόντων φύσιες ἐς τὸ σκεφθῆναι παρέχουσιν, αἵ τε τῶν ἐρευνησόντων ἐς τὴν ἔρευναν πεφύκασιν, 'and it is possible insofar as the natures of the sick submit to examination and the natures of those searching for the non-evident are well suited to the role': here our author considers which medical failures 'are to be attributed to the craftsmen and which to the things being crafted' (8.7). Given the preceding, it would be tempting to gloss the doctor's fight for knowledge of the non-evident as one battle in the war between *technē* and nature, but, on our author's view, this would be a false dichotomy (but see notes on 11.3 below). The doctor's ability to investigate the non-evident is no less natural than the patient's body, which, being a complex of layered tissues, presents a variety of obstacles to the observer. It therefore sets yet another natural limit on the art's potential (cf. 8.2). But if the art is to exist even despite the physician's ignorance, it cannot be identical to his knowledge (i.e., of the correct and incorrect in medicine). Rather, medicine will have to be identified with a method or means for acquiring knowledge, the soundness of which is distinct from the ability of its practitioners to carry it out. This will be the last allusion to the physician's incompetence, however. Henceforth, our author will focus on the obstacles posed by the patient's behavior and the opacity of his body, both of which affect the sick person's submission to examination.

**11.2** μετὰ πλείονος μὲν γὰρ πόνου καὶ οὐ μετ' ἐλάσσονος χρόνου ἢ εἰ τοῖσιν ὀφθαλμοῖσιν ἑωρᾶτο, γινώσκεται, 'for they are known with no less time and with even greater effort than they would have been if seen with the eyes': again, the natural quality required of the researcher is not so much raw intelligence as diligence (cf. 9.4), since knowledge of the non-evident comes by way of a time-consuming effort over and above any relevant observations—Gomperz notes that the pairing of πόνος and χρόνος is commonplace in Greek literature (1910, 133). For the first time in *de Arte*, knowledge and perception come apart: something may be known, even if it is not seen (cf. 2.2).

**11.2** ὅσα γὰρ τὴν τῶν ὀμμάτων ὄψιν ἐκφεύγει, ταῦτα τῇ τῆς γνώμης ὄψει κεκράτηται, 'for what eludes the sight of the eyes is captured by the sight of the mind': here, κεκράτηται, which is contrasted with ἐκφεύγει, 'escape,' must mean captured, not 'conquered' or 'overcome.' The captor is γνώμη, which may know those things that remain hidden to perception through some extra intellectual effort. This pithy and putatively profound exclamation has been compared to similar remarks in the philosophical literature (Introduction 3; cf. especially *Flat.* 106.9–10 = L. 6.94), but it is explicable within the context of the treatise itself.

First and foremost, the noun ὄψις (literally, 'eyesight,' 'vision') must be understood for the metaphor that it is. The etymology of words for knowing (e.g., our author's favorite, εἰδέναι) suggests that, for the Greeks, being seen was at a very primitive level equivalent to, or at least sufficient for, being known. Accordingly, I would recommend that we view the metaphor here in *de Arte* through the lens of this primitive sense, expanding the semantic range of ὄψις to include not just vision, which is one faculty for acquiring knowledge of the sensible world, but any capacity to acquire such knowledge. To paraphrase, then, 'whatever cannot be grasped by the senses nonetheless may be grasped by the mind's capacity for knowing the sensible world.' There is neither implication of, nor need for, an insensible world known only to the mind, and in this way our author closes the gap between seeing and knowing opened in the preceding sentence. Where medical matters are concerned, the mind knows only what is sensible, even if it is not at the moment directly sensed.

**11.3** ἐν τῷ μὴ ταχὺ ὀφθῆναι, 'from a lack of speed in being seen': again, this is 'seen' in the metaphorical sense in which the doctor will come to know, by way of inference, what is happening inside the sick person's body. Our author may also be hinting at a future argument (see 11.6), that the sick do not seek out the doctor, and thus are not 'seen' or 'examined,' until it is too late. While at 11.2 he left open the possibility that the doctor's incompetence was responsible for the failure to diagnose non-evident diseases (though even that failure could be indirectly attributed to nature), he suddenly shifts to a concern with the speed of diagnosis. The shift probably reflects our author's turn to the narrower issue of liability, which is evident in what follows. As a rhetorical tactic, the doctor will ignore even the possibility that he is at fault.

**11.3** οὐχ οἱ θεραπεύοντες αὐτοὺς αἴτιοι, ἀλλ' ἡ φύσις ἥ τε τοῦ νοσέοντος ἥ τε τοῦ νοσήματος, 'it is not those providing treatment who are responsible, but rather nature, specifically, the nature of the sick person as well as the nature of the disease': again, natural limits are blamed for apparent medical failure (cf. 8.2), and it becomes clearer in what way *technē* and nature are genuinely exclusive antitheses. 'Nature' becomes symbolic of the extrinsic factors contributing to technical success or failure (see notes on 7.1), while *technē* will include intrinsic factors—factors that are 'up to' or under the control of the practitioner. Thus, *technē*, though by definition a natural entity with distinctive causal powers and a determinate εἶδος, will be closely connected to νόμος, or convention.

Once again, our author manages to divert an academic concern over epistemic justification into the courtroom, where it assumes the form of a forensic squabble over who is responsible for the patient's death or at least his failure to recover. He deftly converts a disadvantage into an advantage by playing one criticism of medicine against another. To the charge that medicine is poorly equipped to acquire knowledge of internal processes, he stands fast in his conviction that knowledge is possible while conceding that such knowledge is exceedingly difficult to attain due to the non-evidence of the subject matter. Having conceded this, he now puts it forward as the best explanation for patient mortality. The obscurity of most diseases is the cause of death, not any mistake on the part of the physician. He reintroduces into the discussion the natures of patients, but whereas such references are primarily to physical natures, namely the fact that so many regions of the body are difficult to see and explore, we will find that he blames the reluctance of patients to consult a physician for the failure to diagnose and treat diseases in a timely manner (11.6). Thus, the patient's nature will include also his psychological tendencies.

**11.3** ἐπεὶ οὐκ ἦν αὐτῷ ὄψει ἰδεῖν τὸ μοχθέον οὐδ' ἀκοῇ πυθέσθαι, λογισμῷ μετῄει, 'since it was possible neither to see the problem with his sight nor to learn about it by hearing, [he] tried to pursue it using reason': here ὄψις returns to its literal meaning of 'eyesight,' but the meaning of ἀκοῇ πυθέσθαι is not obvious. The immediate context demands that it parallel ὄψει ἰδεῖν. All avenues of potential perceptual access to the disease are closed to the physician, including hearing. Diagnosis by auscultation was a common tool in the Hippocratic repertoire (Langholf 1990, 59), and our author himself regards the quality of a patient's voice as a sign of what ails him (12.2). However, he will shortly complain of the unreliability of patient testimony, claiming that the doctor cannot hear the undistorted truth from their accounts (τὴν ἀναμάρτητον σαφήνειαν ἀκοῦσαι). Probably the development of this argument is anticipated here. Our author will identify three routes to knowledge of the sensible world: direct perception, testimony, and inference. In the case of non-evident disease, direct perception and testimony are insufficient, leaving the doctor to rely on λογισμός alone (cf. *Flat.* 106.9–10 = L. 6.94). Indeed, the usual sense of πυνθάνεσθαι is 'to learn from the testimony of others,' though it can have the simple meaning 'to hear.' It is of note that ὄψις and ἀκοή are paralleled by λογισμός; as sight and hearing are the characteristic functions or capacities of the eyes and ears, respectively, so reasoning is a function of the mind, γνώμη (see also notes on 1.2, 2.1, and 7.1).

Following Jones (1923, 211), I take μετῄει as a conative imperfect. It appears here, I think, because the author stresses the sustained and sincere effort that the physician puts into pursuit of the disease. The word 'pursuit' is chosen deliberately: one pursues those responsible for a murder or other crime (Aeschylus, *Ch.* 273). The diction has the effect of transforming the doctor from defendant to prosecutor. Moreover, insofar as any pursuit involves the use of reasoning to track down what is not present, the verb implicitly compares medicine to forensic investigation, legitimizing the doctor's *technē* by association. Indeed, the verb's past tense, along with the sudden transition to the singular, gives our author's account the feel of a legal narrative (see my introductory comments on this chapter, above).

11.4 ἀπαγγέλλειν, 'the reports': here, reporting is first and foremost a speech act aimed at communicating accurately a non-evident state of affairs. It is in this sense that signs or symptoms will later take on the metaphorical role of messengers or reporters (12.3, 12.6; cf. 2.1).

11.4 δοξάζοντες μᾶλλον ἢ εἰδότες, 'based on opinion rather than on knowledge': the patient's reports are opinions, but not necessarily false opinions, though necessarily some of them will be false (see following note). More important is that the doctor cannot count on the truth of the opinions, since they are not secured in the proper way (i.e., either through direct observation or by carefully reasoned inference from observed fact). The distinction between opinion and knowledge goes back at least to Xenophanes (DK 21 B34, B35), extending through the work of Parmenides (DK 28 B1.28–32) and sophists such as Gorgias (82 DK B11a § 24) and Antiphon (F44(a)II.21–23). The Xenophanean precedent is especially applicable.

> No man has seen (οὔτις ἀνὴρ ἴδεν) nor will anyone know (οὐδέ τις ἔσται εἰδὼς)
> the truth (τὸ σαφές) about the gods and all the things of which I speak.
> For even if a person should in fact say what is absolutely the case,
> still he himself does not know, but opinion (δόκος) is woven into the
> structure of all things. (DK 21 B34)

Our author respects the basic distinction drawn by Xenophanes. Even if the patient holds a true opinion about non-evident matters, he cannot know these things are true because he cannot confirm them by direct perception. (Note that the patients' lack of knowledge becomes an issue specifically with respect to τὰ ἀφανέα.) They can have only opinions about what they cannot perceive.[74] However, on our author's view, there are some privileged few who can break through the Xenophanean barrier. The doctor may grasp facts about non-evident diseases through reason.

Jouanna senses our author's anticipation of the critic's objection that 'the sick person knows his disease insofar as he feels it' (1988, 262 n. 1), but it seems to me rather that he is simply emphasizing the difficulty of diagnosing non-evident diseases. The doctor is utterly alone in his pursuit, since not even the patient is a reliable informant. Some of the patient's reports may be true, but since the patient does not have genuine knowledge of the matter, such reports will be true only, as it were, coincidentally (cf. the fragment of Xenophanes above). The doctor's only rational course of action will be to treat all the patient's reports as potentially false. Only after he has made his own diagnosis will it become clear which among them were true.

Is our author's claim too strong? Surely there are some patient reports that we could call knowledge, and the point is not to discredit the patient's report that, for example, he feels pain, feels hot, feels numb, etc. Instead, our author means that a patient's account of his illness, especially when the problem is internal, and thus non-evident, invariably involves assumptions about internal anatomy, physiology, and even pathology. The patient is unlikely to report simply that he is in pain. More likely, instead, he will report that his stomach hurts, and that he ate something that caused it to hurt. It is not at all implausible that this account of *what* is happening and *why* will turn out to have had little diagnostic value outside of having communicated the fact that the patient was suffering some sort of abdominal pain. Patient reports about internal diseases necessarily refer to, at least implicitly, a picture of anatomy, physiology, and pathology. These pictures are inevitably distorted. They are incomplete, incorrect, or at least poorly understood, and even when there is some grain of truth in the report, there are no grounds for taking the patient's description at face value. (On the ignorance of patients, see also 5.2 and 7.3. Cf. *Flat.* 103.5–8 = L. 6.90.)

11.4 εἰ γὰρ ἠπίσταντο, οὐκ ἂν περιέπιπτον αὐτοῖσι, 'for if they had knowledge, they would not have run afoul of these diseases': it was a standard—and unchallenged—bit of dogma that whoever had mastered the art of medicine would be himself healthy. As Jouanna notes (1988, 262 n. 2), the

[74] My understanding of Xenophanes' skepticism follows the outlines of Barnes's interpretation (1982a, 138–141), which has since become mainstream.

criticism of doctors who fall ill can be found in Aeschylus' (*Pr.* 472–475), but traces of the idea are found also in the *Corpus* (e.g., *Medic.* 20.4–7 = L. 9.204). One assumes, perhaps, that the practitioner will take care in his own case to exercise his expertise to the fullest extent, so that the doctor will be expected to be in excellent health.

This is an unfair expectation, to be sure, and it is no fairer if indeed our author turns it on the sick. It would ignore what writers across the *Corpus* routinely acknowledge: disease can arise from factors outside of one's control (e.g., from environmental or climactic conditions, though perhaps our author's myopic treatment, at 5.4–5, of dietetic elements as the causes of benefit and harm signals a disregard for such factors). Moreover, in the present context it would appear to commit our author to denying weakness of will, since such weakness would explain a person's ill health even in the event that he had genuine knowledge of his disease and how to cure it. A diabetic doctor might know a dessert will have deleterious effects but devour it nonetheless. Does our author deny this is possible? At 7.1, he blames the ἀκρασίη, or weakness, of the patient for his own death, and it is clear at 7.3 that this weakness is primarily (though not exclusively) weakness of will. He will concede, then, that weakness of will exists, at least in the sick person. Perhaps his description of the doctor as being of 'healthy mind and body' (7.3) suggests a correlation between self-control and physical health such that illness is a necessary condition of weakness of will. An imbalance in the appetites, for example, might be thought to supervene on an imbalance of the basic humors. Such a postulate, though vulnerable to obvious counterexamples, would explain why weakness of will could not be responsible for disease. A healthy person could not be weak and so would never become ill—except through ignorance.

If all this seems too conjectural, it may be that we are scrutinizing too closely a casual claim thrown out in the course of an argument whose rhetorical force is concentrated elsewhere. Our author may not consciously rule out climactic conditions and weakness of will as explanations of disease, but he may expect this to be understood. On this interpretation, the sentence lies within the scope of an implicit *ceteris paribus* qualification: 'barring any unusual circumstances—e.g., extreme climactic conditions or a profound weakness of will—if he had knowledge, he would not have fallen ill.' To explicitly enumerate such exceptions, while intellectually integrous, would be rhetorically redundant and ultimately counterproductive to his aim of showing that patients describing their non-evident diseases do not really know what they are talking about.

Furthermore, it is possible that our author does not commit himself to the claim that a person with knowledge will never get sick, but rather that he is making a more subtle turn. The knowledge in question is not general knowledge of medicine (though certainly some of this will be required) but knowledge of what in particular is wrong with the patient. It is this sort of knowledge—knowledge of his own internal, pathological condition—that the patient lacks, and it makes no sense to say that, if he had it, he would not have fallen ill. In fact, the verb περιπίπτειν means not just 'fall in with,' but 'fall in with something bad or evil,' that is, 'run afoul of,' in the sense of to 'collide with, especially so as to cause injury' (cf. περιπίμπτειν τοῖσι θανάτοισιν, 7.5). It is more often than not part of an idiom: one 'falls in with' bad luck, misfortune, or evil (usually great evil) generally (κακοῖς που περιπέσῃ, Aristophanes, *Ra.* 969; τὸν δυστυχίαις μεγάλαις περιπίπτοντα, Aristotle, *EN* 153b; τοιαύτῃ συμφορᾷ περιπέπτωκεν, Demosthenes 21.96). Even when the author of *VM* writes that human beings suffer greatly from consuming foods that are raw, unblended, and possessing great powers, 'falling into strong pains and diseases' (πόνοισί τε ἰσχυροῖσι καὶ νούσοισι περιπίπτοντες, 121.19–20 = L. 1.576), the verb appears to be chosen chiefly to express the severity of the consequences. I can find no examples, either in the *Corpus* or in the literature more broadly, of περιπίπτειν with the simple meaning 'to fall ill' regardless of the severity of the disease. Accordingly, perhaps our author is claiming not that someone knowledgeable about his condition will avoid falling ill altogether, but rather that he will know how to manage his illness such that it does not threaten serious harm.

The real argument, then, would amount to this: if a patient possessed knowledge (or even true opinion) about his disease, he would have been able to catch the disease before his condition had become so critical as to require medical attention. The very fact that he has called in a doctor proves he is at a loss about the nature of his condition. This is a much stronger (though still not uncontestable) argument, one that completely denies a pathogenic role neither for external circumstance (e.g., climactic changes) nor for weakness of will.

11.4 τῆς γὰρ αὐτῆς συνέσιός ἐστιν ἧσπερ τὸ εἰδέναι τῶν νούσων τὰ αἴτια, καὶ τὸ θεραπεύειν αὐτὰς ἐπίστασθαι πάσῃσι τῇσι θεραπείῃσιν αἳ κωλύουσι τὰ νοσήματα μεγαλύνεσθαι, 'since knowing the causes of diseases and knowing how to treat them by all the means that hinder their progress belong to the same intellect': knowing a disease's αἴτια is a necessary and almost singularly sufficient step in correctly determining the course of treatment. The claim is a common one in the *Corpus* (see Introduction 1). However, it is prohibitively strong unless the αἴτια are understood not as just any cause whatsoever (e.g., proximate triggering causes, circumstantial contributing causes, some of which the patient may discern himself) but as explanatory causes. The αἴτια must be those fundamental natural regularities in virtue of which one event causes another and which must be known both to predict the course of a disease and to determine correct treatment in a particular case (cf. notes on 5.2–5, 6.4). If I know a patient has diabetes, and if I have a reasonably complete grasp of the biochemical and physiological explanation of diabetes, then I will know, *ceteris paribus*, what will follow from modifying his blood sugar in various ways, and certainly this is a non-trivial component of devising treatment for him in case of a diabetic episode. (It will not suffice, by contrast, to know simply that he is feeling faint from eating a donut, even though this is one way of knowing the cause of his condition.)

The phrase πάσῃσι τῇσι θεραπείῃσιν αἳ κωλύουσι τὰ νοσήματα μεγαλύνεσθαι tends to confirm the suggestion made earlier that our author is claiming only that a person with knowledge of his disease would be able to treat himself, not that he would not have fallen ill in the first place. There is the further significant implication that a disease develops according to a principle of increase in its power (μεγαλύνεσθαι) to harm the patient, which I will refer to as its 'progression.' This shortens considerably the doctor's window of opportunity and makes diagnosis yet more urgent, if such progress is to be hindered—κωλύειν is encountered for the second time (cf. 1.3) and is probably intended to revive the martial connotations that attended its first occurrence.

**11.4** ὅτε οὖν οὐδ' ἐκ τῶν ἀπαγγελλομένων ἔστι τὴν ἀναμάρτητον σαφήνειαν ἀκοῦσαι, 'now as it is impossible to achieve perfect clarity by listening to these reports': again, the patient's inability to treat himself successfully shows that he holds at least some false beliefs about his condition, which does not imply that the patient's reports are completely false, though it does imply that they involve opinion and are not error-free (ἀναμάρτητον). Thus, patients cannot, on the whole, be considered knowledgeable (εἰδότες).

The use of σαφήνεια as a metonym for truth is somewhat unusual (though recall the similar formulation τὸ σαφές in Xenophanes DK 21 B34, cited above). Meaning literally 'clarity' or 'distinctness,' the term has obvious connections to perception as a source of knowledge. Here it is utilized to refer to knowledge of what cannot be perceived and so must be known either through testimony or inference. We find a parallel in a courtroom speech prepared by Antiphon ('to hear the truth of what was done,' τῶν πραχθέντων τὴν σαφήνειαν πυθέσθαι, 1.13). The parallel is especially intriguing since in *de Arte* the verb ἀκοῦσαι must have the same meaning as Antiphon's πυθέσθαι, 'to learn from oral testimony.' Our author again likens the doctor's task to that of the prosecutor in a law court trying to determine who or what is responsible for the injury sustained. But whereas the prosecutor can often rely on the testimony of the victim, the doctor cannot, which makes diagnosis all the more difficult. He is forced to rely on reasoning or inference (cf. 12.2, 12.4). Thus, it is fitting that the other illuminating instance of σαφήνεια comes to us in a fragment of Alcmaeon of Croton, who uses the term, paradoxically, for divine knowledge of the non-evident, as opposed to what human beings are left to infer (DK 24 B1; cf. Xenophanes DK 21 B34). Jori contends (1996, 252 n. 111) that our author is alluding to the doctrine of Alcmaeon in an attempt to subvert it. Truth or clarity seems to be something available not just to the omnipercipient gods but also to human *technitai* through testimony and inference. I address the significance of this and other fragments in the Introduction (section 3), but here it will suffice to say that Jori's representation of the passage is exaggerated. Our author is more likely pointing out that, in a case of non-evident disease, no one, not even the person closest to the phenomenon, has direct perceptual knowledge (or σαφήνειαν) of the disease and its causes. Thus, he, like any other human being, must make recourse to inference.

That perfect clarity is our author's standard shows that, on his model, medicine will not accommodate cognitive imprecision, making *de Arte* a poor vehicle for the articulation of an alternative, 'stochastic' conception of *technē* (see further Appendix 3).

11.4 τῷ θεραπεύοντι, 'the doctor': literally, 'the one providing treatment.' Concerns for style and clarity prevent me from giving this translation consistently in c. 11, where our author often uses this participle to refer to what in modern vernacular we might call a 'medical provider.' It is unlikely, though not impossible, that he uses the more generic term in order to make his defense applicable to practitioners besides doctors (e.g., midwives). Probably our author depends on the participle to emphasize that, even when the doctor has not yet begun to treat the patient, he is nevertheless actively engaged in providing therapy (see notes on ὑπερβατῶς at 11.7 below). Patients, meanwhile, are portrayed as passive. Referred to mostly as 'the diseased' (οἱ νοσέοντες) or 'the troubled' (οἱ κάμνοντες), they 'are examined' (τὸ ὀφθῆναι), 'are treated' (θεραπεύεσθαι) and 'are healed' (τὸ ὑγιανθῆναι) by the doctor, while they 'are gripped by' (λαμβανόμενοι) and 'suffer from' (πάσχουσιν) their diseases. They are several times characterized by what they do wrong or do not do at all: they do not know (μᾶλλον ἢ εἰδότες), they try (πειρῶνται) but fail to give an accurate report of their diseases, and they bring their own negligence upon themselves (τὴν τῶν καμνόντων ὀλιγωρίην ⟨ἣν⟩ ἐπιτίθενται).[75]

**11.5** ταύτης οὖν τῆς βραδυτῆτος οὐχ ἡ τέχνη, ἀλλ' ἡ φύσις αἰτίη ἡ τῶν σωμάτων, 'thus, it is not the art that is responsible for slowness, but rather the nature of human bodies': the chiasmus of ἡ τέχνη, ἀλλ' ἡ φύσις reinforces the τέχνη-φύσις antithesis (see notes on 11.3 above), as does the isocolon of the sentence as a whole.

**11.5** ἡ μὲν γὰρ αἰσθομένη ἀξιοῖ θεραπεύειν, 'for the art sees fit to provide treatment only after it has perceived the problem': the aorist participle establishes a firm timeline. First, the doctor makes a diagnosis (again, 'perceiving' by way of inference). Only then does he treat the patient. The justification for this approach is left unspoken: to treat before the diagnostic process has been completed is to risk harming the patient further, either by unwittingly exacerbating the existing condition or vainly subjecting the patient to the potentially significant discomforts of treatment. Thus, the author establishes the doctor's motive, which is of the noblest form. Though he works slowly, he does so not out of incompetence, but rather out of concern for the patient's wellbeing.

We may use the timeline to reconstruct the temporal structure of therapeutic interventions as follows.

1. Examination and diagnosis (τὸ ὀφθῆναι): the doctor examines the patient, listens to his complaints, and draws inferences about the underlying causes of the non-evident disease.
2. Treatment (τὸ θεραπεύειν or τὸ ἐγχειρεῖν, 'therapy' in the strict sense): the doctor applies remedies that remove or neutralize the causes of disease.

[75] The distinction between the active doctor and passive patient is made already by Jori on purely conceptual grounds (1996, 100), without citing the linguistic evidence I adduce here. However, one ought not overemphasize the point. Surely patients have a role to play, and many do so successfully. Thus, we should be cautious about accepting Jori's argument (1997) that *de Arte* represents a view of the doctor-patient relationship as an essentially one-sided information exchange in which the knowledgeable doctor issues orders to the ignorant patient without attempting to educate or persuade him. Nothing in *de Arte* would prevent the doctor from taking an 'educational' approach to therapy, but this is somewhat beside the point, which is just to explain what has gone awry when patients die from non-evident disease.

3. Cure (τὸ ὑγιανθῆναι): the causes of disease are destroyed or removed, and so its effects abate.

It is worth noting that this trajectory of therapy, since it describes an intentional act, is organized teleologically around the goal of curing the patient. The teleological structure of the trajectory allows our author to frame the account of its development—to plagiarize Aristotle—as an organically unified narrative with beginning, middle, and end. The story of the doctor is woven together with that of the disease (see notes on the trajectory of disease at 11.6) to produce an agonistic narrative pitting good against evil (quite literally: recall κακὸν at 8.3) on, or rather in, the battlefield that is the patient's body.

**11.5** μὴ τόλμῃ μᾶλλον ἢ γνώμῃ καὶ ῥᾳστώνῃ μᾶλλον ἢ βίῃ θεραπεύῃ, 'its treatments are applied not rashly, but, rather, thoughtfully, and gently rather than violently': Jouanna (1988, 262 n. 6) connects this passage to Herodotus' story of Democedes, who is said to have cured the ailments of the Persian emperor, Darius, with Greek remedies that used gentleness (ἤπια) instead of the Egyptian's violence (τὰ ἰσχυρά) (3.130.1–3). Herodotus may be referring to an Egyptian predilection for intrusive and painful surgical procedures in contrast to the Greek emphasis on drugs and regimen.[76] Our author, at any rate, mentions drugs and regimen as the central types of therapy employed by good physicians (6.1), and *de Arte* contains only an oblique reference to surgery insofar as it apparently mentions cautery in c. 8. Still, even non-surgical procedures, such as the administration of emetics, required that the physician violate the patient's body, and our author may be trying to allay the patient's fear of such measures by assuring him that the treatment will be gauged so as to cause no more discomfort than necessary. The physician, who is 'pursuing' the non-evident diseases (11.3) in an attempt to 'overcome' them (11.2), now shuns the qualities that the Greeks typically prized in their heroes, courage (τόλμη) and physical strength (βίη), which in this context take on a pejorative sense. Instead, the physician uses good judgment (γνώμη) to fight the disease; his easy approach (ῥᾳστώνη, which I translate here as 'gently,' though this does not do full justice to the idea—the Greek word has no elegant English equivalent) delivers an equanimity that gives him an edge in battle. A dichotomy is drawn: do we as patients, attacked by disease, want an ally who rushes into the fray before he knows

[76] On the Hippocratic value of gentleness in treatment, see Jouanna 1999, 131–133. Cf. *Artic.* 4.266.13–19.

the nature of his enemy, who metes out deadly force at random? Or would we prefer someone wise and prudent, who holds his fire until he sees his enemy clearly, who adapts his strategy to the foe at hand and uses no more force than is necessary? The success of the former will be haphazard at best and is liable to inflict irreversible damage on friend as well as foe. The latter is obviously preferable, though even his victory is not guaranteed. An especially swift enemy, or a delay in calling for help, can mean defeat no matter how canny the captain (see following notes).

The tone of concern for the patient's physical comfort marks a sudden shift from preceding lines, in which our author blamed the body, as nature's representative, for the disease's triumph. Perhaps not surprisingly, the respect for nature that informs his metaphysics and theory of language (see 2.2–3) resurges here, bringing *de Arte* into contact with established themes in Greek political and philosophical thought (see also 12.3).

**11.5** ἡ δ' ἢν μὲν διεξαρκέσῃ ἐς τὸ ὀφθῆναι, ἐξαρκέσει καὶ ἐς τὸ ὑγιανθῆναι, 'while the nature of the human body, if it can hold out until it is seen, will hold out long enough to be healed, as well': credit goes to Jouanna (1988, 262 n. 7) for realizing that the prepositional phrases ἐς τὸ ὀφθῆναι and ἐς τὸ ὑγιανθῆναι are temporal and that the verbs διεκαρκεῖν and ἐξαρκεῖν are used in the sense of 'endure,' in close keeping with the original meaning of the root, ἀρκεῖν. The martial metaphor recaptures the high ground here. The patient's body is compared to a besieged city or embattled warrior awaiting help from its allies. The logic of the claim, and its practical implications for medical practice, are vague. Probably it depends on the earlier claim that knowing the causes of a disease and knowing how to treat it are of a piece. Once the patient has been properly diagnosed, the correct treatment will be obvious (at least to the doctor—see 12.3) and may commence forthwith. Thus, if the patient holds out long enough to be diagnosed—not just survives, but resists being overcome by the disease so that he is beyond help (cf. 3.2, 8.5)—his odds of being healed are high. His ability to resist will be a function of his physical strength but perhaps also of his strength of will (cf. 7.3). Either way, his ability to resist will be determined partly by his nature (cf. 11.3).

**11.5** διὰ τὸ βραδέως αὐτὸν ἐπὶ τὸν θεραπεύσοντα ἐλθεῖν ἢ διὰ τὸ τοῦ νοσήματος τάχος, 'whether on account of his slowness in going to the doctor or the speed of the disease': our author formally introduces the excuse, adumbrated at 11.3, that will occupy him for the next several lines: the patient's procrastination (cf. *Prog.* 2.112.6–11). He also mentions, without elaborating, a new excuse, what I will refer to as the 'acceleration' of the disease (τὸ τοῦ νοσήματος τάχος, in contrast to ἐν τῷ μὴ ταχὺ ὀφθῆναι at 11.3), which is just the temporal measure of its progression (μεγαλύνεσθαι, 11.4). Probably, the acceleration of a disease will be neither absolute nor uniform, since it will depend in part on the patient's ability to resist (see preceding note).

**11.6** ἐξ ἴσου μὲν γὰρ ὁρμώμενον τῇ θεραπείῃ οὐκ ἔστι θᾶσσον, προλαβὸν δὲ θᾶσσον, 'for if it starts the race from the same mark as treatment, disease is not the swifter, though it will be swifter if given a head start': athletic imagery of a footrace is layered onto the military imagery of pursuit. Jouanna sees also the possibility of a hunting metaphor (1988, 263 n. 8), citing Xenophon *Cyn.* 7.7, where the verb προλαμβάνειν is used of a hare that has nearly run out of view (recall also ἔρευναν at 11.1 and μετῄει at 11.3). This would be especially fitting given that the non-evident disease is 'hiding' from the doctor.

**11.6** προλαμβάνει δὲ διά τε τὴν τῶν σωμάτων στεγνότητα ἐν ᾗ οὐκ ἐν εὐόπτῳ οἰκέουσιν αἱ νοῦσοι διά τε τὴν τῶν καμνόντων ὀλιγωρίην ⟨ἣν⟩ ἐπιτίθενται, 'and it gets a head start both from the impenetrability of human bodies, which diseases occupy without being seen, and from the negligence of the sick, which they impose upon themselves': the text here is uncertain. Both MSS read ἐπιτίθεται, with the correcting hand of A giving ἐπιτίθενται. Editors have disagreed widely on what should be done with ἐπιτίθεται. Littre (ἐπεὶ ἔοικε·) and Gomperz (ἐπεὶ τί θῶμα;) make radical emendations on the assumption that the text as we have it is nonsensical and hopelessly corrupt. More optimistic editors have tried to make sense of ἐπιτίθεται. Daremberg proposed no changes whatsoever, arguing that the author is straining to produce a balanced chiasmus in which προλαμβάνει governs the first διά-phrase and ἐπιτίθεται the second (1855, 46 n. 51), an ingenious but unsatisfactory idea. The sense is compromised, and, as Jouanna points out (1988, 263 n. 10), we would want in that case for the two prepositional phrases to be connected by a single καὶ, not the conjunctive pair τε ... τε.

I follow in spirit Jouanna's conservative instinct, which is to retain ἐπιτίθεται and include ἣ immediately before. The principle of balance demands that the relative pronoun refer to ὀλιγωρίην to preserve symmetry with στεγνότητα ἐν ᾗ. It is left to tease out a defensible sense for this emendation, which Jouanna locates in a fragment of Antiphon (cited already in my notes on 2.3).

> For those things belonging to convention are impositions (ἐπίθετα), while those that belong to nature are necessary. Further, the agreements of convention are not natural growths, while the growths of nature are not agreements. (F44(a)I.23–33)

As noted earlier, the principal contrast involves nature, which operates from necessity, and convention, which varies according to the whim of those adopting it. The corresponding point in *de Arte* would be that such negligence (and hence the resulting death) could have been avoided had the patient not put off consultation with his doctor.

However, I worry that the force of the verb is weakened by the passive voice employed. Our author looks to round out his indictment of the patient as the cause of his own death. The patient is responsible by nature insofar as his body gives cover to the enemy (the combat metaphor yet again). But he is responsible by convention in that he chooses to delay his examination, unnecessarily adding a further complication to the physician's already insuperable task. The full effect is realized if we take our cue from A$^{corr}$ and read ⟨ἣν⟩ ἐπιτίθενται, taking the verb as the middle form with the meaning 'to bring upon one's self.' Dead patients have no one to blame but themselves. As a final consideration, it should be noted that the understood subject of the next sentence is οἱ καμνόντες, though this understanding is more difficult for the audience to obtain if ὀλιγωρίη intervenes as subject of ἐπιτίθεται.

On a final note, I confess sympathy with Diels' desire to insert something more than a relative pronoun: ⟨οἷσι τὰ λυπεῦντα ἔσωθεν οὔτε προφανῶς οὔτ' ἐξαπίνης⟩ ἐπιτίθεται (1914, 399). The style, namely, our author's obsession with balance throughout the treatise and in this sentence in particular (we should note, though Diels and Jouanna do not, the paromoiosis and parisosis of the two prepositional phrases), calls for a second relative clause to mirror the first. Diels' fantastic confection goes too far, but he is probably right that the original text had more than ᾗ ἐπιτίθεται or ἣν ἐπιτίθενται.[77] The author's sensitivity to syntactical and metrical balance would have demanded it. My own conjecture meets these demands, I think, while building upon the thematic contrasts between seeing and knowing, knowledge and opinion, and technical knowledge and lay ignorance:

Προλαμβάνει δὲ
διά τε τὴν τῶν σωμάτων στεγνότητα
    ἐν ᾗ οὐκ ἐν εὐόπτῳ οἰκέουσιν αἱ νοῦσοι
διά τε τὴν τῶν καμνόντων ὀλιγωρίην
    ⟨ἣν ἐν ἀνεπιστημοσύνῃ⟩ ἐπιτίθενται·

[77] Jori prints ⟨τῆς νούσου, ᾗ αὐτοῖς⟩ ἐπιτίθεται (1996, 66) and translates 'because of the negligence of the sick in confronting the disease that attacks them' ('a motivo della negligenza dei malati nei confronti del male che li aggredisce,' 1996, 82), which strikes me as improbable on several accounts.

The etymological kinship felt between ἀνεπιστημοσύνη and words for attention and inattention (e.g., ἀνεπιστασία) makes it a doubly attractive option, since patient negligence is at issue. Its occurrence in Thucydides (5.7) vouches, I think, for the claim of this conjecture—or something very much like it—to historical and stylistic plausibility. Still, mere plausibility is a low standard on which to base textual decisions, and so I resist printing the conjecture in the main text.

It may be that the term ὀλιγωρίη holds significance for our author as a legal and military term, and so the translation of it as 'negligence' may be particularly apt, though 'neglect of duty' is an attractive alternative. According to the decree of Eubulus in Demosthenes' *On the crown*, a military officer could be punished for his ὀλιγωρίη if he acted outside his orders (18.74). The concept of negligence or neglect does crucial work if our author is employing the legal strategy of blaming the patient. Surely the patient does not intend to kill himself; negligence explains how he could be held responsible nonetheless. In the indictment of the victim and the praise of the physician's gentleness, we hear echoes of cc. 7 and 8, in which our author testified to the physician's soundness of mind while chastising the patient for his weakness of will, which he blamed for the apparent failure of medicine to cure.

**11.6** οὐ λαμβανόμενοι γὰρ ἀλλ' εἰλημμένοι ὑπὸ τῶν νοσημάτων ἐθέλουσι θεραπεύεσθαι, 'for they consent to treatment only once their diseases have taken hold, and not before': as with αἰσθομένη at 11.5 above, the tense and aspect of the participles are employed carefully so as to yield a clear timeline for the narrative. It is not clear, however, whether εἰλημμένοι refers to the therapeutic 'tipping point' indicated by the verb κρατεῖν. If so, then our author's claim here will have to be construed rather loosely. If it were true without exception that the sick waited to consult a doctor until they had been overcome by their diseases, no patient would ever be cured. Alternatively, our author may be introducing a more complicated temporal structure into his nosology, which would include the following phases in the typical disease's development:

1. Start of disease (ὁρμώμενον): presumably through a disruption in physical equilibrium (7.1–3), usually something a person has done or not done (5.5).
2. Onset of disease (λαμβανόμενος): the disease develops according to the interdependent principles of progression (μεγαλύνεσθαι, 11.4) and acceleration (τὸ τοῦ νοσήματος τάχος, 11.5). Shifted into modern idiom, the person is not yet sick but is 'getting sick.'

3. Establishment of disease (εἰλημμένος): the disease, which continues its development, now dominates the body.
4. Point of overcoming (κεκρατημένος): the disease has become so powerful (τὴν δύναμιν τοῦ πάθεος, 8.5) that none of the physician's tools are capable of slowing or reversing its progress.
5. Death (ἀποθνῃσκών): the disease disrupts the body's essential functions to such an extent that the patient dies.

Like the trajectory of therapy outlined above (11.5), the trajectory of disease exhibits a teleological structure. It is organized around the destruction of the sick person in death, as though the disease were a genuine agent performing an intentional act. It is unlikely, I think, that our author conceives of all diseases as susceptible to teleological explanation. More important is the resultant potential for personification and narrative. The disease has its own story, as it were. In c. 11, it is a story of conquest, as the disease defeats the patient despite the doctor's best efforts to defend him. Indeed, in the case of non-evident diseases, defeat is the rule rather than the exception. The closer to phase 1 that examination occurs (ἐξ ἴσου μὲν γὰρ ὁρμώμενον τῇ θεραπείῃ; exact contemporaneity is, as Jori remarks, a limiting case, 1996, 259 n. 123), the better the odds that diagnosis (and the opportune moment for therapeutic intervention) will be reached before phase 4. However, patients do not typically consult the doctor until phase 3, leaving him with only the brief window between phases 3 and 4 in which to make his diagnosis. Given the difficulty of diagnosing non-evident diseases, this is hardly adequate. The patient, more likely than not, will be lost.

**11.7** εἶτα τῆς γε τέχνης τὴν δύναμιν ὁπόταν τινὰ τῶν τὰ ἄδηλα νοσεύντων ἀναστήσῃ θαυμάζειν ἀξιώτερον ἢ ὁπόταν μὴ ἐγχειρήσῃ τοῖσιν ἀδυνάτοισιν, 'so then the power of the art is worthier of admiration when it restores those sick with non-evident diseases than when it does not handle impossible cases?': the text is problematic. Both MSS have ἐπὶ, while their derivatives give ἐπεὶ. But ἐπὶ makes little sense, so some editors, including Jouanna, have turned to ἐπεὶ. However, I have seen no defense of the meaning that results from reading ἐπεί, though perhaps one could infer it from the translations of those who adopt it. Jones translates it 'now' (as in 'now, then,' 1923, 213) while Jouanna gives 'eh bien donc' (1988, 238), that is, both take it as a mundane transitional adverb, which does not, to my knowledge, accord with normal usage. A better solution would be to follow Gomperz, whose paleographically attractive emendation of ἐπὶ to ἔτι is further recommended by the sense it makes of the text. Our author has just finished explaining that patients often wait until the disease has gained the upper hand before consulting a physician. 'Still,' he continues (by which he means to complain: 'this obvious and decisive fact notwithstanding'), people think that success in cases of non-evident disease are testaments to the power of the art, while refusal to undertake cures is a sign of incompetence. But, in fact, such refusals are rational reactions to real situations, requiring the same medical acumen (at least so far as diagnosis is concerned) as successful treatment.

This point of interpretation, too, requires some textual defense, as most have concluded that either the μὴ must be excluded (Littré, Jones, Jori) or a lacuna must be posited (Gomperz, Heiberg, Diels 1914, 400). I will not reconstruct the debate here, except to probe the two most recent contributions, that of Jouanna and Jori. Jouanna argues forcefully for conserving the text as it stands (1988, 263 n. 1). The refusal of impossible cases is built into the very definition of medicine and portrayed as an expression of its power (3.2), while it is argued later that the practice of refusing impossible cases does not impugn the art's power in any way (8.5). Thus, the power of the art is present when a doctor refuses a hopeless case no less than when he cures a non-evident disease, though it is considered (granting a subjective flavor to ἀξιώτερον, which, I think, it can tolerate) more remarkable by the general public. However, in the other handicrafts, no one criticizes a craftsman either for failures due to external factors or for the slowness of his work; instead, they praise his meticulousness.

Jori accepts the validity of Jouanna's argument but objects that it is not plausible to attribute to our author the view that the art merits admiration for its refusal of incurables, since, in the final analysis, these represent limits on the power of the art and so cannot serve as examples of the power of the art itself (1996, 83 n. 9). But again, this overlooks the salient issue, which is that the limits are extrinsic to the *technē*, not intrinsic (see my comments on 7.1). Medicine, when properly practiced, applies the same sound method in each case, and its potential to heal is the same, so long as all relevant external factors are favorably aligned. This is the significance of stressing the power of the art to 'be swifter' when it 'starts from the same place' as the disease while lamenting patients' procrastination. There is a counterfactual lurking between the lines: if only the procrastinating patient had consulted the doctor sooner, the art *could* have saved him. The power is there even when the patient is not.

But many of these disputes dissolve if we conjecture that the original text contained not ἐπὶ, ἐπεὶ, or even ἔτι, but an inferential particle, εἶτα (or the Ionic variant εἶτεν), a paleographically plausible emendation. At the close of the next chapter, our author writes that 'it is no surprise (οὐ θαυμάσιον) that the time spent coming to some conviction about [the signs of non-evident diseases] exceeds that allotted to action' (12.6). This remark may be intended to echo 11.7, and its meaning is clear: it is no surprise that successful treatment of non-evident diseases is often impossible, given the difficulty of making a timely diagnosis. The same sentiment could inspire our author here. It is not at all surprising that non-evident diseases are usually untreatable. Indeed, it is surprising that doctors are ever successful in treating non-evident diseases, given the considerable obstacles. The particle itself is quite capable of standing in the sentence-initial position with an inferential function (Aristophanes, *Av.* 1424). Alternatively, εἶτα is found frequently in sarcastic questions (for εἶτα accompanied by θαυμάζειν, see Demosthenes, 55.2 and 21.203, 204), and that might be its function here. This will require that θαυμάζειν is taken to express admiration, honor, or respect, as at 8.6. Since the object of θαυμάζειν is the power of the art, this strikes me as especially apt. The theme of honor is revived by προτιμᾶται some lines later.

**11.7** οὔκουν ἐν ἄλλῃ γε δημιουργίῃ τῶν ἤδη εὑρημένων οὐδεμιῇ ἔνεστιν οὐδὲν τοιοῦτον, 'surely such is not the case in any of the other crafts that have been discovered up to now': the phrase τῶν ἤδη εὑρημένων connects this passage to c. 1 and the larger narrative of technological progress. That narrative takes on special meaning here, since it is the story of humankind's self-extrication from a state of nature through the development of practical or productive arts (e.g., metalworking), as opposed to theoretical or edifying arts (e.g., astronomy), a distinction implicit in our author's sudden preference for the term δημιουργίη instead of τέχνη. Some have drawn from 11.7 the lesson that there are two different types of *technē*, one precise and the other less so, each of which deserves an independent standard by which to judge its successes and failures.[78] However, the opposite seems true. Our author is faulting the critics for applying different criteria to different *technai*. The handicrafts are in many respects less constrained by the contingencies of nature than is medicine, yet the expectations for their success in the face of contingency is, reasonably enough, low. But expectations for medicine under comparable circumstances remain unreasonably high. Our author asks only that the critics level their expectations.

---

[78] This is asserted, for example, by Roochnik, who sees here an implicit distinction between precise *technai* and so-called stochastic *technai* (1996, 46, 51). For more on the distinction and its applicability to *de Arte*, see Appendix 3.

**11.7** ἀλλ' αὐτέων ὅσαι πυρὶ δημιουργεῦνται, τούτου μὴ παρεόντος, ἀεργοί εἰσι, 'instead, those that work with fire cannot function when it is not present': the phrase ὅσαι πυρὶ δημιουργεῦνται is a deliberate echo of ἃ γὰρ πῦρ οὐ δημιουργεῖ at 8.4, where our author claims that fire is one of the principle instruments of medicine (ὄργανα; cf. ἢν ἀπῇ τι τῶν ὀργάνων later on in 11.7). In its reliance on fire, it is like many of the other handicrafts. Every handicraft depends on nature to produce its effect and so, like medicine, its work is vulnerable to nature's vagaries. When fire is not available, the ironsmith's work ceases; likewise, when the patient's body is unavailable for examination, the doctor's work cannot go forward.

**11.7** καὶ ὅσαι μετὰ τοῦ ὀφθῆναι ἐνεργοὶ καὶ τοῖσιν εὐεπανορθώτοισι σώμασι δημιουργεῦνται, 'and those that work with materials that are visible and malleable': literally, 'however many operate with help from seeing and work with bodies that are easily made right,' probably a sort of hendiadys, as I translate. The doctor cannot see or directly perceive the objects he works on (i.e., the non-evident diseases and internal regions of the body), nor may he simply pull apart or cut through the obscuring layers to improve his view, since the patient is a living organism. Moreover, as Jori notes, the doctor's actions, including his mistakes, are, at least relative to many handicrafts, irrevocable, leaving less room for error (1996, 266–270).[79] Thus, while medicine is assimilated to the handicrafts (both, it turns out, work 'with bodies,' σώμασι), it labors under distinct natural disadvantages. If indeed non-evidence was a feature usually associated with edifying arts such as cosmology (cf. *VM* 119.4–7 = L. 1.572), then medicine emerges as a sort of hybrid, non-evident (like the edifying arts) but productive (like the handicrafts).

**11.7** αἱ δὲ [γραφῇ] χαλκῷ τε καὶ σιδήρῳ καὶ τοῖσι τούτων ὁμοίοισι χύμασιν αἱ πλεῖσται, 'the numerous others that work with bronze or iron or similar metals': Jouanna suppresses the grammatically, syntactically, and thematically

---

[79] On the whole, however, my interpretation of 11.7 is at odds with Jori's (1996, 260–271). On his view, the comparison with the other arts is made to emphasize medicine's differences with the handicrafts. So, he argues (see his table on 270), medicine is superior to the handicrafts in that it uses the 'sight of the mind' to know the non-evident, whereas the handicrafts are dependent on vision and are suspended when their material is insufficiently visible. I see no support for this in the text. Further, medicine puts a premium on speed (at the expense of correctness?), whereas speed is less important to the handicrafts than is correctness. This strikes me as a gross misunderstanding of the text, but the finer points of my disagreement with Jori should be obvious from my comments on 11.7.

awkward γραφῇ (painting or writing), though the conspicuous use of painting and writing as examples of *technē* in the *Corpus* and beyond may weigh (lightly) in favor of its retention (*VM* 146.9 = L. 1.620; *Vict. I* 140.17–23 = L. 6.494–496; *Loc. Hom.* 76.15–20 = L. 6.330–332; Plato, *Statesman* 277c, *Timaeus* 19b, *Gorgias* 450c; Isocrates, 13.10). It is attested in both MSS, and Jori objects that there is no decisive reason for overruling them (1996, 84 n. 10). Though they seem out of place alongside bronze and iron and similar metals, he argues, the point is that modifications to all these media are, as it were, reversible, so that mistakes are easily corrected.

The unusual use of χύμα to refer to metal ingots, and so to metals or alloys generally, may be intended to evoke the word χυμός, or humor. Further, it may be significant for the assimilation of medicine to other handicrafts that 'iron' is sometimes used in the *Corpus* as shorthand for surgery. There is perhaps a hint of wry humor, too, in the assertion that, in comparison to the human body, iron is easy to work with.

**11.7** οὐδ' ὑπερβατῶς, 'without skipping any steps': if medicine exists in virtue of the doctor's manipulation of natural causes and effects to achieve his end, then nature will place obvious constraints on how things must be done, including what steps must be taken and in what order. To put it in familiar terms, there is a determinate correct procedure, distinguishable from what is incorrect (cf. 5.5–6). Most importantly in the case of medicine, diagnosis of the problem must precede any attempt at treatment (see notes on αἰσθομένη at 11.5 above).

**11.7** πρὸς τὸ λυσιτελέον ἀσύμφορον, 'an obstacle to turning a profit': the craftsman cares more about the quality of his work than about money, as does the doctor, who, by analogy, is motivated by concern for the patient (cf. 11.5 above), not greed. This contrasts with the antagonist of 4.3–4, who, after submitting to treatment and recovering, denies the doctor his due. It is not that the craftsman has no interest in money, and thus no care for the speed of his operations. Rather, both the craftsman and the doctor care first about correctness and only then about speed (pace Jori 1996, 270), the doctor because the progression of the disease demands it, the craftsman because it conduces to his personal financial stability.

**11.7** ἀλλ' ὅμως προτιμᾶται, 'nonetheless it is paid greater respect': προτιμᾶται echoes the earlier θαυμάζειν. The ignorant honor cures over refusals, thereby dishonoring the deliberate slowness and care of the physician. However, this is inconsistent with their treatment of the other crafts, whose practitioners are praised for their concern for the quality of their product—though this requires that they work slowly or not at all—rather than the speed of their work.

## 12

The therapeutic narrative is transformed from a story of failure (c. 11) to one of success. The doctor can overcome his disadvantages to formulate an accurate and useful diagnosis that will guide treatment. Still, the doctor's task is not easy, and our author continually stresses (most explicitly in 12.6) that the diagnosis of non-evident diseases is a protracted process. Whereas in c. 11 the negligence of the patient and the speed of the disease are blamed for the slowness of diagnosis, two additional challenges are identified in c. 12: the complexity of sign-inference and the diseased body's 'natural' resistance to therapy. The doctor's encounter with the disease is again characterized metaphorically, both as a military battle replete with espionage (12.3) and a legal prosecution (12.4).

In its style, c. 12 provides further evidence of our author's penchant for euphony, symmetry, and vivid imagery, not to mention his love of oxymoron and paradox. Other figures of note include an instance of hysteron-proteron in 12.3 and the 'legal tautology,' typical of sophistic rhetoric, at 12.6.

**12.1** ἰητρικὴ δέ, 'but medicine': after his digression on the handicrafts at 11.7, our author returns to focus on medicine in particular.

**12.1** τοῦτο μὲν τῶν ἐμπύων, τοῦτο δὲ τῶν τὸ ἧπαρ ἢ τοὺς νεφρούς, 'the abscesses, whether of the liver or the kidneys': abscesses, or 'suppurations,' receive special attention from our author, though he has no problem acknowledging that there are many other diseases that affect the body's interior (see following note). It may be that τοῦτο μὲν τῶν ἐμπύων is meant to parallel τὰ μὲν ἐξανθεῦντα ἐς τὴν χροιὴν at 9.3. The same types of diseases that occur on the body's surface affect its interior, as well. They differ only in their location.

**12.1** τοῦτο δὲ τῶν συμπάντων τῶν ἐν τῇ νηδύι νοσεύντων, 'any of all those diseases located in the bodily cavity': again, the generic use of νηδύς, as at 10.1. Non-evident diseases can be characterized locatively as those in the body's cavity, to be contrasted with evident diseases, which are located at the surface (ἐς τὴν χροιὴν, 9.3).

**12.1** ἀπεστερημένη τι ἰδεῖν ὄψει, 'though deprived of seeing ... with the eyesight': the language echoes 4.2 and has the same juridical edge. Medicine is the victim, unfairly deprived of the privileges afforded other handicrafts, specifically, direct perceptual access to the material it works on.

**12.1** ᾗ τὰ πάντα πάντες ἱκανωτάτως ὁρῶσιν, 'by which all people see all things most adequately': a pleonasm that appears tautological, though it is not. The relative pronoun ᾗ refers back to ὄψει, eyesight or perception more generally. The verb ὁρῶσιν, literally 'see,' exploits the close connection (in Greek and especially in *de Arte*) between seeing and knowing. To paraphrase: 'by perception all people know all things most adequately.' The empiricism is striking (see Introduction 3), as are the implications of the superlative form ἱκανωτάτως. There are other ways of 'seeing' (probably testimony and inference—see notes on 11.3), but these are somehow inferior. In what way are they inferior? Our author does not identify his criteria. We know that both are slower than perception. We know that testimony is less reliable (11.4), and certainly inference (at least in the kinds of cases our author is concerned with) leaves more room for error than does perception.

**12.1** ὅμως ἄλλας εὐπορίας συνεργοὺς εὗρε, 'nonetheless discovered other resources to work with': the aorist again is used to create a narrative feel, continuing the particular 'war story' begun in the previous chapter (or even as early as c. 1—cf. εὐπορέων δὲ διὰ τὴν τέχνην ᾗ βοηθεῖ at 1.3). The connotations attending the term συνεργός ('ally in battle' at Aristophanes, *Eq.* 588; 'partner in crime' at Thucydides 8.92) may be relevant to the combat and courtroom conceits. Like a great warrior, the doctor rallies his allies to defeat the disease. Like a prosecutorial lion, he tracks down the disease's accomplices and presses them into service as informants to determine what is responsible (τὸ αἴτιον) for harming the patient.

The verb εὗρε echoes occurrences of εὑρίσκειν at 1.2 and 6.4 to revive the themes of progress and experience. By closely observing and analyzing the phenomena, doctors gain new advantages over non-evident diseases.

**12.2** φωνῆς τε γὰρ λαμπρότητι καὶ τρηχύτητι καὶ πνεύματος ταχυτῆτι καὶ βραδυτῆτι, καὶ ῥευμάτων ἃ διαρρεῖν εἴωθεν ἑκάστοισι δι' ὧν ἔξοδοι δέδονται ὧν τὰ μὲν ὀδμῇσι τὰ δὲ χροιῇσι τὰ δὲ λεπτότητι καὶ παχύτητι διασταθμωμένη τεκμαίρεται, 'from the clarity or scratchiness of voice, from the speed or slowness of breath, and from each of the fluids regularly discharged through the orifices (gauging some on the basis of their smell, others by their color and still others by their thinness and thickness), it makes an inference': letting ὧν stand before τὰ μὲν ὀδμῇσι, where most editors, including Jouanna, seclude it. The types of phenomena used as the basis for inference—voice, breath, and bodily fluids—share a common origin, namely, the body's interior (cf. the list of secretions at *Alim.* 142.7–10 = L. 9.104). Our author's priority is to demonstrate the usefulness of such phenomena for determining contemporaneous internal conditions. Surprisingly, however, we are not told which conditions they signify. We may guess with some confidence that scratchiness of voice would indicate throat inflammation (though it is asserted at *Loc. Hom.* 58.28 = L. 6.308 that hoarseness of voice is a sign of abscess), but the exact significance of a patient's rate of respiration is more difficult to fathom. Still less informative is our author's enumeration of the relevant powers of bodily fluids (odor, color, and relative density), which may represent the final elements in a deliberate progression from the familiar to the abstruse.

As though to impress upon his audience the variety of resources at the doctor's disposal, our author is careful to include phenomena that appeal to every major sense except taste: hearing, sight, touch, and smell. His primary interest, in this and following passages, seems to be in applying these last three to the bodily fluids, perhaps another indication that *de Arte* depends on a broadly humoral theory of health and disease. Consistent with this is our author's focus not on the identity of the fluids (e.g., urine, phlegm, perspiration, probably even feces—anything that can 'flow out') but on the causal-phenomenal powers they possess.

**12.2** ὧν τὰ σημεῖα ταῦτα ἅ τε πεπονθότων ἅ τε παθεῖν δυναμένων, 'the conditions of which these things are signs, including what has already been suffered and what it is possible yet to suffer': reading τὰ σημεῖα on a suggestion from Lesley Dean-Jones, against the MSS and Jouanna, who have τε σημεῖα. Sometimes translated as 'symptoms,' τὰ σημεῖα must have a broader scope here in *de Arte*, since 'symptom' denotes a phenomenon that is related to (usually as an effect of) the underlying causes of a disease but itself is not a cause. Though, given declarations like that at 11.4 ('knowing the causes of diseases and knowing how to treat them by all the means that hinder their progress belong to the same intellect'), we may suppose that the doctor's main concern is to discern the underlying causes of a disease, the language here in 12.2 is more general. Signs correlate to 'things' or 'conditions' (my rendering of the neuter plural relative pronouns), not necessarily causes, and they do so not only to present conditions, but also to conditions in the past and future (cf. 7.3). Thus, it would appear that signs in *de Arte* are characterized by their logical, not causal, relations: a sign is any empirically derived fact that may be used (presumably as a premise in a syllogism of some kind) to derive further facts that are not, at least not under the current conditions, empirically evident. The text suggests also that these further facts can fail to be non-evident in two ways: spatially or temporally. A disease may be non-evident to the doctor because it is hidden in the interior regions of the body. Alternatively, a past symptom of the disease may be non-evident because the doctor was not present at the time when the patient experienced it.

**12.3** ταῦτα τὰ μηνύοντα, 'these informants': the verb μηνύειν and its cognates have overtly juridical connotations; Attic forensic rhetoric is replete with the term. A μηνύτης is an informant who, by providing an eyewitness account, divulges previously unknown information and verifies the truth of the charges against a suspect, sometimes in exchange for immunity from prosecution (e.g., Lysias 6.21–23). In a military context, a μηνύτης gives away the secret position or strategy of an army (Thucydides 8.39).

Signs are, figuratively speaking, allies and accomplices of the disease who have betrayed its hiding spot (i.e., its location within the body; cf. 11.6, where the disease is said to 'occupy' the body) and plans (i.e., its nature and causes, and thus its past and future course of development). Literally, they are carriers of information regarding the disease—information that they carry in virtue of their direct involvement or contact with the disease. In epistemological terms, our author blurs the lines between knowledge by inference and knowledge by testimony: signs provide a kind of eyewitness testimony to what goes on beneath the surface of the patient's body.

**12.3** μηδ' αὐτὴ ἡ φύσις ἑκοῦσα ἀφιῇ, 'nature herself does not willingly relinquish': nature is personified as the enemy of both the doctor and the patient insofar as it either shelters or simply is the non-evident disease (cf. ἡ φύσις ἥ τε τοῦ νοσέοντος ἥ τε τοῦ νοσήματος at 11.3; also ἡ φύσις αἰτίη ἡ τῶν σωμάτων at 11.5). Either way, there are cases in which she does not afford the doctor the information necessary to make a diagnosis by way of inference.

**12.3** ἀνάγκας εὕρηκεν, 'has discovered devices of compulsion': what is to be done when informants are not willing to talk? A speech prepared by Antiphon describes how such situations are to be handled in a law court (6.25). Free men will be compelled (ἀναγκάζειν) by oaths. Slaves, on the other hand, will be subjected to 'other devices of compulsion (ἑτέραις ἀνάγκαις), by which, even if about to die for their denunciations, they will be compelled to speak the truth (ἀναγκάζονται τἀληθῆ λέγειν).' These 'other devices' amount to inquisition under torture, or βάσανος. The truth is extracted from nature by forcing a confession. There is some question as to whether such torture was actually carried out in the course of Athenian legal proceedings,[80] but there is no question that the threat of slave-torture at least became a rhetorical *topos* routinely employed by Attic forensic speech-writers as a mode of proof. With his metaphorical allusion to βάσανος as a way of extracting reliable information about a 'perpetrator,' our author places himself firmly in the same rhetorical tradition.

In the philosophical and medical traditions, of course, nature is the mother of necessity, specifically, causal necessity, and the connection is made emphatically in the fragments of Antiphon (especially F44(a)I.23–33), with which *de Arte* has a strong affinity (see notes on 2.3). The special role of causal necessity in our author's argument will be addressed shortly. For now it is enough to draw attention to the irony of a necessity that is used against nature. The doctor uses nature against herself, harnessing her effects to intervene in natural processes and to change the 'natural' outcome.

**12.3** ἀζήμιος βιασθεῖσα μεθίησιν, 'is forced—without injury—to surrender them': irony is compounded by paradox. In the speech of Antiphon quoted directly above, free men and slaves are subjected to different 'devices of compulsion' because it would have been outrageous to torture a free man. Again, Antiphon's views on nature are relevant insofar as he characterized nature as intrinsically free and conventions as restrictions on nature (F44(a)IV.1–7; see my notes on 2.3). The sophist Hippias, too, is reported to have taken issue with convention on the grounds that it 'does violence' (βιάζεσθαι) to nature (DK 86 C1 = Plato, *Protagoras* 337d). It is against this sophistic background, and the views of Antiphon especially, that the detail ἀζήμιος becomes salient. If nature is somehow the source or archetype of freedom, and if freedom is a guiding ideal, then it is intolerable that the physician should treat nature like a slave.[81] The scandalous suggestion is softened by characterizing the torture and violence applied to nature as harmless, as something that will not have any lasting, deleterious effect on either nature or freedom—or, for that matter, the patient. Part of our

---

[80] Gagarin 1996 argues that slave-torture was a legal fiction employed in forensic rhetoric, not a genuine practice.

[81] For an entertaining digression on the ubiquity of the image in the developing stages of Western science, see Gomperz 1910, 140–141. Von Staden suggests that here *de Arte* breaks radically with a Hippocratic tradition that views the art exclusively as an ally, not enemy, of nature (2007, 28 ff.); however, he either fails to notice or ignores the ambivalent language of the passage.

author's message is that the doctor can 'see' beneath the concealing layers of the body without peeling them back—that is, without cutting the patient open and doing irreparable damage.

*De Arte* preserves the only unequivocal reference to the procedure of sign-provocation in the *Corpus* (see Introduction 4), thus raising the question whether his treatment is a product of medical innovation or mere imagination. Jori conjectures that the topic is broached in anticipation of an objection to diagnosis by inference (1996, 279): what if the body offers no external signs on which to base an inference? Is the doctor then at a complete loss with respect to non-evident diseases? This opens up the possibility that our author's recourse to sign-provocation reflects rhetorical exigencies rather than real medical practices.

**12.3** ἀνεθεῖσα, 'she is released': most editors and translators have been troubled by the reading ἀνεθεῖσα given by the MSS. How is nature free if she is being tortured? Accordingly, Ermerins thought that the correct reading should be ἀνεθέντα or the active ἀνεῖσα; either the informants should be freed, or nature should be doing the freeing. Reinhold's μεθεῖσα is paleographically plausible and avoids this objection but at the cost of textual integrity. Moreover, as Jouanna recognizes (1988, 266 n. 6), the euphony of the series βιασθεῖσα μεθίησιν ἀνεθεῖσα speaks, however weakly, against such an emendation. Jouanna strives to make sense of the sentence by identifying two distinct moments: 'one at which the signs are provoked, and the other at which they are observed' (1988, 266 n. 6). This may be correct, though the logic of the metaphor is lost. A better solution, on my view, is to construe the sentence as an instance of hysteron-proteron, reversing the temporal order of the finite verb and participle: once she has revealed what she knows, nature is released.[82] Another, but less comfortable, option is to accord to ἀνεθεῖσα the sense of 'remit,' that is, 'abate' or 'go slack' (cf. Thucydides 8.63; Euripides, *Or.* 941). Nature gives up the fight over the informants and, relaxing her resistance, releases them. Giving this sense to ἀνεθεῖσα also heightens the vivacity of the imagery: nature, exhausted from torture, goes limp.

**12.3** δηλοῖ τοῖσι τὰ τῆς τέχνης εἰδόσιν ἃ ποιητέα, 'once she has made it evident to those knowledgeable in the art what should be done': it is no accident that the verb δηλοῦν is found in the middle of our author's defense of medicine's ability to attain knowledge of τὰ ἄδηλα. The signs, being themselves evident

---

[82] Such a construal of the Greek appears to be preferred also by von Staden (2007, 29).

to the senses, render the unseen disease evident to the mind by providing grounds for drawing conclusions, though the diseases themselves remain non-evident. Nor is it an accident that such knowledge is available only to the already knowledgeable. As always, our author is eager to build a wall between experts in a craft and laypersons. Not just anyone can use symptoms to diagnose and treat disease. One must already have some store of medical knowledge in order to read the signs correctly and know in advance what will result from certain courses of treatment.

More than a reiteration of the ignorance of laypersons, however, this remark suggests a crude analysis of medical sign inference itself. An observation of the particular sign-event, together with the special general knowledge of human physiology, allows the doctor to draw a conclusion as to what kind of treatment should be applied. Though here our author makes it sound as though the inference is made from the sign and the general knowledge directly to the appropriate treatment, his remarks should be considered in the light of 11.4. Any ultimate conclusions about treatment are drawn via an inference from signs to the aetiology of the disease.

12.4 βιάζεται δὲ τοῦτο μὲν πῦρ τὸ σύντροφον φλέγμα διαχεῖν σιτίων δριμύτητι καὶ πωμάτων, 'for example, using acrid food and drink the art forces fever to melt the congealed phlegm': a highly contested passage, the majority of editors accept M's πῦρ, taking πῦρ τὸ σύντροφον to refer to the innate heat of the human body. This was Littré's preference: 'medicine forces the innate heat to dispel forth the phlegmatic humor' (6.24). Jouanna detects an echo of the chapter's opening sentence (ἰητρικὴ δέ, τοῦτο μὲν τῶν ἐμπύων) and so adopts A's πυοῦ (reading πύου), translating: 'the art first compels phlegm, an innate humor, to pour forth pus' (1988, 240). Jones dismisses πῦρ τὸ σύντροφον as a gloss (1923, 214 n. 1), and one can surely sympathize with such a drastic measure. Neither πῦρ, πύου nor φλέγμα is an ideal companion for τὸ σύντροφον, at least not on the standard meanings of these words.[83]

Perhaps, then, we should look to the less standard. In his notes on this sentence, Gomperz points out (1910, 141) that the verb τρέφειν, the root of σύντροφον, has the primary meaning 'to thicken a liquid,' i.e. 'to coagulate.' He translates τὸ σύντροφον φλέγμα as 'verdickter Schleim' (thickened phlegm), and this strikes me as the correct approach (cf. *Loc. Hom.* 50.28–29 = L. 6.296, where we find a reference to coagulated phlegm, and 66.15–20

[83] The second and third correcting hands of A give ποιοῦσα in an apparent attempt to bring the passage in line with πώματα καὶ βρώματα ἃ τῶν θερμαινόντων θερμότερα γινόμενα τήκει τε ἐκεῖνα καὶ διαρρεῖν ποιεῖ at 12.5.

= L. 6.318, where fevers are said to be caused by excessive phlegm). It is a peculiar proclivity of our author to employ compound words in ways that reflect a heightened sensitivity to the main root. Thus, where the lexicon tells us that ὑπερβατῶς at 11.7 means 'inverted' or 'miraculous,' Jouanna sees through to the root βαίνειν and understands that our author is talking about skipping steps in a procedure. Similarly, when at 12.2 medicine is said to διασταθμωμένη, Jouanna rightly rejects the lexicon's 'separate' and returns again to the root, σταθμᾶσθαι, 'to apply as a criterion.' Likewise, I argue that here we should refer σύντροφον back to τρέφειν.

This does not in itself solve all the textual problems. Do we choose pus or fire as an accomplice to the sign-expulsion? Again, Gomperz' reasoning is helpful in sorting out the issues involved.

> This is the author's thought: the doctor induces the sick person to take bitter, heating foods and drinks, which increases the strength of the internal heat of the body. The elevated body heat in turn melts the thickened phlegm, makes it more fluid and enables it to be expelled, and the phlegm's condition provides the examining doctor with the desired information. (1910, 142)

In the Greek, of course, there is nothing about hot food and beverages, much less about innate heat, but there is Hippocratic precedent for belief in the heat-inducing properties of acrid substances, most significantly in *VM*, where the author writes of unusually acrid discharge from the nostrils, which 'causes the nostril to swell and inflames it, making it hot and extremely fiery' (142.8–15 = L. 1.614). Our author himself treats solidity, liquidity, heat and cold as fundamental pathological qualities (9.3), perhaps increasing the likelihood that the present passage describes processes of liquefaction and solidification through the actions of cold and heat. We might eliminate the reference to innate heat by supposing that the patient has a πῦρ, which is a way of saying that he suffers from fever. The fever is not intense enough to melt phlegm (the cold humor) on its own, and so the doctor applies a device of compulsion to the disease to force it, by elevating its heat with acrid food and drink,[84] to give up information in the form of melted phlegm.

---

84 Compare Jori's claim that our author intends to affirm that the doctor can stir up the 'internal fire,' that is, the innate heat, at will (1996, 85 n. 11). Still, some caution is in order. It is not obvious that the food and drink stirs up the 'fire,' and there are other plausible interpretations. If we take seriously Gomperz' insight into σύντροφον, it may be worth pointing out that the root verb, τρέφειν, is used frequently of milk, where it means 'to curdle' (e.g., *Od.* 9.246). Accordingly, the noun τροφάλις refers to freshly made cheese. Could our author have in mind a process of curdling? This might be dismissed as so much etymological fantasy if it were not for the fact that the process envisioned is said to involve acrid food and

Once we accept πῦρ as the correct reading, then, some sense can be made of the text. If we do not accept it, our options are limited. Jouanna's adherence to A has insuperable difficulties. First, the grammar of the sentence clearly demands two direct objects: one as the object of βιάζεται, and one as the object of διαχεῖν. Reading πύου does not deliver. Second, it is difficult to assign the genitive form an intelligible function in the sentence. Jouanna (1988, 266 n. 8) asks it to serve as a partitive genitive complement of διαχεῖν, but this, it must be admitted, is a difficult request.[85]

However one prints, and then construes, the text here, there is no doubt that it is intended to illustrate those 'devices of compulsion' (ἀνάγκαι) mentioned earlier. The necessity at issue is some form of causal necessity: such necessity holds between things of distinct physical types (e.g., acrid food and fever, congealed phlegm, etc.). It is also hypothetical. Descriptions of changes or interactions of one type are thought to underwrite an inference, presumably by way of a logical relation of implication, to a description of change or interaction in the corresponding type. (So it is that an ontology with a place for natural types or kinds—in our author's language, εἴδεα—is crucial to 'seeing' the non-evident). If the doctor administers acrid foods to a patient with fever, then the fever will become more intense. Thus it is that technical procedure is parasitic upon the network of causal regularities—in short, upon nature. Indeed, the doctor must already be familiar with these regularities if his attempt to diagnose the non-evident disease is to be anything but haphazard. He must already know what will happen if he administers an acrid drink. It is in precisely this sense that medicine must involve 'things known in advance' (6.4). Further, by mastering these necessities (the expression 'natural laws,' while anachronistic, might be apt), he will be able to make inferences (τεκμαίρεσθαι) regarding 'things that come to be 'because of something'' (6.4), that is, the non-evident disease and its causes.

---

drink. Distinctively acrid compounds—for example, rennet—are today and were then what is used to curdle milk into cheese (Dalby 2003, 80–81). Acrid substances curdle non-acrid liquids, thinks our author, and he does not need to rely just on his observations of cheese-making for this insight. Anyone who has ever drunk an insufficiently dilute glass of lemonade knows that such imbibitions are followed shortly by the accumulation of mucus in the mouth, throat and esophagus. The parallel between phlegm and milk is suggested, too, by the fact that the Hippocratics thought the characteristic color of the humor was white (Langholf 1990, 148 n. 68). Our author may imagine that liquid phlegm is curdled into a solid form and then melted by fever just enough to allow for expectoration.

[85] Compare the similarly perplexing use of διαχεῖν at *Flat.* 116.16 = L. 6.104 and Jouanna's comments (1988, 144 n. 5). The adjacent discussion of phlegm and its mixture with acrid humors (*Flat.* 117.5 = L. 6.106) is compelling but not especially helpful in deciphering *de Arte*.

**12.4** ὧν αὐτῇ ἐν ἀμηχάνῳ τὸ ὀφθῆναι ἦν, 'what it was unable to see': or, more literally, 'the things whose being seen by [medicine] was unworkable,' a tortured paraphrastic construction that once again locates the relevant incapacity in the patient's body, not in the doctor. The unusual phrase ἐν ἀμηχάνῳ reminds us that the conditions in question are not impossible to see (that is, they are not categorically invisible); rather, they are placed where the natural mechanism for their being seen (i.e., direct perception by the eyes) is circumstantially inadequate. The medical *technē*, in its recourse to inference, thus supplements and exceeds nature.

**12.4** τό τ' αὖ πνεῦμα, ὧν κατήγορον, ὁδοῖσί τε προσάντεσι καὶ δρόμοισιν ἐκβιᾶται κατηγορεῖν, 'in turn, by means of steep roads and running the art forces breath to bring a charge against those things of which it is the accuser': another hendiadys. The doctor makes the patient run uphill, presumably to increase the rate and volume of respiration, though we are not told what is to be gleaned therefrom. Ducatillon (1977b, 151–158) compares this passage to descriptions of the methods of the trainer-physician Herodicus of Selymbria found in Plato (*Republic* 406a, *Phaedrus* 227d) and the Hippocratic *Corpus* (*Epid. 6* 5.303.1–7). These methods purportedly emphasized the importance of exercise and gymnastic training for the maintenance of health as well as for curing diseases such as fever. However, our author mentions therapeutic exercise here only as a diagnostic measure and, though vigorous exercise (πόνοι) is mentioned at 5.4 as a possible cause of a person's 'spontaneous' recovery, it is only one on a long list of dietetic cures.

**12.4** τεκμαίρεται, 'the art makes an inference': the verb, in precisely this form, occurs for the third time in this chapter, becoming a sort of refrain. In no case does the author divulge the specific content of the inference, though one might expect that doing so would impress the audience.

**12.5** ἔστι δὲ ἃ καὶ διὰ τῆς κύστιος διελθόντα ἱκανώτερα δηλῶσαι τὴν νοῦσόν ἐστιν ἢ διὰ τῆς σαρκὸς ἐξιόντα, 'there are things that, in passing also through the bladder, are better suited for making the disease evident than when they pass out through the flesh': the things that 'pass out through the flesh' are the fluids associated with the perspiration induced as described at 11.4. The author does not explain why urinalysis is superior in some cases to the analysis of perspiratory excretions. Urinary sediment was used as a sign in Hippocratic medicine (see, for example, *Prog.* 2.138.15–142.15, and *Alim.* 143.15–22 = L. 9.106–108, where sweat and urinary sediment are listed among the τεκμήρια), and the underlying idea is probably that such sediment often will not be fine enough to pass through pores in the skin, whereas it may pass more easily through the bladder and urethra.

**12.5** ἐξεύρηκεν οὖν καὶ τοιαῦτα πώματα καὶ βρώματα ἃ τῶν θερμαινόντων θερμότερα γινόμενα, 'accordingly, medicine has discovered food and drink that become hotter than the sources of heat': this final example shows how the physician exploits heat to gain a better understanding of a patient's internal disease. Heat may be the prime causal mechanism in all our author's examples. First, acrid food and drink is used to stoke a fever. Then, the patient is made to run uphill, which brings on sweats, as does immersion of the patient in a hot bath. Finally, hot food and drink is used to melt the fever-producing substances in the body. (Recall also his remarks on skin eruptions at 9.4, which may give some theoretical priority to the causal powers of heat and cold.)

In this passage, the physician harnesses the heat of certain foods and drinks that he has discovered. However, his notion of discovery is not without its problems. In the case of 'hot' food and drink, as in the earlier case of acrid ones, our inclination is to suppose that our author means hot in a straightforward sense: food that feels hot. But would hot food need to be discovered? Could any food not simply be heated up through cooking? It would seem that we are dealing here not with the phenomenal quality of hotness, but rather with elemental heat, the kind of 'heat' that can be present in an object irrespective of its apparent temperature.

Heat and cold as purely medical-theoretical constructs are criticized at length in *VM* (cc. 13–19), a criticism of which our author is either unaware or unconcerned. But if *de Arte* runs afoul of *VM*'s critique, and even if his physics is wrong, it does not follow that he is wrong to rely on physics. From his knowledge of physics, the physician is familiar with the constituents of the body and their causal powers. He knows what effect moistness, dryness, heat, cold, acridness, etc. have on the various things that are exposed to them. He has discovered various foods, drinks, and other substances that possess these powers to certain degrees. That is, he has come to discover their natures or forms. Knowing, then, what the causes of the disease were exposed to (e.g., hot liquid), and knowing what the externalized effect was, he can deduce some facts about the internal states of the patient. In fact, in the cases of expectorated phlegm and sediment in the urine, and perhaps in all such cases, the physician can make the stronger claim that he actually observes the cause of the disease itself, since he forces to the outside the entity or substance causing the condition under investigation. In the case of τῶν θερμαινόντων, especially, diagnostic procedures may do double work as treatment, since the hot food and drink eliminate (homeopathically—a striking divergence from the standard Hippocratic approach) the fever's cause.

The virtue of this type of account is that it stages an effective defense against an attack on the possibility of gaining knowledge about the internal processes of the body. The physician can force the body to expel things that it contains, and so he knows at least, for example, that patient's lungs contain phlegm. He knows also the nature of phlegm insofar as it is open to observation. However, it remains to be shown that such knowledge is at all useful to the physician. Why should the physician think that phlegm has something to do with the causes of the disease in question? How does he know that the sediment passing through the urine is the dissolved remains of what caused the patient's fever? It becomes clear that in order for him to make such claims, he will have to know quite a bit about the structure, composition, and function of the internal organs and systems. The limited anatomy and physiology he gives in c. 10 certainly cannot do that work.

**12.5** τήκει τε ἐκεῖνα καὶ διαρρεῖν ποιεῖ, ᾗ οὐκ ἂν διερρύη μὴ τοῦτο παθόντα, 'melting them and causing them to pass from the body along a route by which they never would have passed had they not been subjected to this': the efficacy of the doctor's diagnostic interventions is demonstrated by a counterfactual. Had the doctor not taken these steps, the sources of heat would not have been eliminated. Perhaps our author is responding to persistent pressure from critics who charge that doctors take credit for recoveries that would have occurred even without their intervention.

**12.6** ἕτερα μὲν οὖν πρὸς ἑτέρων καὶ ἄλλα δι' ἄλλων, 'differ with respect to the different routes they take and the different information they carry': I give to δι' ἄλλων a locative sense corresponding to the prefix in τὰ διιόντα and to πρὸς ἑτέρων a generic sense of relation that conveys the contextual variability of signs (τὰ ἐξαγγέλλοντα) and their signification. The awkward phrasing expresses the 'relativism' typical of sophistic declamations (cf. Gorgias, *Helen*, DK 82 B11 §1; Plato, *Protagoras* 334a–c; and *Flat.* 102.1–4 = L. 6.90, 110.3–6 = L. 6.98, but especially *Alim.* 142.11–13 = L. 9.104).[86] Here

[86] For a repudiation of the traditional view that the Sophists (excepting Protagoras) were radical relativists, see Bett 1989. Bett dubs such sophistic expressions of the variability of relational properties 'relationalism,' which should be kept wholly distinct from genuine relativism.

our author employs the rhetorical flourish to underscore the complexity of diagnosis, which explains his vagueness regarding the conditions indicated by the provoked signs. The possible signs, and the underlying conditions they indicate, are too numerous to list.

**12.6** τά τε διιόντα τά τ' ἐξαγγέλλοντα, 'the things that escape the body and betray its secrets': military imagery persists. The exotic diction suggests that the signs are to be compared to informants betraying a city under siege. They must 'go through' the body's protective layers in order to 'get their reports outside' (cf. Holmes 2010, 124).

**12.6** οὐ θαυμάσιον, 'it is no surprise': given the many barriers to his success, one ought rather to expect failure from the doctor trying to treat non-evident diseases (cf. 11.7).

**12.6** αὐτῶν τάς τε πίστιας χρονιωτέρας γίνεσθαι τάς τ' ἐγχειρήσιας βραχυτέρας, 'the time spent coming to some conviction about them exceeds that left for action': literally, '(coming to some) conviction about them becomes more time-consuming and (the time for) handling them becomes shorter.' The stylistically striking sequence (note the paromoiosis and isocolon of τάς τε πίστιας χρονιωτέρας and τάς τ' ἐγχειρήσιας βραχυτέρας) compresses the basic argument of the last two chapters into the space of a sentence.

**12.6** δι' ἀλλοτρίων ἑρμηνειῶν πρὸς τὴν θεραπεύουσαν σύνεσιν ἑρμηνευομένων, 'their interpretation must pass through foreign translators on its way to the intellect that provides treatment': the genitive participle ἑρμηνευομένων modifies αὐτῶν while the prepositional phrases δι' ἀλλοτρίων ἑρμηνειῶν and πρὸς τὴν θεραπεύουσαν recall δι' ἄλλων and πρὸς ἑτέρων from earlier in the sentence, though the meanings of the prepositions themselves have shifted slightly. It is not clearly specified in what sense the translators (i.e., the signs, which make the disease intelligible to the doctor) are foreign, though the idea must be at least that they are foreign to the doctor in that he must translate the 'physical language' of their 'reports,' which they give in the form of the various phenomenal qualities they exhibit, into propositional knowledge of the non-evident disease. Further, they are foreign insofar as they are hostile; they put up resistance to the doctor and so must be coerced.

## 13

With respect to its compositional structure, perhaps the most conventional feature of *de Arte* is its epilogue, which briefly summarizes the main points of the speech and comments on its persuasiveness. Note especially the echoes of the prooimion proper, including the references to public displays of skill and the reemergence of the λόγος-ἔργον antithesis.

**13.1** λόγους ἐν ἑωυτῇ εὐπόρους ἐς τὰς ἐπικουρίας ἔχει ἡ ἰητρική, 'medicine has well equipped arguments of its own to help in its fight': our author fuses the two operative combat metaphors. Medicine is under siege from its critics, and our author rushes to its defense with the arguments contained in *de Arte*. Thus, the epilogue opens with an echo of the prologue (εὐπορέων δὲ διὰ τὴν τέχνην ᾗ βοηθεῖ) and an air of paradox. The arguments belong to medicine, and yet they rally to its aid (ἐς τὰς ἐπικουρίας) as allies or even mercenaries. What does it mean, in the first place, to say that these arguments belong to medicine? It means, at least, that there are such arguments and that they are effective (εὐπόρους). It means, too, that medicine in an important sense has the resources for such arguments already at its disposal. Its principles and practices are effective and self-sufficient; they are not parasitic upon some other *technē* or inquiry (e.g., physics, mathematics, or philosophy). Medicine stands on its own. But in what sense, then, are the arguments mercenary? They are foreign to medicine insofar as their formulation and articulation are not properly the work of the doctor, whose task is to practice medicine in the service of others, not to defend the legitimacy of those practices through argument. That is not to say that a doctor could not undertake such a defense, but it will not be in the course of fulfilling his role as doctor that he undertakes it.

But there is another battle raging as well: the patient is under attack from the disease. Accordingly, many commentators have taken the phrase λόγους ἐν ἑωυτῇ εὐπόρους in connection with the εὐπορεῖν-ἀπορεῖν antithesis as employed at 10.1 with respect to medicine's ability to conquer disease.[87] Medicine possesses effective rational principles by which doctors, in exchange for money, help its patients (ἐς τὰς ἐπικουρίας) in their fight against sickness. Thus, there is a certain ambiguity in our author's use of the

[87] Jouanna's translation is representative of the majority who take λόγους to mean primarily 'reasoning,' 'principles,' 'method,' *vel sim.*: 'la médecine renferme en elle-même des raisonnements pleins de resource pour porter secours' (1988, 241). As Jori notes (1996, 291 n. 4), the majority includes also Littre, Gomperz, Jones, Diller, Vegetti, and Jori himself.

word λόγος. It refers both to the arguments presented in *de Arte* and to the rational principles upon which medicine is based. The ambiguity, however, is no equivocation, since the two meanings of λόγος are essentially related: the rational structure (λόγος) of the *technē* makes possible its defense by rational argument (λόγος).

13.1 οὐκ εὐδιορθώτοισι δικαίως οὐκ ἂν ἐγχειρέοι τῇσι νούσοισιν, 'it rightly does not handle diseases that cannot be remedied': in his summation, our author identifies two specific threats to medicine's existence that he believes himself to have neutralized with the discourse. The first of these is the physician's refusal to intervene in cases deemed 'impossible' (11.7), namely, where patients have been 'overcome by their diseases' (3.2, 8.1). Here he refers to such cases by way of the disease's character: they are irremediable, the adjective εὐδιορθώτοισι echoing the expression τοῖσιν εὐεπανορθώτοισι σώμασι at 11.7 to remind us of the argument absolving the doctor of responsibility for that irremediability.

13.1 ἐγχειρευμένας ἀναμαρτήτους ἂν παρέχοι, 'when it does handle a disease, it does so without making mistakes': the second specific threat is medicine's apparent failures, cases in which the doctor attempts to intervene and yet the patient does not recover. Though at first it may sound as though our author is asserting, implausibly, that doctors cure every patient they treat, he means only that medical treatment is free from error, not that it is always successful. The claim is made not of doctors but of their *technē*—note that the subject of the sentence is medicine itself. Doctors may make mistakes insofar as they fail to follow the methods and precepts of the art, but the methods and precepts themselves are reliable (cf. τὰς ἀκέσιας ἀναμαρτήτους at 9.4). Unreliable are the reports given by patients of their non-evident diseases (οὐδ' ἐκ τῶν ἀπαγγελλομένων ἔστι τὴν ἀναμάρτητον σαφήνειαν ἀκοῦσαι, 11.4), just one of the many extrinsic factors affecting the doctor's success.

There is some question as to whether the proper object of ἐγχειρευμένας ('when it does handle') is οὐκ εὐδιορθώτοισι τῇσι νούσοισιν ('diseases that cannot be remedied') or simply τῇσι νούσοισιν ('diseases').[88] The doctor will

[88] Littré is representative of those who take οὐκ εὐδιορθώτοισι τῇσι νούσοισιν as the object: 'ou bien, y touchant, elle n'y commet aucune faute' (6.27). Jouanna, following Daremberg (1855, 37) and Diels (1914, 399 n. 1), takes our author to be concerned only with curable diseases ('pour les maladies traitées,' 1988, 241). See discussions of the problem by Jouanna (1988, 268 n. 5), who complains that Littré's interpretation puts our author at odds with himself, specifically with his remarks at 8.6, and Jori (1996, 292 n. 7), who sides with Littré, arguing that our author is addressing the problem that arises in cases of unsuccessful therapy

justifiably refuse to intervene in cases in which he has discovered the disease to be incurable, though he may still provide therapy, by way of diagnosis, to patients whose conditions he does not yet know to be incurable, even though they are or will inevitably become so. This would establish the plausibility of taking οὐκ εὐδιορθώτοισι τῇσι νούσοισιν as the object of ἐγχειρευμένας if it were not for the fact that ἐγχειρεῖν is used elsewhere always to refer specifically to treatment or its refusal (3.2, 7.3, 8.1, 8.6, 11.7), not to therapy broadly conceived to include diagnosis (for which the verb θεραπεύειν is employed: 11.3, 11.4). Moreover, the hyperbaton places a substantial space between the modifying adjective and the modified noun, resulting in a syntactical distance between οὐκ εὐδιορθώτοισι and ἐγχειρευμένας that suggests a corresponding semantic difference. Finally, there is the problem, from a rhetorical standpoint, of motivating a restriction to the class of irremediables. Why would our author want to claim that medicine makes no errors only in cases of incurable disease? Does he want to leave open the possibility that it makes mistakes with curable conditions? The answer should be both obvious and decisive.

**13.1** οἵ τε νῦν λεγόμενοι λόγοι δηλοῦσιν, 'the discourse given here makes it evident': or, alternatively, 'the words (or arguments) said just now make it clear,' which certainly gives *de Arte* the feel of a speech, though this does not necessarily mean that it was intended for public recitation. These words 'make evident' the existence of medicine insofar as they impart to the audience a cognitive clarity on the matter. Moreover, they literally 'make evident' the fact that medicine has good arguments in its defense by producing those very arguments for all to 'see.'

**13.1** αἵ τε τῶν εἰδότων τὴν τέχνην ἐπιδείξιες, 'this is made evident also by the displays of those knowledgeable in the art': the occurrence of ἐπιδείξιες echoes ἐπίδειξιν at 1.1, and it is remarkable that *epideixis* is attributed both to the critics and to doctors but never, at least not explicitly, to the author or speaker of *de Arte*. The treatise itself would certainly qualify as an *epideixis* by Aristotle's standards (see Introduction 2), though it is not immediately obvious whether it would qualify by its own. In 1.1 and 13.1, an *epideixis* is a public demonstration or display of *technē* or pseudo-*technē*. The critics

where failure cannot be attributed to the patient's lack of composure. Jori cites in defense the fact that in c. 11 'i malati possono soccombere durante il trattamento (e in particulare nella fase dell'indagine diagnostica),' but my own observations show that this is not the sort of case our author has in mind here at 13.1.

publicly attack the arts with speeches, and this is called an *epideixis* of their self-styled 'skill' of rhetorical refutation. Doctors heal the sick while friends and family (and perhaps others) watch. In this, they give an *epideixis* of their skill in medicine.

By this standard, too, *de Arte* would qualify as an *epideixis* of τὸ λέγειν, or speaking (see notes below), but more specifically of constructing well equipped arguments and logical demonstrations (τὴν ἀπόδειξιν ποιήσομαι, 3.1). It is puzzling that our author withholds this designation from his own work. Perhaps his decision is merely an accident of composition. If not, we can only speculate about his motives, though it is worth considering the consequences had he affirmed the epideictic character of *de Arte*. Since an *epideixis* is given usually by an expert professional, to have referred to *de Arte* itself as an *epideixis* would have been to give the impression that our author or the speaker (supposing these might not have been identical) was a professional speaker. This would certainly contravene the common rhetorical convention of denying one's skill at speaking and perhaps other interests of our author.

If an *epideixis* demonstrates a point through action, while an *apodeixis* makes its point through language and logic, then we should detect in the contrast between the 'discourse given here' and the 'displays of those knowledgeable in the art' traces of the λόγος-ἔργον antithesis. Traditional Greek conceptions gave to λόγοι a secondary status in relation to ἔργα, and our author exploits at 1.2 the perceived inferiority of words (λόγων οὐ καλῶν τέχνῃ) to actions. Here, however, he puts the two on an equal footing: both arguments and actions make evident that medicine is well equipped. In this, he follows the lead of Gorgias, who in his *Helen* hailed the power of λόγοι to influence and control ἔργα and, according to Plato, boasted that the skilled speaker was more persuasive than experts when talking about the arts, while he himself claimed to have helped doctors by persuading reluctant patients to submit to treatment (456a–457c; see also Introduction, sections 2 and 5). As Jori observes, this raises the possibility that our author conceives of rhetoric and medicine, or any productive *technē*, for that matter, as symbiotic or collaborative (1996, 295). While the doctor demonstrates the existence of medicine by its therapeutic results, the expert in λόγοι provides an auxiliary support for medicine's foundations and, ultimately, for its existence (1996, 296). But why should medicine need such support? Or, to put it another way, what is it that the actions of medicine lacks that the words of rhetoric can supply? If medicine is, as our author has already suggested, self-sufficient, then *de Arte* is a work of mere words whose demonstrative parity with medicine is a mere appearance.

**13.1** ἅς ἐκ τῶν ἔργων ἥδιον ἢ ἐκ τῶν λόγων ἐπιδεικνύουσιν, 'for whom it is easier to give a display in action rather than in word': a belated variation on the standard plea of legal or rhetorical inexperience, typically a feature of the *prooimion*, not the *epilogos* (cf. Antiphon 5.1; Lysias 12.3; Plato, *Apology* 17b). The λόγος-ἔργον antithesis already in play is made explicit in a remark that reveals our author's motive for writing *de Arte*. It is difficult (though not impossible) for those knowledgeable about medicine to give an *epideixis* in words. This is an indication that *de Arte* is meant to give guidance to doctors who would have difficulty devising comparable discourses on their own. Still, this does not show conclusively that they are in great need of such discourses, as their own demonstrations may be sufficient.

**13.1** οὐ τὸ λέγειν καταμελετήσαντες, 'since they have not made a study of speaking': Jouanna (1988) corrected the long-standing and unfortunate tradition of emending the text to καταμελήσαντες ('neglecting;' see Jouanna's justification on 268 n. 2). The claim is not that doctors know nothing about speaking, nor that they are incapable of giving a good speech. Rather, they have not studied τὸ λέγειν with the discipline required to become experts, which follows simply from the fact that they have cultivated expertise in another area. It is this lack of sustained study that explains their general ineptitude with λόγοι.

**13.1** ἀλλὰ τὴν πίστιν τῷ πλήθει, ἐξ ὧν ἂν ἴδωσιν, οἰκειοτέρην ἡγεύμενοι ἢ ἐξ ὧν ἂν ἀκούσωσιν, 'instead, they hold that the majority of people are more apt to be convinced by what they see rather than by what they hear': Jouanna compares the last lines of *de Arte* to passages in Heraclitus ('for the eyes are more accurate witnesses than the ears,' DK 22 B101) and Herodotus ('for the ears turn out to be less trustworthy for men than their eyes,' 1.8), and there is evidence that the sentiment was a recognized rhetorical formula even later in antiquity (cf. Dio Chrysostom, 12.71; see also *Flat.* 125.1–4 = L. 6.114).[89] Indeed, Empedocles' apparent attempt to subvert it might be evidence that it was clichéd already by his time.

> but come, consider, by every device, how each thing is clear
> not holding any vision as more reliable than what you hear (ἀκουή),
> nor the echoes of hearing than the clarities of the tongue,

---

[89] Further examples are given in Cherniss 1952, 202 n. 9.

> and do not in any way curb the reliability (πίστις) of the other limbs by
> which there is a passage for understanding,
> but understand each thing in the way that it is clear.
>
> (DK 31 B3 = Inwood 14, trans. Inwood)

For Empedocles, some truths are better comprehended by argument than through direct apprehension by the senses, just as, for our author, some diseases are better known through reasoning (λογισμῷ, 11.3). As he has insisted all along in his defense of medicine, sight has its limitations.

All this suggests that our author's attitude toward this 'formula' may be more complex than has generally been acknowledged. If construed as a judgment about the relative reliability of perception as compared to inference, he might be sympathetic (cf. 12.1). But, strictly speaking, the formula concerns not the ideal method of acquiring knowledge but rather the cognitive psychology of conviction (πίστις). Which is more persuasive, actions seen or words heard? Doctors are committed to the former, but our author does not explicitly endorse their view; rather, he offers it simply as an explanation for the fact that 'those knowledgeable in the art' have never made a study of speaking. This leaves open the possibility that their view is, by his account, wrong. Moreover, since he has gone to the trouble of so painstakingly crafting his speech, there is good reason to ask whether our author would have accepted without qualification the proposition that actions are more convincing than arguments. For if they were, there would have been little need for *de Arte* and even less point in writing it.

Thus, we should not conclude, as Jori does, that our author retreats from the appearance of relative parity in power of λόγοι and ἔργα (1996, 296). Nor is there anything that prevents him from adopting the Gorgianic position that λόγοι are superior insofar as the expert speaker can speak more persuasively about a *technē* than can its *technitēs*. Indeed, if the purview of τὸ λέγειν includes also reasoning, λογισμός, as it well may (cf. 8.6), the doctor will depend on the art of discourse for more than just its persuasive power (cf. 7.3, 11.3; see also the relevant discussions in the Introduction, sections 2 and 5).

## APPENDIX

# *DE ARTE* AND THE HELLENISTIC DEBATE

### 1. *Introduction*

The close relationship between medicine and philosophy in early Greek thought, evident especially in works from the Hippocratic *Corpus* and fragments of the pre-Socratics, persisted for centuries. The issues surrounding medicine's legitimacy addressed in *de Arte*, that is, the legitimacy of medicine's practices and methods, as well as its very existence, were alive and well into the Hellenistic period. There is little to suggest that *de Arte* influenced the later Hellenistic debates directly; still, it will be productive to examine the extent to which *de Arte* does or does not anticipate the Hellenistic treatment of these issues.

This essay will focus on three themes of the Hellenistic debates over *technē* with which *de Arte* might be thought, prima facie, to make contact. First, given that our author responds to a general attack on all *technai* (cc. 1 and 2), we might expect some thematic continuity between *de Arte* and Hellenistic attacks on the *technai*, specifically that of Sextus Empiricus' *Against the professors*. Second, since one of our author's main objectives is to defend the integrity of medicine in the face of obvious failure (cc. 4, 7, 8, and 11), we might look in *de Arte* for seeds of the emerging notion of a stochastic *technē*, that is, an art that tolerates a certain level of inherent error or imprecision. Third, our author dedicates significant space to defending the doctor's ability to know the non-evident causes of most diseases (cc. 10, 11, and 12), and we might ask whether his discussion prefigures any of the Hellenistic views on the non-evident and the means—epistemological and therapeutic—for coping with it. I do not think that in all of these cases *de Arte* is a window into the subsequent history of medicine and philosophy, but certainly the points of discontinuity between the Hippocratic and Hellenistic may be just as illuminating as their continuities.

## 2. *Traces of a Lost Text?*

In the Introduction (5), I voice skepticism about the conjecture that Sextus' account of Anacharsis' argument against technical criteria (M 7.55) preserves an original element of the Protagorean attack on *technē*. But even if it does, I find it doubtful (though plausible) that *de Arte* contains a roughly contemporary response. Yet there are other passages in Sextus that may preserve elements of Protagoras' attack that provoked reactions from the author of *de Arte*. I have in mind specifically the first book of πρὸς μαθηματικους, or *Against the professors*, the structure of which Sextus lays out as follows:

> It is necessary for present purposes to point out that of the arguments made against the professions, some are quite general, being made against all the professions, while others are specific and are made against each art independently (τὰ μὲν καθολικῶς πρὸς πάντα τὰ μαθήματα τὰ δ' ἰδίως πρὸς ἕκαστα). For example, that the profession does not exist (τὸ περὶ τοῦ μηδὲν εἶναι μάθημα) is a more general argument, while more specific is the argument against, say, the grammarians concerning the elements of speech, or against the geometers on the grounds that it is wrong to assume their axioms by hypothesis, or against the musicians on the grounds that neither tone nor time exists. First, then, let us look at the more general refutation. (1.8)

As promised, Sextus treats (albeit briefly) the more general arguments against the professions as a whole before moving on to consider the individual arts of grammar, rhetoric, geometry, arithmetic, astrology, and music. Thus, the structure of *Against the professors* fits Plato's description of the Protagorean work in which the sophist laid out for the benefit of anyone wanting to learn, 'the points one ought to raise in a debate against each craftsman himself, concerning all *technai* in general and each *technē* specifically (τά γε μὴν περὶ πασῶν τε καὶ κατὰ μίαν ἑκάστην τέχνην)' (Plato, *Sophist* 232d–e; see also Introduction 5). Indeed, *de Arte* and *Against the professors* exhibit the same structure. Both begin by addressing general arguments for and against the very existence of *technē* before moving on to individual *technai*.

I cannot believe that these similarities are mere coincidences. Their most plausible and economical explanation is that *de Arte* in its preliminary argument is responding to an attack made by Protagoras, an attack that is preserved in some form by Sextus. How much does Sextus preserve? That is difficult to say. Most of *Against the professors* draws upon, rather transparently, later Epicurean and Pyrrhonist traditions, a fact about which Sextus himself is forthright in his introductory remarks (M 1.1–7). It may well be that Sextus inherited from Protagoras only a broad topical schema. However, there are reasons to think that at least some of *Against the professors* derives ultimately from the Protagorean tract. The general arguments begin at M 1.9 and continue through 1.40, at which point Sextus transitions into his first specific attack (against the grammarians). The general conclusion for which Sextus argues is given in 1.9: art (μάθημα, literally, 'thing learned,' which Sextus uses to refer to the various *technai*; indeed, he uses the terms interchangeably at 1.31ff.) does not exist. The argument itself takes the form of a destructive dilemma: where art exists, one will find also a subject to be taught (τὸ διδασκόμενον πρᾶγμα), a teacher and a learner (τὸν διδάσκοντα, τὸν μανθάνοντα), and a method of learning (τὸν τρόπον τῆς μαθήσεως). But none of these things exists. Therefore, there is no art.

The three subsequent chapters give Sextus' reasons for denying all the above. They are entitled, respectively, 'On what is taught' (περὶ τοῦ διδασκόμενου; 1.10–18); 'On the corporeal' (περὶ σώματος; 1.19–30); and 'On the teacher and learner' (περὶ τοῦ διδάσκοντος καὶ μανθάνοντος; 1.31–40). Of these, 'On the corporeal' cannot be of Protagorean provenance. The subject matter digresses from the basic argument outlined by Sextus at 1.9, and it treats a topic of special interest to Hellenistic, not Pre-Socratic, philosophy. Not only is the chapter riddled with explicit references to Stoic, Epicurean, Sceptical and Platonic ideas, but, more importantly, it depends materially on those doctrines to make its argument.

'On what is taught' is perhaps a better candidate. The chapter contains two distinct but similar arguments (1.10–14 and 1.15–18) intended to show that nothing is taught. Part of the second of these seems to depend materially on Stoic philosophy: "moreover, if something is taught, it will be taught either by means of 'nothings' or by means of 'somethings.' But it is not possible for it to be taught by means of 'nothings,' since these are unreal to reason according to the Stoics" (1.17). Of course, the principle that 'what-is-not' cannot be thought has a history that precedes the Stoics by generations; it is adopted even by the author of *de Arte* (see my notes on 2.2). But the reference to Stoic principles suggests strongly that the argument was designed as an attack on Stoic dogma, and so caution compels me to reject the second argument in 'On what is taught.' The first argument, however, does not depend materially on post-Protagorean ideas. While the technical vocabulary exhibits the sophistication of Hellenistic philosophy (e.g., at 1.11, where we find συμβαίνειν in the sense of 'to have a property' and ὑπάρχειν in the sense of 'to really exist,' as well as φαντασία for 'sense impression' at 1.12), the argument itself is elementary enough—just one of many 'trifling sophisms,' in Barnes' estimation (1988, 60)—to be translated back into the Pre-Socratic idiom. In other words, it is possible that the argument is older than the language in which it is couched.

The last chapter of general argument, 'On the teacher and learner,' is linguistically less indebted to Hellenistic jargon. Again, the chapter contains two main arguments; neither one, surprisingly, endeavors to show that neither the teacher nor the learner exists as such. Instead, both purport to prove, in turn, that the act of teaching is incoherent (1.31–34) and impossible (1.35–38). The first argument is especially remarkable for its reversion to the language of *technē*. The teacher and learner are referred to as the τεχνίτης and the ἄτεχνος, respectively (1.31). Art is τέχνη, not μάθημα (1.33). The argument itself is a destructive dilemma. If teaching and learning exist, then either 1) the non-expert will teach the non-expert, 2) the expert the expert, 3) the non-expert the expert, or 4) the expert the non-expert (1.31). Possibilities 1–3 are dispatched in short order, for obvious reasons. Before tackling 4, however, Sextus interjects that 'the expert, together with the basic principles of his art, has been called into question in our discussion of Skepticism' (1.33). He then drafts into service a particularly fatuous variation on Meno's paradox to show that the expert can become expert neither from a state of expertise nor from one of non-expertise (1.34). Is Sextus drawing on proprietary Sceptical arguments? Probably not. The 'discussion of Scepticism' he has in mind occurs in chapter 29 of *Outlines of Pyrrhonism*, 'Are there any teachers and learners,' specifically sections 3.260–263. There, Sextus reports, 'it is said that generally it is impossible for there to be experts' (P 3.260), and he raises a soritical objection to the standard Stoic definition of *technē* ('a compound of apprehensions that have been exercised together,' 3.188). This is not the paradox laid out in *Against the professors*, which in fact is found also in the *Outlines*, adjacent to, but distinct from, the soritical objection (3.264).[1]

[1] The paradox echoes, albeit superficially, an argument Sextus attributes to Anacharsis the Scythian at M 7.55, and this similarity is used by Untersteiner to bolster his contention that M 7.55 gives us an argument made not by the historical Anacharsis but rather by the character of Anacharsis in the *Antilogy* of Protagoras (1948a 42–43). As mentioned above, I address (and call into question) elements of Untersteiner's thesis in the Introduction (5). Here, it will suffice to point out that, if we grant that the arguments at M 1.34 and M 7.55 are relevantly similar (which I do not), Sextus' attribution of the argument to Anacharsis gives us a strong prima facie reason to deny Protagorean authorship. A plausible conjecture to the contrary will require formidable evidence not adduced, on my view, by Untersteiner.

From the paradox, Sextus transitions to the topic of the method of learning proper. In course, he refers to 'our refutations of the physicists,' but the reference is purely circumstantial and carries no logical weight (1.35). The formal argument against the existence of a method of learning begins at 1.36. Though some of the technical vocabulary is Hellenistic (ἐναργεία to denote evidence to perception at 1.36; σημαίνειν to denote linguistic signification at 1.37; and, at 1.38, compounds of λαμβάνειν for various forms of epistemic apprehension), the argument depends on a primitive conception of natural and conventional theories of the correctness of names, as well as a quaint distinction between the Greek and the barbarian (1.37–38). I am again inclined to suppose that here Sextus preserves the logic of an older argument while updating its language. Indeed, I would rank it relatively high as a plausible candidate for Protagorean origins, filling out the list as follows.

1. 'On the teacher and learner,' first argument
2. 'On the teacher and learner,' second argument
3. 'On what is taught,' first argument
4. 'On what is taught,' second argument
5. 'On the corporeal'

Here, 1 is the most plausible candidate, purely on material and linguistic grounds, while 5 is the least. Admittedly, this list does little more than schematize the intuition, however accurate, that there are moderate to strong reasons for thinking 4 and 5 could not be Protagorean, while there are few if any reasons for thinking 1 through 3 could not be. Lacking are any positive reasons, other than Sextus' conformity to the topical schema of both *de Arte* and the lost work described at *Sophist* 232d–e, for thinking that any of the above have Protagorean origins. Given the paucity of extant material and testimony, I submit that the best evidence for a Protagorean origin in any particular case will be the commonality of logical content between *Against the professors* and *de Arte*. Naturally, the apparent strength of such evidence will be directly proportional to confidence in the hypothesis that *de Arte*, at least in c. 2, is responding exclusively to objections raised by Protagoras in the lost work (see Introduction 5).

Of the top three candidates, 1 is easily excluded since *de Arte* does not address the alleged incoherence of the concept of education. Rather, its coherence is assumed throughout (see especially 1.3, 2.2, and 9.4). One might level the same charge at 3, though the case is less clear. *De Arte*, in its assertion that 'there is no art that is not' (2.1), certainly appears to rebut the charge that there is no *technē* (or, in Sextus' lingo, μάθημα) whatsoever. However, there are few indications that the Hippocratic writer is attempting to exterminate progenitors of the arguments made in *Against the professors*. There Sextus' strategy is to pose a destructive dilemma: that which is taught must be either existent or non-existent, but (it turns out) it can be neither (1.10). Perplexingly, most of his effort is devoted to showing that the non-existent cannot be taught, a thesis that most would regard as trivial or at least unproblematic, and his argument that the existent cannot be taught is unimpressive.

> Nor, indeed, is the existent, insofar as it exists (τὸ ὂν τῷ εἶναι), taught. For, if what exists is evident to all (τῶν ὄντων πᾶσι φαινομένων), then all things will be equally untaught, from which it will follow that nothing is taught. For one must assume something untaught so that the learning of it can come to be from what is already known. (1.14)

The argument turns on multiple modal fallacies and is clearly invalid. What is potentially evident is not necessarily actually evident; nor is the teachable necessarily taught. But while the author of *de Arte* does not himself fall prey to these fallacies, neither does he overtly denounce them, not even in the more general arguments of c. 2.

The second chapter of *de Arte* does contain, however, an argument involving the correctness of names, and it is here that there is greatest promise of overlap with *Against the professors*. When we juxtapose the second argument of 'On the teacher and learner' with *de Arte* 2.2–3, the similarities are especially conspicuous. First, Sextus, whose goal is to show that teaching cannot occur through speech:

> But if [the language used to teach] signifies something, it does so either by nature (φύσει) or by convention (θέσει). It does not signify by nature, since it is not the case that everyone understands everyone else he hears speak, whether it be a Greek listening to a foreigner, or a foreigner listening to a Greek, or even a Greek to a Greek and a foreigner to a foreigner. If it signifies by legislation, it is clear that those who have already grasped that to which the words are applied will also understand them, not because they have been taught, using words, what they did not know, but insofar as they renewed what they already knew. But those who lack learning of what they do not know will not understand. (1.37–38)

Then, the Hippocratic:

> Whereas the things-that-are always are in every case seen and known, the things-that-are-not are neither seen nor known. Accordingly, the arts are known only once they have been taught, and there is no art that is not seen as an outgrowth of some form. In my opinion, they acquire their names, too, because of their forms. For it's absurd—not to mention impossible—to think that forms grow out of names: names for nature are conventions imposed by and upon nature, whereas forms are not conventions but outgrowths.

As I note in my commentary on this passage, there is broad consensus that the author is sketching a theory of the correctness of names that incorporates both 'natural' and 'conventional' elements. Simply put, our author denies the major premise of Sextus' destructive dilemma while attempting to capture the intuitions behind a naïve application of the *nomos-physis* antithesis to the correctness of names. The inherent logical structure of the Hippocratic passage reflects the contours of Sextus' attack. If an art exists or 'is,' then it is knowable. If it is knowable (i.e., if it is knowledge), then it is teachable. With his refutation of the standard dilemma, our author eliminates a threat to the teachability of *technē* and in turn to its very existence.

That Sextus' linguistic argument is the last of the general arguments is suggestive, too, as the exposition of our author's language theory is the final parry in his defense of *technē* generally. This, in conjunction with the other affinities in structure and content between *de Arte* and *Against the professors*, makes it likely that there existed at one time a third and earlier work that informed both. That this work was the 'layperson's guide to technical disputation' attributed to Protagoras at *Sophist* 232d–e cannot be known with certainty, though it certainly seems a likely source.

## 3. *Medicine as a Stochastic* Technē

Every art, craft, or skill is susceptible to error. Pilots sometimes bring their vessels into safety at a time or place other than those appointed and, in especially tragic cases, not at all. Geometers sometimes get proofs wrong. Even the simple act of writing can be foiled by a mechanical malfunction or a nervous tick. Pencils have erasers for a reason.

That every *technē* involves risk was acknowledged by the Greeks and, as noted in the Introduction (section 1), articulated in explicit terms by Solon. The potential for error is ineliminable. However, not all errors are created equal, and error in the practice of a *technē* may or may not threaten someone's claim to expertise. Certain external contingencies, for example, may disrupt or interfere with the execution of technical procedures. So a malevolent pharmacist might systematically pervert a doctor's prescriptions, thereby preventing his patients from recovering. But even if the doctor's success rate were, as a result, relatively low, no one with full knowledge of the situation would question his expertise on the basis of these failures. This is an important point, for it shows that, despite the tendency to use the *frequency* of failure as a criterion of expertise, frequency serves usually as a proxy—sometimes a poor proxy—in making judgments about the *source* of failure.[2] Barring the interference of external contingency, the source of technical error must be internal, either to the professed expert or to the *technē* itself (cf. the distinction between extrinsic and intrinsic factors in my notes on 7.1). In the former case, a practitioner poorly executes otherwise sound procedures or methods that, if practiced properly, would have led to success. In the latter, a practitioner executes with precision procedures or methods that are flawed or imperfect in some way so that the probability of failure is present from the very beginning.

The implications that failure may have for a particular *technē* and its putative experts will vary in accordance with the degree to which that *technē* is insulated by its nature from these external and internal sources of failure. Generally speaking, the geometer's failure will not be attributed to external interference, since externalities play little role in the practice of the *technē*, and then only incidentally. Writing (i.e., correctly writing words or sentences) is also heavily insulated from external interference, if not as heavily as geometry. Further, it is well insulated from failures that originate from within the *technē* itself, since its procedures are relatively simple and largely stipulative.[3] By contrast, the *technē* of piloting would seem to be highly susceptible to failure from all three sources. Moreover, failures due to external interference (e.g., mechanical malfunctions or mistakes made by subordinates) may be more difficult to detect, so that it will often be difficult, if not impossible, to rule out internal sources. And if failure is fairly common to all, even the 'best,' practitioners, one might be still more inclined to look for the source of failure in the procedures and methods of the *technē* itself.

Therein lies the rub. A *technē*, at least in its ideal form,[4] cannot by definition tolerate rules, procedures, or methods that point its practitioners in the wrong direction. Such a *technē*, the Greeks might have said, is no *technē* at all. Perhaps piloting as such does not even exist. Medicine, too, along with many other *technai*, is vulnerable to a similar challenge, a challenge to which one might plausibly respond by distinguishing between procedures or methods that are *incorrect* and those that are irreducibly *vague* or *imprecise*. To illustrate: a set of directions that tells me to head west when the

---

[2] Roochnik tends to see the frequency or very fact of failure alone as the problem to which stochastic theories of *technē* respond (1996, 52), as does, at times, Allen (1993, 84–85).

[3] At least, this was the commonplace in roughly contemporary discussions of the matter. See *Loc. Hom.* 76.15–20 = L. 6.330–332 and Isocrates 13.12.

[4] One could, of course, deny that the *technē* as currently practiced represented its ideal form. This forms part of the defense in *VM* (132.18–133.6 = L. 1.596–598).

correct direction is east is simply wrong. A set that tells me the correct direction lies somewhere between northeast and southeast is imprecise but not simply wrong. It is still of marginal value in finding my way, and I am better off, in any case, than if I knew nothing at all.

Such a *technē* would generate not pinpoint predictions but educated (as opposed to blind) guesses about the best means to a technical end in a particular situation. The Greek verb that captures this notion is στοχάζεσθαι, which Plato uses in the *Gorgias* to characterize the sub-technical practice of rhetoric (463a–b) and again in the *Philebus* to distinguish between precise *technai* that involve a quantifiable (and thus measurable) subject matter and imprecise *technai* that navigate their domains by sense experience alone (55e–56a; see Mann 2008b, 96–97). As James Allen details in a masterly paper on the topic of ancient models of the 'stochastic' arts, philosophers and doctors after Plato developed their own models of an inherently imprecise discipline that nevertheless retained its technical status (1993). On Allen's account, the main models were proposed by Aristotle and later Peripatetics, especially Alexander of Aphrodisias, and by Rationalist and Empiric physicians of the Hellenistic era. For present purposes, the nuances attending each model are less important than their similarities and differences in general approach. Aristotle saw *technē* as dependent on knowledge of the real natures of things, including their causes, powers, and so forth (e.g., at *Metaph.* 981a). But nature itself is not perfectly precise. Natural processes are, on the Aristotelian view, teleological, but in many cases the end of a natural process is realized only 'for the most part' (*Ph.* 198b34–35). Thus, knowledge of nature will reflect nature's vagueness, and the stochastic character of a *technē* will be attributable ultimately to the 'metaphysical imprecision' of the natural entities it handles (Allen 1993, 92).

The Rationalist physicians, like Aristotle, thought that the correct practice of medicine depended on knowledge of nature, specifically on knowledge of the underlying causes of disease (Allen 1993, 95). Unlike Aristotle, however, and consistent with philosophical views of nature expounded by Stoics and Epicureans, the Rationalists did not allow for natural imprecision or irregularity. If experts were unable to translate the precision of nature in theory into perfect accuracy in practice, this was because practice involved particular individuals and their circumstances, and particulars, unlike universals, could not be *known* precisely, at least not by human beings (see, e.g., Galen, *Meth. med.* 10.209). Thus, while medical theory was precise, when used to formulate medical directives applicable to particular cases, this precision was unavoidably and irreversibly compromised. The Empirics, by contrast, denied that there was precision at any level, either general or particular. Eschewing claims to knowledge of underlying causes, they strove to document connections between appearances, the frequency of which fell into four categories: always, for the most part, roughly half the time, and rarely (Galen, *Subfig. emp.* 45, 25–30, 58, 15 ff.). Clearly, these categories are designed to deal with a world far more imprecise and irregular than anything Aristotle would have deemed acceptable, one in which stochastic *technai* were chancy affairs indeed.

Whatever differences there were between Peripatetics, Rationalists, and Empirics on the issue, common to all their models is the conviction that the practitioner of a stochastic *technē* will press on despite the ineliminable imprecision of its directives. The risk that accrues from the art's stochastic character is regarded as an occupational hazard. Importantly, this risk may not be attributed to the technical expert in any way. It stems neither from his error in application of technical principles nor from a defect peculiar to his understanding of the technical domain. Rather, it happens that even the so-called internal sources of failure are subject to externalities for which the expert cannot be held accountable.

While none of this does full justice to the developing concept of a stochastic *technē* or to the specific models proposed, it gives us enough background to begin raising questions about the Hippocratics. While it is probably anachronistic to ask whether any of the Hippocratic authors consciously subscribed to some notion of a stochastic *technē*,[5] we might reasonably ask whether any of their reflections on medicine prefigured the models described above. Some have suggested that traces of stochasticism are evident in *Vict.* and *Loc. Hom.*,[6] and many commentators interpret remarks in *VM* as embracing a stochastic model of some sort.[7] David Roochnik, in his

[5] Whether the question is anachronistic depends on the chronology assigned to a particular treatise, which may itself depend on the question of its stochasticism. Hutchinson, for example, sees the allegedly stochastic elements in *VM* as confirmation of a post-Platonic date of composition (1988, 49; see also Diller 1952, 403). Still, since Plato and Aristotle themselves did not have fully worked-out theories of stochastic *technē*, it will be appropriate to talk of Hippocratic reflection on the matter merely as anticipatory of the later Hellenistic models and theories.

[6] For *Vict.*, see Hutchinson (1988, 34), who cites *Vict.* 124.17–28 = L. 6.470–472 and 194.2–16 = L. 6.592–594. For *Loc. Hom.*, see Allen (1993, 88; cf. *Loc. Hom.* 76.1–84.16 = L. 330–342).

[7] See, e.g., Hutchinson (1988, 26–27; 42–43), Allen (1993, 85, 88), Roochnik (1996, 50–57), and Schiefsky (2005, 186–189, 361–374). But see also the informed dissent in Boudon-Millot (2005, 87–99).

book *Of art and wisdom*, contends that the author of *de Arte*, too, employs a stochastic model of *technē* in his defense of medicine (1996, 50–57), and it is this claim that I will evaluate in what follows. My own view is that *de Arte* contains no discernibly stochastic elements whatsoever. I have come to this view after considering both the weakness of Roochnik's main points and the difficulty of assimilating the position articulated in *de Arte* to the family of models sketched above.

Roochnik's central argument is that, according to the author of *de Arte*, the *technē* of medicine tolerates failure. In making his case, he concentrates on cc. 7, 8, and 11 (50–51). While it is true that our author is concerned in these sections with the problem of the physician's lack of success, the 'failures' he confronts are either failures from an external source or are not failures at all, strictly speaking. In c. 7, our author suggests that patients who die after being treated by a doctor do so because they failed to follow the doctor's orders. While this is certainly suspect as a general explanation of patient mortality, the underlying point is clear and valid. Medical failure cannot be attributed confidently to an internal source unless all external contingencies have been ruled out (see my notes on 7.1–3). Further, medicine is at greater risk of external interference than are many other *technai*. But all this is true regardless of whether or not medicine is stochastic.

In c. 8, our author is ostensibly concerned with futile cases in which non-intervention is deemed the proper medical response. The central argument turns on the coherence of the idea that there are natural limits on the expert's ability to achieve his ends (see especially my notes on 8.2–4). As our author puts it:

> For of those things that we can master using the instruments of art and nature, we can be craftsmen (δημιουργοί). Of other things, we cannot. Thus, whenever a person suffers some evil that is stronger than the instruments of medicine, he should not expect medicine to be able somehow to overcome this. (8.3)

The limitations in question are set by what is physically possible, not by the imprecision of medicine's principles, methods, or subject matter (which is governed, we are told, by discoverable ἀνάγκαι, causal necessities or laws; see my notes on 12.3). Moreover, our author appeals to the generic concept of the δημιουργός to emphasize that all *technai* are constrained by physical possibility. Medicine is not special, nor does it belong to a species of *technē* that requires special accommodation. The same sentiment spurs our author's selection of the word δημιουργίη and its verbal cognate in 11.7, where medicine is compared to other arts, especially handicrafts. Pace Roochnik (51), the point of the passage is to stress the similarity between medicine and these other crafts, not to demand, implicitly or otherwise, a special standard for stochastic arts (see further my notes on 11.7).

Better evidence of stochastic sympathies in *de Arte* comes in the opening lines of c. 11, a fragment of which Roochnik quotes but does not analyze in depth.

> Of course, it is impossible for a person who sees only with his eyes to know any of the things just mentioned. For this reason, I have given them the name 'non-evident,' and so they have been judged by the art. However, they have not prevailed just because they are non-evident; rather, they have been prevailed over where possible. And it is possible insofar as the natures of the sick submit to examination and the natures of those searching for the non-evident are well suited to the role. (11.1)

By 'natures of the sick' our author means the bodies of individual patients, and the phrase evokes the Rationalist model of stochastic *technē*, which held the ineffability of particulars ultimately responsible for the imprecision of technical directives. However, our author will go on to insist that no particular patient or disease is by nature incapable of being known; rather, internal diseases merely take more time to be diagnosed.

> But if, in the time it takes for this to be seen, the sick person is overcome, whether on account of his slowness in going to the doctor or the speed of the disease, he will be lost. For if it starts the race from the same mark as treatment, disease is not the swifter, though it will be swifter if given a head start. And it gets a head start both from the impenetrability of human bodies, which diseases occupy without being seen, and from the negligence of the sick, which they impose upon themselves. (11.5–6)

The last sentence is especially important because it shows that these diseases are not by nature beyond the ken of the finite human intellect. For if the minimum time required for any doctor to diagnose a disease exceeded the maximum time required for the same disease to kill the patient, then treatment of necessity will begin prior to and without the benefit of complete diagnosis, leaving the doctor to fill in any gaps as best he can. But our author clearly believes that complete diagnosis of a disease is always possible, provided the patient does not dawdle on his way to the doctor.

Most problematic for a stochastic reading of *de Arte*, however, is our author's insistence that physicians do not attempt treatment until they have diagnosed the disease.

> Thus, it is not the art that is responsible for slowness, but rather the nature of human bodies. For the art sees fit to provide treatment only after it has perceived (αἰσθομένη) the problem, taking care that its treatments are applied not rashly, but, rather, thoughtfully, and gently rather than violently ....
> (11.5)

Surely the doctor perceives the disease only figuratively, but the image suggests that direct observation sets the epistemic standard for diagnosis. Insofar as it is knowledge of the disease, diagnosis will be as secure and detailed—we might say precise, though our author does not—as that normally afforded by the senses. If the precision of diagnosis by inference is contested anywhere in *de Arte*, it is at 12.1, where our author seems to imply that it is somehow inferior to perceptual knowledge: vision is the faculty 'by which all people see all things most adequately.' Perhaps the 'knowledge' afforded by inference is vague or intrinsically less reliable. This is not impossible, but considered in context it is more likely that our author is emphasizing the fact that inference is more difficult and time-consuming for the doctor. This will make it a tool of last resort, but not an inherently imprecise tool. Alternatively, he may mean that knowledge of objects is more complete when we are directly acquainted with them than when we are limited to the descriptions afforded by inference. But though this *might* mean that there are idiosyncrasies of particular cases that are beyond the reach of inference, thus bringing *de Arte* closer to the Rationalist model of a stochastic *technē*, it need not, and indeed there are no other indications that our author intends his remark to be taken in this way.

But even if *de Arte* is not stochastic, as indeed it is not, it is easy to understand why some are inclined to treat it as proto-stochastic. For it is one of the earliest—perhaps the earliest—sustained investigations into the different sources of technical failure and the relative threat each poses to the credibility of a *technē*. Though he expounds in detail the natural limits of medicine, our author never takes the final step of declaring medicine to be a special kind of art the subject matter of which limits the precision of its rational procedures and methods. It was left to Plato and Aristotle, but especially to Hellenistic physicians and philosophers, to introduce such a distinction.

## 4. *Signs of the Unseen*

In cc. 10 through 12 of *de Arte*, our author attempts to make the case that doctors are not at a loss when it comes to the non-evident (ἄδηλα) parts of the body and the diseases that affect them. As I explain in the Introduction (section 3; see also notes on 11.1), the problematic role of non-evident facts or entities in accounts of the cosmos had become a going epistemological concern in Pre-Socratic thought. And though Plato and Aristotle were markedly less interested in the problem, it would not go quietly into the dark night of historical obscurity. Indeed, by the Hellenistic period, ἄδηλον was a technical philosophical term of importance, as attested by Sextus Empiricus.

> According to the dogmatists, some things are self-evident (πρόδηλον) and some are non-evident (ἄδηλα). Of the non-evident, there are the absolutely non-evident, the temporarily non-evident, and the naturally non-evident. They say the self-evident are those that come to be known by us of their own accord, for example, that it is day. The absolutely non-evident are those that do not by nature allow us to apprehend them, for example, whether there is an even number of stars. The temporarily non-evident are those that have a nature that is directly perceivable but is non-evident to us at the moment because of some external circumstance, as the city of Athens is to me right now. Those naturally non-evident do not have a nature that allows us to directly perceive it, like the intelligible pores. For these are never apparent in and of themselves, but are thought to be apprehended, if at all, from other things, for example, from perspiration or something like it. So, they say, the self-evident does not require a sign (σημεῖον), for they are apprehended in and of themselves. Nor do the absolutely non-evident, since they cannot even begin to be apprehended. But the temporarily non-evident and the naturally non-evident are apprehended through signs, and not through themselves. The temporarily non-evident are apprehended through the 'commemorative' (ὑπομνηστικόν) signs, while the naturally non-evident are apprehended through 'indicative' (ἐνδεικτικόν) signs.
>
> (P 2.97–99)

Sextus makes a distinction between what does not allow us to perceive it (ὑπὸ τὴν ἡμετέραν πίπτειν ἐνάργειαν) and what does not allow us to apprehend it (εἰς τὴν ἡμετέραν πίπτειν κατάληψιν), what we might call the perceptually ἄδηλον in contrast to the epistemically ἄδηλον. Obviously, this latter is a much broader category; it covers those cases in which we cannot attain certainty, where we assume there *must* be a fact of the matter, but we are unable to ascertain it. The precise number of stars would be an example.[8] Sextus' language hints also at a syntactical difference in the way ἄδηλον is to be employed, depending on whether the perceptual or epistemic species is at issue. If the perceptual, then ἄδηλον is predicated of subjects. We say that the pores themselves are imperceptible, or non-evident. In the

[8] In Sextus' taxonomy, there is only one sub-species of the epistemically ἄδηλον, namely that which is by nature inapprehensible. This mirrors his characterization of the naturally ἄδηλον, which is by nature imperceptible. It is worth wondering why Sextus did not round out his categories with a sub-species of the epistemically ἄδηλον that corresponds to the temporary sub-species of the perceptually ἄδηλον, a category that would include, e.g., temporary uncertainty about whether first-order logic is complete because one has forgotten how to prove it.

epistemic case, we are uncertain about a sentence or proposition. We say that it is uncertain whether the number of stars is even or whether first-order logic is indeed complete.

The epistemic species corresponds more or less to the colloquial usage of ἄδηλον. In standard Greek, δῆλον and its alpha-privative, ἄδηλον, were used in much the same way that in modern English we use the pair 'clear' and 'unclear.' Thus, when Hippolytus says 'it is δῆλον that woman is a great evil,' he means that the fact is beyond doubt (Euripides, *Hippolytus* 627). Likewise, when the plaintiff in one of Antiphon's court speeches charges that 'concerning these [slaves], it is not ἄδηλον that they [the defendants] shied away from learning the truth of what was done, for they knew that the evil that was about to come to light belonged to their household,' he is claiming that it is *not uncertain* that the defendants were motivated by their own interests to keep the truth a secret (1.13). And when Aristotle admits that 'it is ἄδηλον whether this distinction of the many compared with the few sincere men can exist in every democracy and every group' (*Pol.* 1281b16), he is expressing his uncertainty about whether the phenomenon he describes is truly universal. In these examples, δῆλον and ἄδηλον are used to indicate the speaker's epistemic relation to various sentences or propositions. It is important to note that if p is ἄδηλον, it does not follow that *not-p* is δῆλον. Rather, ἄδηλον indicates that the subject declines to commit either to the sentence in question or to its contradictory.

If this analysis is correct, then it should be said that Sextus' presentation is somewhat confusing insofar as it gives the impression that he is presenting mutually exclusive categories to be applied to tokens of the same type. He is not. Rather, he is outlining some different ways in which the term ἄδηλον is used by philosophers, principally by the Stoics. In his defense, the taxonomy as a whole is unimportant to his mission. Of primary interest to him are the temporary and natural sub-species of τὸ ἄδηλον, for it is on this ground that he will make his stand against the dogmatists. Sextus, as a Pyhrronian sceptic and Empiric physician, rejects the naturally non-evident and thus the indicative signs that reveal it. His targets are the Epicureans and Stoics. The former especially relied on a notion of the cognizable yet naturally non-evident, since they were atomists, holding that reality was atoms and void, both of which are, according to Sextus' categories, naturally non-evident. According to Diogenes Laertius, Epicurus held that 'one ought to make sign-inferences (σημειοῦσθαι) from the phenomena (τὰ φαινόμενα) concerning the non-evident (τὰ ἄδηλα)' (10.32 = LS 16B). This, of course, is a Hellenistic paraphrase of the Anaxagorean dictum issued over a century earlier (DK 59 B21a; see Introduction 3).

The debate over τὰ ἄδηλα in this special, philosophical sense, goes back to Pre-Socratic philosophy, though it may seem as though the terms of the debate did not acquire genuine conceptual sophistication until the Hellenistic period, when Stoics and other 'dogmatists' began marking the distinctions reported by Sextus. By introducing the notions of sign and inference into his discussion of diagnosis, our author helps himself to a semiotic vocabulary common to many works in the *Corpus*. But what is a sign? The Greek authors of the Hippocratic *Corpus* did not openly analyze the semeiotic concepts they used nor did they as a rule explicitly justify their procedures for acquiring knowledge of τὰ ἄδηλα. We may contrast this with the Stoics, who define a sign as the antecedent in a sound conditional that is revelatory of the consequent (Sextus Empiricus, M 8.245), which suggests that a sign-inference will involve a *modus ponens* syllogism along the following lines.

1. If there is sweating, then there are invisible pores in the skin.
2. There is sweating.
3. Therefore, there are invisible pores in the skin.

In the Stoic example,[9] sweating is the evident sign that grounds a deductive, and therefore necessary and secure, inference to the existence of non-evident pores. The Stoics believed the soundness of this sign-inference to rest on a further argument (Sextus Empiricus, M 8.309):

4. It is not possible for liquid to pass through a solid body.
5. Sweat passes through the body.
6. The body is not solid.

Now recall the general analysis of the inference-pattern used in c. 10 of *de Arte* to justify the anatomical claims about the body's internal structure of 'containers' (see my comments on 11.1):

1'. Fluid is escaping from point A in this body.
2'. As a general rule, fluid does not simply come out of nowhere.
3'. The fluid escaping this body at point A is not coming out of nowhere.
4'. Therefore, the fluid is coming from somewhere, i.e., there is a reservoir of fluid inside the body.

[9] The Stoic example and its significance for Stoic doctrine are recorded in Sextus' *Against the professors*. My account of the Stoic views follows the succinct and well informed analysis given by Hankinson (1998, 233).

The argument given in 1'–4' is readily restructured into a form that parallels the Stoic example,[10] and it is striking that both the Hippocratic and Stoic sign-inferences concern structural discontinuities indicated by the escape of fluid (cf. 10.5). According to the Stoics, such an inference is expressed in the form of a deductively valid argument;[11] thus, logic will play a necessary role in any art, including medicine, that makes recourse to sign-inference. Indeed, the Empirics attacked Rationalist physicians for their dependence on logic (cf. Galen, *Sect. intro.* 5.10–11), an attack they could well have made against the author of *de Arte*, who insists not only that the doctor gains knowledge of non-evident diseases through inference from evident signs (12.2), but also that this involves a process of reasoning (11.3; cf. 7.3). And while *de Arte* lacks an overt commitment to deductive rigor in sign-inference, our author's invocation of perfect clarity (τὴν ἀναμάρτητον σαφήνειαν, 11.4) and evidence (δηλοῖ, 12.3), not to mention the physical necessities (ἀνάγκας) upon which the provocation of signs relies (12.3), suggest that he adopts a high standard for the security of the inferences involved, a standard consistent with deductive validity.

Other elements of our author's attitude toward the non-evident and sign-inference prefigure positions taken by Stoic philosophers and Rationalist physicians. Our author is committed to the idea that diagnosis of the underlying, often non-evident, cause of a disease is essential to its treatment (see

---

[10] E.g., 1'. If fluid is escaping from point A in this body, then there is a reservoir of fluid inside the body; 2'. fluid is escaping from point A in this body; 3'. there is a reservoir of fluid inside the body; 4'. it is not possible for escaping fluid to have come from nowhere; 5'. fluid is not accumulating from a source external to the body; 6'. the fluid is escaping from some source internal to the body.

[11] For the Stoic, sign-inferences, once they have been logically reconstructed, are always deductively valid. This might strike us at first as too rigid a requirement, for Aristotle (e.g., *APr.* 70a30 ff.) and the Hippocratics (see Introduction 3) give the impression that the Greek notion of sign was much looser, that it did not guarantee outright the truth of the conclusions drawn. The Stoics soften this potential objection by distinguishing between two different types of sign: the 'peculiar,' which is an infallible guide to what it reveals (and is therefore a sign in the strict sense), and the 'common,' which is fallible, at least in theory (and so is not a proper sign). Sedley (1982, 256) has argued that sign-inferences involving peculiar signs are made on the basis of strong, logically necessary conditionals, while common signs use material conditionals. As he points out (254), this offers little immediate comfort—exceptions falsify a material conditional no less than a necessary one. However, falsification of a material conditional is less damaging, since, unlike in the case of the logically necessary conditional, it does not include the implicit modal claim that the consequent could not possibly be false given the truth of the antecedent. For a different analysis, see Burnyeat (1982), who believes the distinction between sign-inferences involving material versus necessary conditionals amounts to an originally Stoic distinction between commemorative and indicative signs. For a comprehensive study of sign-inference in antiquity, see Allen 2001.

especially 11.4 and my notes ad loc.). Predictions about what will happen to the patient, with or without treatment, are made on the basis of causal understanding (6.4). Unlike some other Hippocratics (e.g., the author of *Prog.*; see Introduction 3), never does our author advocate a sort of sign-inference that bypasses underlying causes altogether—in Hellenistic jargon, predicting the occurrence of the temporarily non-evident on the basis of commemorative signs. Remarkably, this is so despite our author's implicit recognition of the distinction between the naturally and temporarily non-evident. Indeed, the distinction is built into the structure of the treatise itself, insofar as our author treats in c. 10 the *spatial* impediments to observing the internal anatomy before moving on in c. 11 to address the *temporal* impediments to observation (see my introductory remarks to the commentary on both chapters). The contrast crystallizes in the course of an argument in c. 11 (cited earlier).

> For if it starts the race from the same mark as treatment, disease is not the swifter, though it will be swifter if given a head start. And it gets a head start both from the impenetrability of human bodies, which diseases occupy without being seen, and from the negligence of the sick, which they impose upon themselves. For they consent to treatment only once their diseases have taken hold, and not before. (11.6)

As I point out in the commentary, this passage contains a subtle application of the *nomos-phusis* antithesis. The disease gets a head start both from nature, i.e., the internal structure of human bodies, which cannot be altered by human intervention and is in this sense necessary, and from convention, i.e., the patient's unnecessary decision to delay consultation. The disease's 'head start,' accordingly, is due to two different kinds of non-evidence: 1) the natural non-evidence of the internal disease, which is never evident to anyone at any time; and 2) the temporary non-evidence of the patient to the doctor, who at the critical moment cannot observe the patient and his symptoms, even though they will become evident to him at a later time. Thus, it turns out that, like philosophers and physicians of the Hellenistic period, our author has the capacity to sort the naturally from the temporarily non-evident; he simply finds the latter of little or no use in medical therapy, though it may be applicable to other ends.

## 5. *Concluding Remarks*

The three questions addressed in this essay can be treated in relative isolation, and indeed I have done so above. In reality, they probably were not so independent of each other. The attack on *technē* compiled by Sextus is made, we must remember, by a Sceptical philosopher and Empiric physician. Whoever resists the ambition to acquire knowledge of underlying, non-evident causes will fall back on the evident phenomena of his experience, and the irregularity of that experience will in turn push him away from a model of *technē* that insists on precision. Indeed, insofar as the notion of *technē* proper is thought to require precise knowledge of underlying causes and their future effects, he might be inclined to deny that medicine is a *technē* at all or, rather, that medicine conceived as a *technē* does not exist.

Against this general picture stand the views of 'dogmatic' philosophers and Rationalist physicians; the author of *de Arte* espouses views on *technē* and medicine so similar to theirs that he might reasonably be called a proto-Rationalist. Even on the point of greatest disagreement—the question of stochasticism—*de Arte* maintains many of the same basic commitments of the Rationalists and dogmatists. Indeed, the *recherché*, almost grudging quality of the Rationalists' concession to imprecision in the end may resemble our author's utter denial of medical imprecision more than it does the Peripatetic and Empiric attempts to provide a metaphysical justification for it. That said, there is no easy way of trimming *de Arte* to fit a Hellenistic mold, and our appreciation of it ought not turn on its historical precociousness. It is a child of the fifth century (see Introduction 5), an age with its own problems and priorities, and to judge it in any other way would constitute an abuse of historical privilege.

# BIBLIOGRAPHY


Allen, James. 1993. Failure and expertise in the ancient conception of an art. In *Scientific failure*, ed. Tamara Horowitz and Allen Janis, 81–108. Lanham, MD: Rowman and Littlefield.

———. 2001. *Inference from signs: Ancient debates about the nature of evidence*. Oxford: Oxford UP.

Barnes, Jonathan. 1982a. *The presocratic philosophers*. 2nd ed. Boston: Routledge and Kegan Paul.

———, et al, eds. 1982b. *Science and speculation: Studies in Hellenistic theory and practice*. Cambridge: Cambridge University Press.

———, 1984. *The complete works of Aristotle*. Princeton: Princeton University Press.

———. 1988. Scepticism and the arts. *Apeiron* 21: 53–77.

Bett, Richard. 1989. The Sophists and relativism. *Phronesis* 34: 139–169.

Boudon-Millot, Véronique. 2005. Art, science, and conjecture, from Hippocrates to Plato and Aristotle. In *Hippocrates in Context: Papers read at the XIth International Hipoccrates Colloquium University of Newcastle upon Tyne 27–31 August 2002*, ed. Phillip J. van der Eijk, 87–99. Boston: Brill.

Bourgey, Louis. 1953. *Observation et expérience chez les médecins de la Collection Hippocratique*. Paris: Libraire Philosophique J. Vrin.

Boyd, Richard. 1999. Kinds as the "workmanship of men:" Realism, constructivism, and natural kinds. In *Rationalität, Realismus, Revision: Proceedings of the 3rd International Congress of the Society for Analytical Philosophy, September 15–18, 1997 in Munich*, ed. Julian Nida-Rümelin, 89–104. New York: W. de Gruyter.

Brown, Lesley. 1994. The verb 'to be' in Greek philosophy. In *Language*, ed. Stephen Everson, 212–236. New York: Cambridge University Press.

Burnyeat, M.F. 1982. The origins of non-deductive inference. In *Science and speculation: Studies in Hellenistic theory and practice*, ed. by Jonathan Barnes, 193–238. Cambridge: Cambridge University Press.

Carnap, Rudolf, Hans Hahn, and Otto Neurath. 1929. *Wissenschaftliche Weltauffassung: Der Wiener Kreis*, Wien: Wolf.

Caston, Victor. 2002. Gorgias on thought and its objects. In *Presocratic philosophy: Essays in honor of Alexander Mourelatos*, ed. Victor Caston and Daniel Graham, 205–232. Burlington, VT: Ashgate.

Chadwick, J., and W.N. Mann, trans. 1978. The science of medicine. In Lloyd 1978, 139–147. London: Penguin Books.

Chase, J. Richard. 1961. The classical conception of epideictic. *Quarterly journal of speech* 47: 293–300.

Cherniss, Harold. 1952 Review of *Les Sophistes: Protagoras, Gorgias, Prodicus, Hippias*, by Eugene Dupreel. *The American Journal of Philology* 73: 199–207.

Cochrane, C.N. 1929. *Thucydides and the science of history*. Oxford: Oxford University Press.

Cole, Thomas. 1991. *The origins of rhetoric in ancient Greece*. Baltimore, MD: Johns Hopkins University Press.

Cooper, John, ed. 1997. *Plato: Complete works*. Indianapolis: Hackett Publishing Co.

Craik, Elizabeth M. 1998. *Hippocrates: Places in Man*. Oxford: Clarendon Press.

———. 2009. *The Hippocratic treatise* On glands. Boston: Brill.

Curd, Patricia. 2007. *Anaxagoras of Clazomenae: Fragments and Testimonia*. Toronto: University of Toronto Press.

Dalby, Andrew. 2003. *Food in the ancient world from A to Z*. New York: Routledge.

Daremberg, Charles. 1855. *Œuvres choisies d'Hippocrate*. 2nd ed. Paris: Labe.

Dean-Jones, Lesley. 2003. Literacy and the charlatan in ancient Greek medicine. In *Written texts and the rise of literate culture in ancient Greece*, ed. Harvey Yunis, 97–121. New York: Cambridge University Press.

Deichgräber, K. 1930. *Die griechische Empirikerschule: Sammlung der Fragmente und Darstellung der Lehre*. 2nd ed. Berlin and Zurich: Weidmannsche Verlagsbuchhandlung.

———. 1933. ΠΡΟΦΑΣΙΣ. Eine terminologische Studie. *Quellen und Studien zur Geschichte der Naturwissenschaften und der Medizin* 3: 1–17.

Demand, Nancy. 1996. Medicine and philosophy: the Attic orators. In Wittern and Pellegrin 1996, 91–99.

Demont, P. 1981. Le sens d'ἰχώρ chez Homère (*Iliade* V, v. 340 et 416) et Eschyle (*Agamemnon*, v. 1480) en relation avec les emplois du mot dans la *Collection Hippocratique*. *R.E.A.* 83: 197–209.

Denniston, J.D. 1929. Note on Hippocrates P. TEXNHS 5. *Classical review* 43: 125.

Diels, H. 1914. Hippokratische Forschungen IV (Zu *De Arte*). *Hermes* 49: 378–407.

Diels, H. and W. Kranz. 1951. *Die Fragmente der Vorsokratiker*. 6th ed. Zürich: Weidmann.

Diller, Hans. 1932. ὄψις ἀδήλων τὰ φαινόμενα. *Hermes* 67: 14–42.

———. 1952. Hippokratishe Medizin und attische Philosophie. *Hermes* 80: 385–409.

———. 1971. Zum Gebrauch von εἶδος und ἰδέα in vorplatonischer Zeit. In *Medizingeschichte in unserer Zeit*, ed. Edith Heischkel, Walter Artelt, and Hans-Heinz Eulner, 23–30. Stuttgart: F. Enke.

———. 1975. Das Selbstverständnis der griechischen Medizin in der Zeit des Hippokrates. In *La collection hippocratique et son rôle dans l'histoire de la médecine: Colloque de* Strasbourg *October 23–27, 1972*, 77–93. Leiden: Brill.

Dodds, E.R. 1973. *The ancient concept of progress and other essays on Greek literature and belief.* Oxford: Clarendon Press.

Ducatillon, Jeanne. 1977a. *Polemiques dans la collection hippocratique*. Paris: Atelier reproduction des thèses, Université de Lille III.

———. 1977b. Qui est l'auteur du traite hippocratique De L'Art? In *Corpus Hippocraticum: Actes du Colloque Hippocratique de Mons*, September 22–26, 1975, ed. Robert Joly, 148–158. Mons: Université de Mons.

Dupréel, Eugene. 1948. *Les sophistes*. Neuchâtel: Editions du Griffon.

Edelstein, Ludwig. 1967. *The idea of progress in classical antiquity*. Baltimore: Johns Hopkins University Press.

Ermerins, F.Z. 1862. *Hippocratis et aliorum medicorum veterum reliquiae*. Vol. 2. Traiecti ad Rhenum: Kemink et filium.

Fabrini, P., and A. Lami. 1979. Il problema della lingua nello scritto ippocratico De arte. *Rivista critica di storia della filosofia* 34:123–133.
Gagarin, Michael. 1996. The torture of slaves in Athenian law. *Classical philology* 91: 1–18.
———. 1997. *Antiphon: the speeches*. Cambridge: Cambridge University Press.
———. 2001. Did the sophists aim to persuade? *Rhetorica* 19: 275–291.
———. 2002. *Antiphon the Athenian: Oratory, law, and justice in the age of the Sophists*. Austin: University of Texas Press.
———. 2003. Telling stories in Athenian law. *Transactions and proceedings of the american philological association* 133:2: 197–207.
Gillespie, C.M. 1912. The use of Εἶδος and Εἴδεα in Hippocrates. *Classical quarterly* 6: 179–203.
Gomperz, Theodor. 1910. *Die Apologie der Heilkunst. Eine griechische Sophistenrede des fünften vorchristlichen Jahrhunderts*. 2nd ed. Leipzig: Viet & Comp.
Guthrie, W.K.C. 1971. *The sophists*. London: Cambridge University Press.
Hankinson, R.J. 1987. Evidence, externality and antecedence: Inquiries into later Greek causal concepts. *Phronesis* 32: 80–100.
———. 1995a. "Experience and expertise: Aristotle's conception of Technē" Photocopy.
———. 1995b. Pollution and infection: An hypothesis stillborn. *Apeiron* 28: 25–65.
———. 1998a. *Cause and explanation in ancient Greek thought*. New York: Oxford University Press.
———. 1998b. *Galen, On antecedent causes*. Cambridge: Cambridge University Press.
Hart, H.L.A. 1961. *The concept of law*. 2nd ed. Oxford: Oxford University Press.
Heiberg, I.L. 1927. *Hippocratis opera*. Corpus Medicorum Graecorum Vol. 1, no. 1. Berlin: B.G. Teubner.
Heinimann, Felix. 1945. *Nomos und physis*. Basel: F. Reinhardt.
———. 1961. Eine vorplatonische Theorie der Τέχνη. *Museum Helveticum* 18: 105–130.
Hempel, C., and P. Oppenheim. 1948. Studies in the Logic of Explanation. *Philosophy of Science* 15: 135–175.
Hintikka, Jaakko. 1986. The varieties of being in Aristotle. In *The logic of being*, ed. S. Knuuttila and J. Hintikka, 81–114. Dordrecht: Reidel.
Hirschberg, Julius. 1913. Ärztliche Bemerkungen über die in der hippokratischen Sammlung überlieferte Schrift περὶ τέχνης. *Archiv für die Geschichte der Naturwissenschaften und der Technik* 6: 163–173.
Holmes, Brooke. 2010. *The symptom and the subject*. Princeton and Oxford: Princeton University Press.
Hutchinson, D.S. 1988. Doctrines of the mean and the epistemology of skill in ancient medicine and ethics. In *Method, medicine, and metaphysics: Studies in the philosophy of ancient science*, ed. R.J. Hankinson. *Apeiron* 21:17–52.
Inwood, Brad. 1992. *The poem of Empedocles: A text and translation with an introduction*. Toronto: University of Toronto Press.
Irigoin, J. 1983. Préalables linguistiques a l'interprétation de termes techniques attestés dans la collection hippocratique. In *Formes de Pensée dans la Collection Hippocratique: Actes du IVe Colloque International Hippocratique*, ed. F. Lasserre and P. Mudry, 173–180. Geneva: Université de Lausanne, Publications de la Faculté des Lettres.

Johnson, M.R. 2010. The medical background of Aristotle's concept of nature and spontaneity. Paper presented at the Boston Area Colloquium in Ancient Philosophy, December 2, 2010, Worcester, Massachussetts.

Joly, R. 1956. Notes Hippocratiques. *Revue des études anciennes* 58: 195–210.

———, ed. and trans. 1984. *Hippocrate, Du régime*. CMG 1.2.4. Berlin: Akademie-Verlag.

Jones, W.H.S. 1923. *Hippocrates II*. LCL 148. Cambridge: Harvard University Press.

Joos, P. 1957. Zufall, Kunst, Natur bei den Hippokratikern. *Janus* 46: 238–252.

Jouanna, Jacques, ed. and trans. 1972. *Hippocrates, Du régime des maladies aiguës-Appendice-De l'aliment-De l'usage des liquides*. C.U.F. 6.2. Paris: Les Belles Lettres.

———, ed. and trans. 1975. *Hippocrate, La nature de l'homme*. CMG 1.1.3. Akademie-Verlag.

———. 1984. Rhétorique et médecine dans le collection hippocratique. *R.E.G.* 97: 26–44.

———, ed. and trans. 1988. *Hippocrates, Des vents-De l'art*. C.U.F. 5.1. Paris: Les Belles Lettres.

———, ed. and trans. 1990. *Hippocrates, L'Ancienne médecine*. C.U.F. 2.1. Paris: Les Belles Lettres.

———. 1999. *Hippocrates*. Translated by M.B. DeBevoise. Baltimore, MD: Johns Hopkins University Press.

———, ed. and trans. 2003. *Hippocrates, La Maladie sacrée*. C.U.F. 2.3. Paris: Les Belles Lettres.

Jori, Alberto. 1985. Note per un'attribuzione del *peri technes* pseudoippicratico. Atti dell'Istituto Veneto di Scienze, Lettere ed Arte. 143: 237–267.

———. 1996. *Medicina e medici nell'antica Grecia: Saggio sul peri technes ippocratico*. Bologna and Naples: Il Mulino.

———. 1997. Il Medico e il suo rapporto con il paziente nella Grecia dei secoli V e IV A.C. *Medicina nei secoli*. 9: 189–221.

Kahn, Charles. 1973. *The verb 'be' in ancient Greek*. Dordrecht: Reidel.

Kerferd, G.B. 1981. *The Sophistic movement*. London: Cambridge University Press.

Kirkwood, Gordon. 1952. Thucydides' words for 'cause.' *The American journal of philology* 73: 37–61.

Kripke, Saul. 1972. *Naming and necessity*. Cambridge: Harvard University Press.

Kudlien, F. 1967. *Der Beginn des medizinischen Denkens bei den Griechen*. Zürich: Artemis Verlag.

———. 1973. The old Greek concept of 'relative' health. *Journal of the history of behavioral sciences* 9: 53–59.

Kühn, K.G. [1821–1833] 1964–1965. *Claudii Galeni opera omnia*. 20 vols. 2nd ed. Hildesheim: Olms Verlag.

Langholf, Volker. 1990. *Medical theories in Hippocrates*. Berlin: W. de Gruyter.

Liddell, Henry George, Robert Scott, and Henry Stuart Jones, eds. 1996. *A Greek-English lexicon*. Oxford: Clarendon Press.

Littré, E. [1839] 1961. *Œevres completes d'Hippocrates*. 2nd ed. Amsterdam: A.M. Hakkert.

Lloyd, G.E.R., ed. 1978. *Hippocratic writings*. London: Penguin.

———. 1979. *Magic, reason, and experience*. Cambridge: Cambridge University Press.

———, 1987. *The revolutions of wisdom*. Berkeley: University of California Press.

———, 1991. The medical Τέχνη in the fifth and fourth centuries. In *Science and philosophy in classical Greece*, ed. Alan C. Bowen. New York: Garland Publishing.

Long, A.A., ed. 1999. *The Cambridge companion to early Greek philosophy*. Cambridge: Cambridge University Press.

Long, A.A., and D.N. Sedley. 1987. *The Hellenistic philosophers*. 2 vols. Cambridge: Cambridge University Press.

Longrigg, James. 1989. Presocratic philosophy and Hippocratic medicine. *History of Science* 27: 1–39.

Lulofs, Heindrik J. 1923. Hippocrates over de kunst (De arte). *Bijdragen tot de geschiedenis der geneeskunde* 3: 157–166.

Mackie, J.L. 1974. *The cement of the universe*. Oxford: Oxford University Press.

Maloney, Gilles, and Winnie Frohn, eds. 1986. *Concordances des œuvres hippocratiques*. 6 vols. New York: Olms-Weidmann.

Mann, Joel E. 2008a. On the (distinctively Hippocratic?) Art. Paper Presented at the XIIIth Colloquium Hippocraticum, August 11–13, Austin, Texas.

———. 2008b. Prediction, precision, and practical experience: The Hippocratics on *technē*. *Apeiron* 41: 89–122.

———. 2010. The varieties of spontaneity: A response to Johnson. Paper presented at the Boston Area Colloquium in Ancient Philosophy, December 2, 2010, Worcester, Massachussetts.

McKirahan, Richard. 1994. *Philosophy before Socrates*. Indianapolis: Hackett.

Mondolfo, Rodolfo. 1958. *La comprensione del soggetto uano nell'antichità classica*. Florence: La nuova Italia.

Morrison, J.S. 1976. The truth of Antiphon. In *Sophistik*, ed. C.J. Classen, 519–536. Darmstadt: Wissenschaftliche Buchgesellschaft.

Mourelatos, A.P.D. 1970. *The Route of Parmenides*. 2nd ed. New Haven: Yale UP.

———. 2006. The concept of the universal in some of the pre-Platonic cosmologists. In *The blackwell companion to ancient philosophy*, ed. Mary Louise Gill and Pierre Pellegrin, 56–76. Oxford: Blackwell.

Müri, Walter. 1936. Arzt und Patient bei Hippokrates. *Beilage zum Jahresbericht über das Städtische Gymnasium in Bern*. 1–64.

Nachmanson, Ernst. 1917. *Erotianstudien*. Leipzig: Kommission.

Nutton, Vivian. 2004. *Ancient Medicine*. London and New York: Routledge.

Ostwald, Martin. 1982. *Autonomia: Its genesis and early history*. Chico, CA: Scholars Press.

Parker, Robert. 1983. *Miasma: Pollution and purification in early Greek religion*. Oxford: Oxford University Press.

Parry, Adam. 1981. *Logos and ergon in Thucydides*. New York: Arno Press.

Pearson, Lionel. 1952. Prophasis and aitia. *Transactions and Proceedings of the American Philological Association* 83: 205–223.

———. 1972. Prophasis: A clarification. *Transactions and Proceedings of the American Philological Association*. 103: 381–394.

Pendrick, Gerard. 2002. *Antiphon the Sophist: The fragments*. Cambridge: Cambridge University Press.

Putnam, Hilary. 1972. Explanation and reference. In *Conceptual change*, ed. G. Pearce and P. Maynard. Dordrecht: Reidel.

Rawlings, Hunter R., III. 1975. *A semantic study of prophasis to 400 B.C.* Wiesbaden: Franz Steiner Verlag.

Rechenauer, Georg. 1991. *Thukydides und die Hippokratische Medizin*. Hildesheim: Georg Olms Verlag.

Reinhold, Karl H.Th. 1865. *Ἱπποκράτης*. Athens: C. Antoniadis.

Roochnik, David. 1996. *Of art and wisdom: Plato's understanding of techne*. University Park, PA: Pennsylvania State University Press.

Rosen, Ralph M. 2008. Towards a Hippocratic anthropology? *On ancient medicine* and the origins of humans. Paper presented at the XIIIth Colloquium Hippocraticum, August 11–13, Austin, Texas.

Scarborough, John. 1983. Theoretical assumptions in Hippocratic pharmacology. In *Formes de pensée dans la Collection Hippocratique: Actes du IVe Colloque International Hippocratique*, ed. Lasserre and P. Mudry, 307–325. Geneva: Université de Lausanne, Publications de la Faculté des Lettres.

Schiappa, Edward. 1999. The beginnings of rhetorical theory in classical Greece. New Haven, CT and London: Yale University Press.

Schiefsky, Mark. 2005. *Hippocrates* On ancient medicine. Boston and Leiden: Brill.

Schmidt, V. 1980. Ὑγιαίνομαι im Corpus Hippocraticum und ein Fragment des Musonius. *Würzburger Jahrbücher für die Altertumswissenschaft* 6b: 29–44.

Sedley, D.N. 1982. On signs. In Barnes 1982, 239–272. Cambridge: Cambridge University Press.

———. 2003. *Plato's Cratylus*. Cambridge: Cambridge University Press.

Smyth, Herbert Weir and Gordon M. Messing. 1984. *Greek grammar*. Cambridge: Harvard University Press.

Taylor, A.E. 1911. *Varia Socratica*. Oxford: James Parker and Co.

Untersteiner, Mario. 1948a. 'Le Antilogie di Protagora.' *Antiquitas* 2–3: 34–44.

———. 1948b. *I Sofisti*. trans. by Kathleen Freeman. 1954. *The Sophists*. Oxford: Blackwell.

Van Brock, N. 1961. *Recherches sur le vocabulaire médical du Grec ancien*. Paris: Klincksieck.

Vegetti, Mario. 1964. Technai e filosofia nel Peri Technes pseudo-ippocratico. *Atti della Academia della Scienze di Torino* 98: 308–380.

———. 1965. *Opere di Ippocrate*. Turin: Unione tipografico-editrice torinese.

———. 1999. Culpability, responsibility, cause: Philosophy, historiography, and medicine in the fifth century. In Long 1999, 271–289. Cambridge: Cambridge University Press.

Von Staden, Heinrich. 1990. Incurability and hopelessness: the *Hippocratic Corpus*. In *La maladie et les malades dans la Collection hippocratique*, ed. Paul Potter, Gilles Maloney, and Jacques Desautels, 78–117. Québec: Les Éditions du Sphinx.

———. 2007. Physis and Technē in Greek Medicine. In *The artificial and the natural: an evolving polarity*, ed. Bernadette Bensaude-Vincent and William R. Newman, 21–49. Cambridge, MA and London: MIT University Press.

Weidauer, K. 1954. *Thukydides und die Hippokratische Schriften*. Heidelberg: C. Winter.

West, M.L., ed. 1972. *Iambi et elegi Graeci ante Alexandrum cantati, vol. 2: Callinus. Mimnermus. Semonides. Solon. Tyrtaeus. Minora adespota*. Oxford: Clarendon Press.

Wickkiser, Bronwen. 2008. *Asklepios, Medicine, and the Politics of Healing in Fifth-Century Greece*. Baltimore, MD: Johns Hopkins University Press.

Wittern, Renate and Pierre Pellegrin. 1996. *Hippokratische Medizin und antike Philosophie: Verhandlungen des VIII. Internationalen Hippokrates-Kolloquiums in Kloster Banz/Staffelstein vom 23. bis 28. September 1993*. Hildesheim: Olms-Weidmann.

Woodruff, Paul. 1994. *Eikos* and bad faith in the paired speeches of Thucydides. *Proceedings of the Boston Area Colloquium in Ancient Philosophy* 10: 115–145.

———. 1999. *Paideia* and good judgment. In *Philosophy of education: Volume 3 of the proceedings of the twentieth World Congress of Philosophy*, ed. David M. Steiner, 63–75.

———. 2004. Antiphons, Sophist and Athenian. *Oxford Studies in Ancient Philosophy* 26: 323–336.

Woodruff, Paul, and Michael Gagarin, trans. 1995. *Early Greek political thought from Homer to the sophists*. Cambridge: Cambridge University Press.

# GENERAL INDEX

Note: index does not include the text or translation of *de Arte*

# INDEX LOCORUM

www.ingramcontent.com/pod-product-compliance
Lightning Source LLC
LaVergne TN
LVHW011117300926
849160LV00008B/427
* 9 7 8 9 0 0 4 2 2 4 1 3 1 *